Local Anesthetics for Plastic Surgery

Editor

NASIM S. HUQ

CLINICS IN PLASTIC SURGERY

www.plasticsurgery.theclinics.com

October 2013 • Volume 40 • Number 4

ELSEVIER

1600 John F. Kennedy Boulevard • Suite 1800 • Philadelphia, Pennsylvania, 19103-2899

http://www.theclinics.com

CLINICS IN PLASTIC SURGERY Volume 40, Number 4
October 2013 ISSN 0094-1298, ISBN-13: 978-0-323-26406-8

Editor: Joanne Husovski
Development Editor: Donald Mumford

Clinics in Plastic Surgery (ISSN 0094-1298) is published quarterly by Elsevier Inc., 360 Park Avenue South, New York, NY 10010-1710. Months of issue are January, April, July, and October. Business and Editorial Offices: 1600 John F. Kennedy Blvd., Suite 1800, Philadelphia, PA 19103-2899. Periodicals postage paid at New York, NY and additional mailing offices. Subscription prices are $466.00 per year for US individuals, $693.00 per year for US institutions, $229.00 per year for US students and residents, $529.00 per year for Canadian individuals, $809.00 per year for Canadian institutions, $607.00 per year for international individuals, $809.00 per year for international institutions, and $289.00 per year for Canadian and foreign students/residents. To receive student/resident rate, orders must be accompanied by name of affiliated institution, date of term, and the *signature* of program/residency coordinator on institution letterhead. Orders will be billed at individual rate until proof of status is received. Foreign air speed delivery is included in all *Clinics* subscription prices. All prices are subject to change without notice. **POSTMASTER:** Send address changes to *Clinics in Plastic Surgery*, Elsevier Health Sciences Division, Subscription Customer Service, 3251 Riverport Lane, Maryland Heights, MO 63043. **Customer Service: 1-800-654-2452 (US and Canada). From outside of the United States and Canada, call 314-447-8871. Fax: 314-447-8029. E-mail: JournalsCustomerService-usa@elsevier.com (for print support); JournalsOnlineSupport-usa@elsevier.com (for online support).**

Reprints. For copies of 100 or more of articles in this publication, please contact the Commercial Reprints Department, Elsevier Inc., 360 Park Avenue South, New York, New York 10010-1710. Tel.: (+1) 212-633-3874; Fax: (+1) 212-633-3820; E-mail: reprints@elsevier.com.

Clinics in Plastic Surgery is covered in *Current Contents, EMBASE/Excerpta Medica, Science Citation Index, MEDLINE/ PubMed (Index Medicus), ASCA, and ISI/BIOMED.*

Printed and bound by CPI Group (UK) Ltd, Croydon, CR0 4YY

Transferred to digital print 2012

Contributors

EDITOR

NASIM S. HUQ, MD, FRCSC, MSc, FACS, CAQHS, DABPS
Assistant Clinical Professor of Surgery, Niagara Plastic Surgery Centre, McMaster University, Niagara Falls, Ontario, Canada; Division of Dermatology, Department of Medicine, McMaster University, Hamilton, Ontario, Canada; Private Practice, Plastic, Reconstructive, Hand and Microsurgery, Niagara Falls, Ontario, Canada

AUTHORS

NAWEED AHMED, BSc, MD
Niagara Plastic Surgery Centre, McMaster University, Niagara Falls, Ontario, Canada

KEVIN ARMSTRONG, MD
Associate Professor, Department of Anesthesia and Perioperative Medicine, Schulich School of Medicine and Dentistry, Western University, Ontario, Canada

MICHEL J. BELLIVEAU, MD, FRCSC
Fellow in Ophthalmic Plastic and Reconstructive Surgery, Department of Ophthalmology and Vision Sciences, University of Toronto, Toronto, Ontario, Canada

FRANCES CHUNG, FRCPC
Professor of Anesthesia, Department of Anesthesia, Toronto Western Hospital, University Health Network, University of Toronto, Toronto, Canada

ALEX COLQUE, MD
Private Practice, Waukesha, Wisconsin

MICHAEL L. EISEMANN, MD
Private Practice, Houston, Texas

HANA FARHANGKHOEE, MD, MSc
Resident Physician, Division of Plastic Surgery, Department of Surgery, Faculty of Medicine, McMaster University, Hamilton, Ontario, Canada

JEROD GOLANT, BSc, MD, FRCPC
Department of Anesthesia, Mackenzie Health, Richmond Hill, Ontario, Canada

MICHELLE HARRIS, FANZCA
Anesthesia Fellow, Department of Anesthesia, Toronto Western Hospital, University Health Network, University of Toronto, Toronto, Canada

NASIM S. HUQ, MD, FRCSC, MSc, FACS, CAQHS, DABPS
Assistant Clinical Professor of Surgery, Niagara Plastic Surgery Centre, McMaster University, Niagara Falls, Ontario, Canada; Division of Dermatology, Department of Medicine, McMaster University, Hamilton, Ontario, Canada; Private Practice, Plastic, Reconstructive, Hand and Microsurgery, Niagara Falls, Ontario, Canada

DIMITRI J. KOUMANIS, MD, FACS
Private Practice, Capital Area Plastic Surgery of New York, Saratoga Springs, New York

LOUISE CAOUETTE LABERGE, MD, FRCSC
Professor of Surgery, Chief of Plastic Surgery, Department of Surgery, CHU Ste Justine, University of Montreal, Montreal, Quebec, Canada

SAMUEL M. LAM, MD, FACS
Director, Willow Bend Wellness Center, Plano, Texas

ERIC YU KIT LI, MD
Division of Plastic Surgery, Department of Surgery, Faculty of Medicine, McMaster University, Hamilton, Ontario, Canada

ALA LOZINSKI, MD, FRCPC, DABD
Assistant Clinical Professor Adjunct, Division of Dermatology, Department of Medicine, McMaster University, Hamilton, Ontario, Canada

DOUGLAS R. MCKAY, MD, MBA, FRCSC
Assistant Professor, Departments of Surgery and Oncology, Hotel Dieu Hospital, Queens University, Kingston, Ontario, Canada

SONUL MEHTA, MD
Fellow in Ophthalmic Plastic and Reconstructive Surgery, Department of Ophthalmology and Vision Sciences, University of Toronto, Toronto, Ontario, Canada

AQIB NAKHOODA, MD
Niagara Plastic Surgery Centre, McMaster University, Niagara Falls, Ontario, Canada

TARIQ I. NAKHOODA, MD, BSc
Niagara Plastic Surgery Centre, McMaster University, Niagara Falls, Ontario, Canada

JAMES H. OESTREICHER, MD, FRCSC
Director of Fellowship in Ophthalmic Plastic and Reconstructive Surgery, Professor of Ophthalmology, Department of Ophthalmology and Vision Sciences, University of Toronto, Toronto, Ontario, Canada

CHRIS OFFIERSKI, MD, FRCS
Orthopedic Surgery, Greater Niagara General Hospital, Niagara Falls, Ontario, Canada

MEHDI RAZEGHI, MD
Niagara Plastic Surgery Centre, McMaster University, Niagara Falls, Ontario, Canada

MICHAEL SKLAR, BSc, MD
Resident Physician, Department of Otolaryngology-Head & Neck Surgery, University of Toronto, Toronto, Ontario, Canada

JENNA SMITH
Glens Falls Hospital, New York, New York

PHILIP SOLOMON, BSc, MD, FRCSC
Division of Facial Plastic and Reconstructive Surgery, Department of Otolaryngology-Head & Neck Surgery, Chief of Surgery, Mackenzie Health, Staff Surgeon, St. Michael's Hospital, University of Toronto, Toronto, Ontario, Canada

ACHILLEAS THOMA, MD, MSc, FRCS (C), FACS
Clinical Professor, Division of Plastic Surgery, Department of Surgery, Faculty of Medicine, McMaster University; Associate Member, Department of Clinical Epidemiology and Biostatistics, McMaster University, Hamilton, Ontario, Canada

KING H. WONG, MB BCh, FRCS
Toronto, Ontario, Canada

Contents

identify the nerve. Blocking nerves in the distal extremity is safe with low risk of toxicity. The effect of the nerve block is limited to the distribution of the nerve. The distal nerves in the lower extremity are sensory branches of the sciatic nerve. This provides a sensory block only. This has the advantage of allowing the patient to actively contract tendons in the foot and ambulate more quickly after surgery.

varied anatomic sites are discussed, as well as other indications for tumescent anesthesia.

Hair Transplant and Local Anesthetics   615

Samuel M. Lam

 Video of technique for donor and recipient tumescence for hair transplant accompanies this article

Hair restoration is an art and a science that requires an experienced and dedicated surgeon and team to achieve consistently superior outcomes. In addition to discussion of local anesthetic in use for hair restoration, this article emphasizes the pearls and pitfalls that are involved at every phase of the procedure including judgment, hairline design, donor harvesting, recipient-site creation, graft preparation, and graft placement. Two recent advances in the field are highlighted: the use of regenerative medicine (platelet-rich plasma and ACell), and developments in follicular-unit extraction as an alternative to traditional linear donor harvesting.

Rhinoplasty with Intravenous and Local Anesthesia   627

Michael Sklar, Jerod Golant, and Philip Solomon

 Videos of Local Anesthesia; Cartilage Delivery; Dorsal Exposure; Dorsal Reduction; Osteotomies; Caudal Septoplasty; and Retrograde Cephalic Trim accompany this article

Procedural sedation for a rhinoplasty, like any procedure, relies on careful patient selection and patient and surgeon compliance. Patients should have an American Society of Anesthesia (ASA) score of 1 or 2, with a possibly well-controlled 3 also acceptable, and should be devoid of certain comorbidities, including obstructive sleep apnea, gastroesophageal reflux disease, and obesity (body mass index ≥35). Before the procedure begins, clinicians must explicitly communicate to patients that they will feel no pain; however, because they are being sedated, they may know what is occurring during surgery, but they should not care. A common misconception about sedation is that it involves general anesthesia without an airway. Clinicians must reassure patients that the anesthetist will be with them the entire time, and any discomfort can be dealt with immediately and the anesthesia titrated to an acceptable level.

Oculoplastic Surgery   631

Sonul Mehta, Michel J. Belliveau, and James H. Oestreicher

Esthetic and functional surgery in the periocular region falls into the domain of oculoplastic surgeons, as well as plastic surgeons and otorhinolaryngologists with training in facial plastic surgery. This article provides a description of 8 common eyelid procedures that are routinely performed under local anesthesia, with or without mild intravenous sedation. Serious complications are rare. The rate of postoperative infection in the highly vascularized eyelid tissues is less than 1% in our experience.

Cosmetic Face, Neck, and Brow Lifts with Local Anesthesia   653

Nasim S. Huq and Tariq I. Nakhooda

The sections on the face, neck, and brow include descriptions of facelift, neck lift, and open brow lift techniques, anesthesia, treatment goals, procedural approaches, complications, management, preoperative and postoperative care, rehabilitation, recovery, and outcomes. The approach to facial rejuvenation the midface and periorbital area is detailed. These operations are often and easily performed entirely with the use of local anesthesia and mild oral sedation. There are very high satisfaction rates.

Otoplasty can be performed safely and effectively under local anesthesia in children as young as 5 years of age. Child preparation, local anesthetics, detailed infiltration technique, surgical procedure, and complications are discussed.

CLINICS IN PLASTIC SURGERY

RELATED INTEREST

Neck lift General Anaesthesia Versus Thoracic Paravertebral Block for Breast Surgery: A meta-analysis Review Article, Volume 64, Issue 10, October 2011, Pages 1261–9
Journal of Plastic, Reconstructive & Aesthetic Surgery
Youssef Tahiri, De Q.H. Tran, Jeanne Bouteaud, Liqin Xu, Don Lalonde, Mario Luc, and
Andreas Nikolis, *Editors*

DOWNLOAD Free App!

Review Articles
THE CLINICS

NOW AVAILABLE FOR YOUR iPhone and iPad

Preface

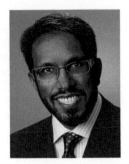

Nasim S. Huq, MD, FRCS(C), MSc, FACS, CAQHS, DABPS
Editor

I am very honored to be the guest editor of this edition of *Clinics in Plastic Surgery* with a focus on local anesthetics.

For many years, my staff has humored me each and every time I said, "I have an idea!" I have performed many operations using local anesthesia, from bilateral breast reductions, abdominoplasties, full face and open brow lifts, to microsurgical digital replantation. Plastic surgery is almost by definition an innovative field that inevitably changes with the times. Today, much cosmetic surgery is performed by non-plastic surgeons. This issue of *Clinics in Plastic Surgery* has a great group of diverse authors with tremendous experience in their respective fields, including anesthesia, dermatology, ophthalmology, orthopedic surgery, otolaryngology, business, and, of course, plastic surgery. The first few articles focus on the use and benefits of local anesthesia procedures. The remaining articles describe, in detail, select surgeries without general anesthesia, in various fields.

It seems as if we have silos of information and experience, which are separated only by geography. Recently, in the 21st Century, with the Internet, social media, video conferencing, eBooks, and virtual assistants, the world has become flattened. It is so much easier to learn our own field and everyone else's with a gentle embrace of technology. Efficient logistic systems of knowledge are now enjoyed by many fields even outside of medicine as some patients are sometimes more aware of current developments than their doctors.

Patients want surgical care that is fast, high quality, and inexpensive. Unfortunately, most health systems can only provide two of these

three. In order to maintain consistency with a high quality of care, the American Association for Accreditation of Ambulatory Surgical Facilities has helped to establish the expected standard of care in over 2000 facilities. As to cost, economics will always play a role in the practice of medicine. As to time, in a world where there is an economy of time and movement, there are many fixed commodities. We all have the same number of hours in a day. We cannot bank or deposit our time, so we should focus on how we spend it. The entire paradigm shifts, however, when we leave the confines of a hospital setting for a privately run facility. The scheduling, staff cooperation, stresses, and overall friendly environment are all important considerations. Ultimately, patient care should be the final factor. There are tradeoffs in every practice decision or career decision.

The hardest practice decision, in my opinion, is really in the change in yourself. A few years ago I took my first golf lesson, as I never learned to play properly. I was the "Happy Gilmore" of golfers. The 85-year-old golf pro asked me a question in the end, "You spent your first 40 years golfing left. Do you want to spend the next 40 golfing 'right'?" From this, I knew he meant, "correctly." We are creatures of habit, especially after years of training and even more years of practice. To actually convince an established surgeon to change his practice without a serious impetus is like changing handedness. You really have to want to change.

I am deeply indebted to Elsevier for this wonderful opportunity to be a contributor and guest editor to this volume of *Clinics in Plastic Surgery*. I greatly appreciate all of the authors'

Clin Plastic Surg 40 (2013) xi–xii
http://dx.doi.org/10.1016/j.cps.2013.09.006
0094-1298/13/$ – see front matter © 2013 Elsevier Inc. All rights reserved.

and assistants' contributions through their unique experiences and expertise. I would also like to thank Ms Joanne Husovski for her tremendous guidance and support in the preparation of this issue. I would like to acknowledge the assistance of my staff, especially, Kim, Vikki, Patti, and Sarah, for keeping the practice together. I thank my loving wife, Dr Sarah Danial, and three sons, Musa, Eesa, and Yousuf, for their unconditional love and continued support during this and many other on-going projects. I thank God, for the ability to see and learn from my teachers and patients and to deliver ideas in this issue that may grow to a significant contribution to surgical literature.

Nasim S. Huq, MD, FRCS(C), MSc, FACS, CAQHS, DABPS
McMaster University
Niagara Plastic Surgery Centre
5668 Main Street, Suite 1
Niagara Falls, Ontario L2G 5Z4, Canada
www.niagaraplasticsurgery.com

E-mail address:
niagaraplasticsurgery@gmail.com

Complications of General Anesthesia

Michelle Harris, FANZCA, Frances Chung, FRCPC*

KEYWORDS

• General anesthesia • Complications • Morbidity • Risk • Incidence • Perioperative medicine

KEY POINTS

• General anesthesia has potential complications that may contribute to perioperative morbidity.
• Cardiorespiratory complications are the most common in the perioperative period.
• Thorough preoperative assessment is essential to identify patients at risk of complications.
• Minor complications such as sore throat and dental damage are common and can lead to patient dissatisfaction.
• Delayed discharge and unplanned admission as a result of perioperative complications are important quality outcome measures, particularly in ambulatory surgery.

INTRODUCTION

Each year, increasing numbers of people are undergoing surgery. Many of these patients are older and have multiple comorbidities. General anesthesia is a reversible state of unconsciousness that allows patients to undergo surgical procedures in a safe and humane way. Although it is increasingly safe, general anesthesia is not without risks and complications. Anesthesia-related mortality is rare and has declined significantly over the past 5 decades.[1,2] Morbidity associated with general anesthesia ranges from minor complications that affect the patient's experience with no long-term consequences to complications with long-term repercussions resulting in permanent disability.

Cardiovascular and respiratory complications are the most common. Myocardial infarction, interference with lung mechanics, and exacerbation of preexisting comorbidities can all occur. Other serious complications include acute renal impairment and the development of long-term postoperative cognitive dysfunction. Minor but important complications of general anesthesia include postoperative nausea and vomiting, sore throat, and dental damage. All these complications can have a significant impact on patients and may result in prolonged hospital stay and expense.

By being aware of potential complications related to general anesthesia, many can be predicted and prevented. Thorough preoperative assessment is the key to identifying risk factors and stratifying patients so that optimization and planning can occur preoperatively.

CARDIOVASCULAR COMPLICATIONS WITH GENERAL ANESTHESIA

Perioperative cardiac complications include myocardial ischemia or infarction (MI), heart failure (HF), and cardiac arrest.

Myocardial Infarction

Recent studies suggest up to 5% of patients undergoing elective noncardiac surgery have MI.[3] In the presence of 1 cardiac risk factor, the incidence is 4.4%, with the risk of cardiovascular death approximately 1.6%.[4] Most perioperative

No disclosures by either author.
Department of Anesthesia, Toronto Western Hospital, University Health Network, University of Toronto, 399 Bathurst Street, McL 2-405, Toronto ON M5T 2S8, Canada
* Corresponding author.
E-mail address: frances.chung@uhn.ca

Clin Plastic Surg 40 (2013) 503–513
http://dx.doi.org/10.1016/j.cps.2013.07.001
0094-1298/13/$ – see front matter © 2013 Elsevier Inc. All rights reserved.

ischemic events are silent and may have no clinically appreciable signs or symptoms. The true incidence of ischemia in the perioperative period is likely underestimated.

Perioperative MI is common but can be hard to predict and prevent. It usually occurs in the first 48 hours postoperatively.[5] Most perioperative MIs result from oxygen supply-demand mismatch. Anesthesia and surgery confer a physiologic stress test to the patient that increases O_2 demand. Hypotension, anemia, and coronary artery disease prevent this demand from being met. Thrombus formation or plaque rupture account for only one-third of events.[6]

Several risk indices allow the stratification of patients according to the likelihood of perioperative cardiac complications. The most commonly used is the Revised Cardiac Risk Index (RCRI). This identifies 6 independent predictors of major cardiac complications: high-risk surgery, history of ischemic heart disease, history of HF, history of cerebrovascular disease, diabetes requiring insulin, and chronic renal impairment.[7] Risk increases with the presence of each additional risk factor.

The American Heart Association devised a stepwise approach to help manage patients undergoing noncardiac surgery. Their recommendations incorporate assessment of patients for risk factors, rational use of investigations that influence patient treatment, and provision of recommendations for preoperative optimization.[8]

Certain drugs in the perioperative period can influence cardiac outcomes. β-Blockers have been shown to decrease the incidence of perioperative MI but the potential for harm (most notably stroke) means no recommendations can be made at present.[4,8] There is also insufficient data on the potential benefit of commencing statins perioperatively. Use of nitrous oxide can lead to impairment of methionine synthase and inhibition of folate synthesis resulting in hyperhomocysteinemia, which has been associated with myocardial ischemia and infarction.[9,10] Studies are ongoing to determine whether the use of clonidine and aspirin are effective in reducing the incidence of major cardiovascular events perioperatively.

Heart Failure

HF occurs in 1% to 6% of patients after major surgery.[11] It is most common in patients with underlying cardiovascular disease.[11,12] Negative pressure pulmonary edema results from high-pressure respiratory effort in the setting of an obstructed airway. It occurs in approximately 0.1% of patients undergoing general anesthesia and complete recovery occurs in most patients.[13]

Arrhythmia

Bradyarrythmias and ventricular arrhythmias are rare in the perioperative period. Less than 1% of all surgical patients (including cardiac surgery) experience a bradyarrhythmia or ventricular arrhythmia that is severe enough to require treatment.[14] Atrial fibrillation is the most common perioperative arrhythmia with an incidence of 0.37% to 20% in noncardiac surgery patients.[15] The incidence is highest in patients undergoing major vascular and open abdominal surgery and least in those having ophthalmic or superficial minor surgery. Preoperative risk factors for development of atrial fibrillation include increasing age, male gender, preexisting heart disease, American Society of Anesthesiologists Class 3 or 4, and preoperative electrolyte disturbances.[15]

New-onset arrhythmias in the perioperative period are usually self-limiting with more than 80% reverting to sinus rhythm before discharge.[15] Management consists of recognizing the arrhythmia and instituting rate and rhythm control methods under expert medical guidance.

Thromboembolism

Venous thromboembolism (VTE) includes both deep vein thrombosis (DVT) and pulmonary embolism (PE) and is a significant cause of morbidity and mortality in the perioperative period. In patients undergoing plastic surgery, the overall incidence of VTE is 1.69%, however this varies according to the presence of risk factors.[16] Several tools exist to help assess and stratify the risk of VTE for each patient. The Carprini Risk Assessment Model (**Fig. 1**) has been validated for use in plastic surgery patients[16] and endorsed by the American Society of Plastic Surgeons.[17] Current recommendations on thromboprophylaxis in surgical patients are based on the calculated risk of VTE and consideration of the risk of bleeding associated with any intervention. These recommendations are summarized in **Table 1**.[18]

Cardiac Arrest

The risk of anesthesia-related cardiac arrest is 1.86:10,000.[6,19] It is more likely in patients at the extremes of age (neonates, elderly), patients with poor physical function, and emergency surgery. General anesthesia is a risk factor for cardiac arrest. More than 90% of anesthesia-related cardiac arrests are related to airway management or medication administration. Respiratory causes are more common in the pediatric population, whereas cardiac arrest after administration of

Each Risk Factor = 1 point
Age 41-60 years
Minor surgery planned
Prior major surgery (<1 month)
Varicose veins
History of inflammatory bowel disease
Swollen legs
Obesity (BMI>25)
Acute myocardial infarction
Congestive heart failure (<1 month)
Sepsis (<1 month)
Serious lung disease (<1 month)
Abnormal pulmonary function (e.g. COPD)
Medical patient currently at bed rest
Other risk factors

Each Risk Factor = 2 points
Age 60-74
Arthroscopic surgery
Malignancy (present or previous)
Major surgery (>45minutes)
Laparoscopic surgery (>45minutes)
Patient confined to bed (>72 hours)
Immobilizing plaster cast (<1 month)
Central venous access

Each Risk Factor = 3 points
Age > 75 years
History of DVT/PE
Family history of thrombosis
Positive Factor V Leiden
Positive Prothrombin 20210A
Elevated serum homocysteine
Positive lupus anticoagulant
Elevated anticardiolipin antibodies
Heparin-induced thrombocytopenia
Other congenital/acquired thrombophilia

Each Risk Factor = 5 points
Elective major lower extremity arthroplasty
Hip, pelvis or leg fracture (<1 month)
Stroke (<1 month)
Multiple trauma (<1 month)
Acute spinal cord injury (<1 month)

For Women Each Risk Factor = 1 point
Oral contraceptives or hormone replacement therapy
Pregnancy or postpartum (<1 month)
History of unexplained stillborn infant, recurrent spontaneous abortion (>3), premature birth with toxemia or growth-restricted infant

Fig. 1. Thrombosis risk assessment tool. (*Data from* Murphy RX, Schmitz D, Rosolowski K. Evidence-based practices for thromboembolism prevention: a report from the ASPS Venous Thromboembolism Task Force. Arlington Heights (IL): American Society of Plastic Surgeons; 2011.)

medications causing cardiovascular depression occurs more commonly in adults.[19]

RESPIRATORY COMPLICATIONS

Perioperative respiratory complications are an important predictor of morbidity and mortality and affect the financial burden of health care by increasing the length of hospital stay.[20] The incidence is similar to that for perioperative cardiac complications at 6.8%; serious complications occur in 2.6%.[21] Anesthesia-related complications include atelectasis, aspiration, and bronchospasm; exacerbation of existing lung disease and infection are less relevant in the intraoperative period.[22]

Atelectasis

Atelectasis accounts for up to 70% of severe postoperative hypoxemia and is a risk factor for the development of pneumonia and acute lung injury.[20] Within minutes of induction of general anesthesia, mechanical compression of alveoli, reabsorption of alveolar gases, and paralysis cause diaphragm displacement. Functional residual capacity and lung compliance is reduced, increasing airway resistance. These changes can progress throughout general anesthesia and manifest clinically as V/Q mismatch (or shunt), impaired gas exchange, hypoxemia, diaphragm dysfunction, decreased respiratory drive, inhibition of cough, and impaired mucociliary clearance.[23]

Several patient and surgical factors increase the risk of perioperative respiratory complications; these include advanced age, an American Society of Anesthesiologists status greater than 2, functional dependence, congestive cardiac failure, and a history of chronic obstructive pulmonary disease.[21] Risk increases with emergency surgery and procedures in close proximity to the diaphragm.[21,24] Cigarette smoking has recently been shown to be associated with increased 30-day mortality and perioperative respiratory complications.[25]

Table 1
Incidence of VTE and recommendations for thromboprophylaxis based on Caprini Risk Assessment Model (RAM) score

Caprini RAM Score	Risk of VTE (%)	Recommended Thromboprophylaxis
0	<0.5	Nil/ambulate early
1–2	1–5	Mechanical prophylaxis (IPC)
3–4	3.0	If not high risk for major bleeding: LMWH or LDUH or mechanical prophylaxis (IPC) If high risk for major bleeding: mechanical prophylaxis (IPC)
>5	6.0	LMWH or LDUH and mechanical prophylaxis (IPC)

Abbreviations: IPC, intermittent pneumatic compression; LDUH, low dose unfractionated heparin; LMWH, low molecular weight heparin.
Data from Gould MK. Prevention of VTE in nonorthopedic surgical patients: antithrombotic therapy and prevention of thrombosis. Chest 2012;141:e227S–77S.

Prevention of perioperative complications is facilitated by accurate risk stratification and preoperative optimization with a multidisciplinary team approach. Intraoperative ventilatory strategies to reduce atelectasis including postinduction recruitment maneuvers and minimizing intraoperative inspired oxygen concentrations are beneficial.[23] Preoperative respiratory muscle training, incentive spirometry, and chest physiotherapy may confer some benefit although this has not been proved.[26,27] Smoking cessation for 4 to 8 weeks preoperatively reduces the risk of respiratory complications to baseline and cessation for shorter periods is likely to decrease risk.[28]

Aspiration

Aspiration of gastric contents into the airway is the most common cause of airway-related death during anesthesia.[29] It occurs in 1:4000 patients undergoing general anesthesia, increasing to 1:900 in emergency surgery. The highest risk is at intubation and extubation.[29,30] Identifying patients at risk of aspiration is key to its prevention.[29] Risk factors and methods to modify them are outlined in **Table 2**.

Bronchospasm

Bronchospasm is caused by the constriction of bronchial smooth muscle and edema, which untreated can result in hypoxia, hypotension, or death.[31,32] It occurs in 0.2% of patients undergoing general anesthesia. Preexisting airway disease, recent or active upper respiratory tract infection, smoking history, and atopy all increase risk.[32,33] The key triggers are airway instrumentation or delivery of inhalational anesthetic agents. Early surgical stimulation without adequate depth of anesthesia, airway soiling, and medications (eg, β-blockers, neostigmine, morphine, atracurium) can also induce bronchospasm.[32] Prevention relies on the optimization of underlying airway disease, being aware of drug sensitivities, encouraging smoking cessation, delaying surgery if recent upper respiratory infection, and avoiding unnecessary airway manipulation. Algorithms exist for the management and diagnosis of bronchospasm, the mainstay of which consist of removing the trigger, supplying high flow oxygen, and administering bronchodilators to facilitate the relaxation of airway smooth muscle relaxation.[31]

NEUROLOGIC COMPLICATIONS
Postoperative Cognitive Dysfunction

Postoperative cognitive dysfunction (POCD) is defined as a decline in cognitive levels from preoperative function as detected by changes on neuropsychological testing.[34] It occurs in approximately 9.9% of patients.[35] Postoperative delirium is defined as an acute change in cognition and attention, which may include alterations in

Table 2		
Risk factors and interventions for aspiration		
	Risk Factor	Intervention
Patient	↑ gastric contents • Not fasted • Delayed gastric emptying • Bowel obstruction Lower esophageal sphincter dysfunction • Hiatus hernia • Gastroesophageal reflux • Pregnancy • Obesity • Neuromuscular disease Abnormal laryngeal reflexes	Routine preoperative fasting Empty stomach with oro/nasogastric tube Administer prokinetic premedication
Surgical	Abdominal surgery Emergency surgery Position • Trendelenburg • Lithotomy	
Anesthetic	Difficult intubation Gastric insufflation Inadequate depth of anesthesia	Avoid general anesthesia; consider regional Rapid sequence induction Monitor depth of anesthesia Ensure paralysis reversal

consciousness and disorganized thinking.[36] The incidence varies according to the type of surgery and is highest (35%–65%) in patient's undergoing hip fracture surgery.[36]

Patient factors may be the most important in the development of POCD.[35] Advanced age is an independent risk factor both acutely and in the long term. Recent studies demonstrate that the development of POCD is independent of major changes in blood pressure and oxygenation. Cardiac surgery is associated with an increased incidence at 7 days postoperatively, but this difference does not exist by 3 months suggesting the development of POCD is independent of the type of procedure or anesthetic.[35]

The exact mechanisms of POCD are yet to be elucidated and no specific treatment exists for either POCD or postoperative delirium. Neuroinflammatory mediators such as tumor necrosis factor α may play a role and are potential therapeutic targets.[37] Screening patients postoperatively, minimizing analgesic medications, early reestablishment of routines, and early mobilization and discharge may help.[36]

Awareness

Awareness is defined as consciousness under general anesthesia with subsequent recall of the events experienced.[37] It has been reported to occur in 0.03% of patients.[38] In a recent survey of anesthesiologists, it was reported as 1 in 15,000 implying that many cases of awareness are not identified nor reported.[39] Up to 26% of patients have significant long-term sequelae after an episode of awareness. The sequelae include anxiety, depression, and, in severe cases, posttraumatic stress disorder.[40]

Awareness results from an inadequate depth of anesthesia. Several risk factors have been identified for the development of awareness and are listed in **Box 1**.[41] Most cases occur at induction/emergence when the anesthetic is being titrated to surgical conditions. Risk is highest when neuromuscular blocking drugs are used.

Use of bispectral index monitoring has been shown to decrease awareness in high-risk patients.[41] However, subsequent studies did not demonstrate a difference in the incidence of awareness with bispectral index monitoring compared with protocols that use measured anesthetic agent targets to ensure depth of anesthesia.[42,43] This is also true for non–high-risk patients.[44] Electroencephalography-based monitoring techniques do not constitute routine care; however, there may be a role when total intravenous anesthesia is used.

> **Box 1**
> **Risk factors for development of awareness**
>
> *Patient Factors*
> - Alcohol
> - Opioid use
> - History of awareness
> - Elderly (when anesthetic depth is compromised for hemodynamic stability)
>
> *Surgical Factors*
> - Emergency surgery
> - Obstetrics
> - Ear, nose, and throat/airway surgery
> - Cardiac surgery
>
> *Anesthetic Factors*
> - Total intravenous anesthesia
> - Use of muscle relaxants

RENAL COMPLICATIONS

Perioperative renal dysfunction occurs in 1% to 5% of patients admitted to hospital.[45] The lack of a universally accepted definition of renal dysfunction or injury means the true incidence is difficult to quantify. Working definitions that aim to classify renal injury based on serum creatinine level and urine output have now been developed.[46–48] The importance of this complication is its association with increased morbidity and mortality.[48,49]

Prerenal and intrinsic causes account for up to 90% of perioperative renal injury.[50] General anesthesia contributes to renal dysfunction in several ways; the most common physiologic derangement is hypoperfusion. Fluid depletion from preoperative fasting, anesthetic agent–induced hypotension and positive pressure ventilation all impair renal blood flow. These hemodynamic perturbations are exacerbated by the physiologic stress response to surgery with release of catecholamines and activation of the renin-angiotensin-aldosterone system.

Pharmacologic agents can cause direct cellular insult or impair intrinsic autoregulatory mechanisms responsible for maintaining constant renal blood flow. These include nonsteroidal antiinflammatory drugs (NSAIDs), aminoglycoside antibiotics, angiotensin-converting enzyme inhibitors/angiotensin receptor blockers, and contrast media. Metabolism of the volatile anesthetic agent sevoflurane produces a nephrotoxic metabolite. However, no renal injury has been shown to occur in humans.[51]

Most healthy patients with normal preoperative renal function can withstand minor alterations in renal blood flow associated with general anesthesia and surgery.[52] Risk of renal injury is increased in the setting of existing renal impairment, advanced age, diabetes, hypertension and cardiovascular disease, and hepatic dysfunction.[49]

Maintenance of adequate renal perfusion and oxygen delivery are the mainstay of preventing perioperative renal injury.[48] This is achieved by maintaining normovolemia, normotension, and cardiac output. Awareness of the patient's risk factors and avoidance of nephrotoxins is essential. At present, there is no strong evidence that any other strategies are effective in the prevention of anesthesia-related renal dysfunction.[45,48,53]

POSTOPERATIVE NAUSEA AND VOMITING

Postoperative nausea and vomiting (PONV) is experienced by 20% to 30% of patients. The incidence can be as high as 70% to 80% in high-risk individuals.[54] PONV can result in significant patient distress and additional health care costs. A summary of risk factors for PONV is shown in **Box 2**. Four factors (female sex, nonsmoking status, history of PONV or motion sickness, and opioid use) have been well validated. The incidence of PONV is estimated at 10%, 20%, 40%, 60%, and 80% depending on the presence of none, 1, 2, 3, or 4 risk factors, respectively.[55] General anesthesia is a significant risk factor, resulting in an 11-fold increased risk for PONV compared with those receiving regional anesthesia.[54]

Up to 37% of patients may experience postdischarge nausea and vomiting.[56] The most important predictors for this complication are female gender, age less than 50 years, history of PONV, opioids administered in the postanesthesia care unit, and nausea in the postanesthesia care unit.[56]

A summary of the management recommendations for PONV[54] is presented in **Fig. 2**. As the cause of PONV is multifactorial, a multimodal approach to its treatment is recommended. Dexamethasone, ondansetron, droperidol, and total intravenous anesthesia with propofol have all been shown to independently decrease the risk of PONV by approximately 26%.[57] The absolute risk reduction with these interventions is greatest in patients with a high baseline risk and routine use should be reserved for these patients.

Evidence also exists for the reduction in baseline risk by avoidance of volatile anesthetic agents and nitrous oxide, maintenance of anesthesia with propofol, and minimization of intraoperative and postoperative opioids.[58] Minimizing preoperative anxiety, ensuring adequate patient hydration, and ensuring adequate pain management while minimizing the use of opioids may also have a role in reducing the incidence of PONV.[59]

SORE THROAT

Sore throat is a common postoperative complaint and affects up to 12.1% of patients at 24 hours after surgery.[60] Rates seem directly related to the degree of airway instrumentation with up to 50% of patients intubated with an endotracheal tube experiencing sore throat symptoms. Use of a laryngeal mask airway (LMA) reduces the incidence to between 17.5% and 34%.[60,61]

The main mechanism of injury related to intubation is mechanical trauma such as epithelial loss, glottic hematoma, glottic edema, submucosal tears, and contact ulcer granuloma.[61] The most common injury attributed to LMA use is pharyngeal erythema, and uncommonly, nerve palsies, artyenoid dislocation, and epiglottic and uvular bruising.[61] Sequelae of such injuries are pain, hoarseness, and dysphagia.

The incidence of sore throat increases with the diameter of the endotracheal tube, as a result of increased pressure at the tube-mucosal interface.[62] High-volume low-pressure cuffs have been associated with a higher incidence of sore throat as there is a greater area of cuff-tracheal contact and superficial mucosal damage.[61] Uncuffed endotracheal tubes are also associated with a higher incidence of sore throat as is the use of lidocaine gel for lubrication.[61,63]

When laryngeal mask airways are used, larger size, multiple attempts at insertion, and longer duration of surgery are all associated with an

---

Box 2
Risk factors for PONV

Patient Factors

Female gender

Nonsmoking status

History of PONV/motion sickness

Anesthetic Factors

Use of volatile anesthetics

Use of nitrous oxide

Use of intraoperative/postoperative opioids

Surgical Factors

Duration of surgery >30 min

Type of surgery (laparoscopic, breast, strabismus, plastic surgery, maxillofacial, gynecologic, abdominal, neurologic, urologic)

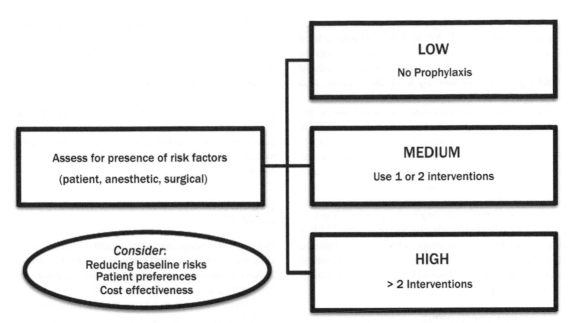

Fig. 2. An approach to management of PONV.

increased incidence of sore throat.[60] Reduction of LMA intracuff pressure to less than 44 mm Hg lowers the incidence of postoperative sore throat, dysphagia, and dysphonia.[64]

Limiting mechanical trauma to the airway through the course of the patient's anesthetic decreases but does not eliminate the risk of sore throat. Avoidance of intubation if appropriate, use of smaller endotracheal tubes, limitation of endotracheal cuff pressure to 20 to 30 cm H_2O and avoidance of uncuffed tubes and lignocaine lubricants may limit sore throat. Routine measurement of LMA pressure after insertion, and reduction to less than 44 mm Hg should be recommended as anesthetic best practice.[64] The technique used to insert an LMA is also important. Partially inflating the LMA or using an insertion aid may limit sore throat.[61]

Inhaled steroid, topical NSAIDs, or premedication with antibacterial lozenges may have a role in reducing the incidence of sore throat.[63] In most cases, a sore throat is a self-limiting complication that does not require specific treatment and responds well to simple analgesia.

DENTAL DAMAGE

Dental trauma occurs in 0.04% to 0.05% of patients undergoing general anesthesia.[2,65] Enamel fracture is the most common injury followed by loosening or subluxation of teeth, avulsion, and crown fracture.[66]

Dental damage can occur either from direct trauma or biting. Biting can generate significant force on the incisors resulting in dental trauma especially when oropharyngeal airways are used as bite blocks.[66] Poor laryngoscopic technique is a common iatrogenic cause; the culprit maneuver is use of the upper teeth as a fulcrum. Almost half of all anesthesia-related dental injuries occur during laryngoscopy for tracheal intubation.[2] Difficult intubation magnifies the risk 20-fold.[65]

There are also several patient factors that make teeth more susceptible to dental trauma, including dental caries, periodontal or gum disease, protruding upper incisors (buck teeth), veneers, crowns, bridgework and implants, isolated teeth, and previously traumatized teeth.[66]

Avoiding unnecessary airway instrumentation and taking due care with airway equipment is key to preventing dental damage. Specifically designed bite blocks or ones made of gauze should be used in favor of hard oral airways to reduce the risk of trauma due to biting.[66] Preoperative optimization of dental integrity may be useful. The use of mouth guards in the setting of poor dentition has not been shown to decrease the incidence of dental trauma.[65]

In the event of dental damage, all missing fragments need to be accounted for; the patient should be provided with a full explanation and referral should be made for dental assessment.

DRUG REACTIONS
Anaphylaxis

Anaphylaxis is a type 1 hypersensitivity reaction resulting from antigen-triggered histamine release.

The incidence of anaphylaxis in patients undergoing anesthesia is 1:10,000 to 1:20,000 and is fatal in up to 10% of cases.[67] In anesthesia, up to 60% of anaphylaxis is caused by neuromuscular blocking drugs followed by antibiotics, latex, and chlorhexidine.[67,68]

Anaphylaxis can manifest in many ways including cardiovascular (tachycardia, hypotension), cutaneous (rash), and respiratory symptoms (bronchospasm, hypoxia), and rarely, cardiovascular collapse or cardiac arrest. Treatment consists of removing the causative agent, administering vasopressors, bronchodilators, and intravenous fluids. Adrenaline is the mainstay of treatment. There is no evidence that steroids change outcome.[68] After any suspected case of anaphylaxis, it is essential to refer patients for allergy testing. The gold standard is skin testing, which should be done 6 weeks after the event.[67]

Malignant Hyperthermia

Malignant hyperthermia (MH) is an autosomal dominant, pharmacogenetic disorder of skeletal muscle. When exposed to a trigger agent, patients susceptible to MH have disordered regulation of calcium within skeletal muscle leading to a hypermetabolic state. This potentially fatal state results in tachycardia, muscle rigidity, hypercapnea, and hyperthermia. All volatile anesthetic agents and depolarizing muscle relaxants are triggers for MH. The incidence of MH is in the order of 1:40,000 to 1:100,000, however the prevalence of MH is up to 1:3000 patients.[69,70] Many people who have suspected MH susceptibility who present for surgery have not had formal testing to confirm the diagnosis and a family history of this disorder should always be elicited. Patients with known or suspected MH susceptibility can still be safely anesthetized with a nontriggering anesthetic that ensures strict avoidance of triggering agents.[70] Treatment consists of early recognition, removal of the trigger agent, and administration of dantrolene.[69] MH is a true anesthesia emergency and protocols exist to provide team members with explicit roles should it occur.

Succinylcholine Apnea

Succinylcholine is a depolarizing neuromuscular blocking drug with a rapid onset and short duration of action because the drug is metabolized by plasma cholinesterase. Variations in plasma cholinesterase can result in decreased metabolism of succinylcholine and prolonged duration of action. This condition can be inherited or acquired. Inherited forms result in decreased or absent plasma cholinesterase. Acquired forms result in normal levels of plasma cholinesterase but with reduced activity and can occur in hypothyroidism, pregnancy, liver or renal disease, or as a result of other medications such as methotrexate or anticholinesterases.[71] If succinylcholine apnea occurs, the patient needs to remain anesthetized and ventilated until neuromuscular function returns. They should be advised to avoid succinylcholine in the future and formal testing should be arranged for themselves and their families.

DELAYED DISCHARGE AND UNPLANNED ADMISSION

Delayed discharge and unplanned hospital admission are potential complications of any anesthetic. They are measures of quality of care and important markers in assessing outcomes.[72]

Delays can occur when discharging patients from the postanesthesia care unit or to home. Risk factors for delayed discharge and unplanned admission are outlined in **Box 3**.[73,74] Both delayed discharge and readmission can have significant costs attached.

One to two percent of ambulatory surgical patients are unable to be discharged home after

---

Box 3
Risk factors for delayed discharge and unplanned admission

Patient
- Increased age
- Intraoperative cardiac event
- Lack of escort
- Comorbidities (ischemic heart disease, diabetes, obstructive sleep apnea)

Surgical
- Ear, nose, and throat, strabismus surgery, urologic procedures, orthopedic surgery
- Long duration
- Inexperience of surgeon
- Bleeding

Anesthetic
- General anesthesia
- Spinal anesthesia
- PONV
- Pain
- Drowsiness
- Inexperienced recovery nurse

surgery as planned, resulting in an unplanned admission. One to three percent of ambulatory surgery patients who have been discharged appropriately require readmission to hospital within 30 days of surgery. This is commonly due to surgical complications such as bleeding, infection, and pain. Anesthesia is rarely a factor in hospital readmission.[73]

SUMMARY

General anesthesia is safe and uneventful in most patients. Some perioperative morbidity and mortality is inevitable, especially as more surgical procedures are now performed on older, sicker patients. Some anesthesia-related complications such as PONV, sore throat, and dental damage cause significant patient distress but no long-term morbidity, whereas cardiac, respiratory and renal perioperative complications are associated with long-term morbidity and mortality. All complications have associated costs to patients and the health system. By appropriately assessing patients preoperatively, risk factors for general anesthetic complications can be identified and modified.

REFERENCES

1. Bainbridge D, Martin J, Arango M, et al. Perioperative and anaesthetic-related mortality in developed and developing countries: a systematic review and meta-analysis. Lancet 2012;380:1075–81.
2. Jenkins K, Baker AB. Consent and anaesthetic risk. Anaesthesia 2003;58:962–84.
3. Devereaux PJ, Xavier D, Pogue J, et al. Characteristics and short-term prognosis of perioperative myocardial infarction in patients undergoing noncardiac surgery: a cohort study. Ann Intern Med 2011;154:523–8.
4. Devereaux PJ, Yang H, Yusuf S, et al. Effects of extended-release metoprolol succinate in patients undergoing non-cardiac surgery (POISE trial): a randomised controlled trial. Lancet 2008;371:1839–47.
5. Landesberg G, Beattie WS, Mosseri M, et al. Perioperative myocardial infarction. Circulation 2009;119:2936–44.
6. Devereaux PJ. Perioperative cardiac events in patients undergoing noncardiac surgery: a review of the magnitude of the problem, the pathophysiology of the events and methods to estimate and communicate risk. Can Med Assoc J 2005;173:627–34.
7. Lee TH, Marcantonio ER, Mangione CM, et al. Derivation and prospective validation of a simple index for prediction of cardiac risk of major noncardiac surgery. Circulation 1999;100:1043–9.
8. Fleisher LA, Beckman JA, Brown KA, et al. ACC/AHA 2007 guidelines on perioperative cardiovascular evaluation and care for noncardiac surgery: a report of the American College of Cardiology/American Heart Association task force on practice guidelines. Circulation 2007;116:e418–500.
9. Myles PS, Leslie K, Peyton P, et al. Nitrous oxide and perioperative cardiac morbidity (ENIGMA-II) trial: rationale and design. Am Heart J 2009;157:488–94.e1.
10. Beattie WS, Badner NH. The enigma of ENIGMA-I. Anesth Analg 2011;112:255–7.
11. Valchanov KP, Arrowsmith JE. The role of venodilators in the perioperative management of heart failure. Eur J Anaesthesiol 2012;29:121–8.
12. Priebe HJ. Preoperative cardiac management of the patient for non-cardiac surgery: an individualized and evidence-based approach. Br J Anaesth 2011;107:83–96.
13. Bhaskar B, Fraser J. Negative pressure pulmonary edema revisited: pathophysiology and review of management. Saudi J Anaesth 2011;5:308.
14. Amar D. Strategies for perioperative arrhythmias. Best Pract Res Clin Anaesthesiol 2004;18:565–77.
15. Walsh SR, Tang T, Wijewardena C, et al. Postoperative arrhythmias in general surgical patients. Ann R Coll Surg Engl 2007;89:91–5.
16. Pannucci CJ, Bailey SH, Dreszer G, et al. Validation of the Caprini Risk Assessment Model in plastic and reconstructive surgery patients. J Am Coll Surg 2011;212:105–12.
17. Murphy RX, Schmitz D, Rosolowski K. Evidence-based practices for thromboembolism prevention: a report from the ASPS Venous Thromboembolism Task Force. Arlington Heights (IL): American Society of Plastic Surgeons; 2011.
18. Gould MK. Prevention of VTE in nonorthopedic surgical patients: antithrombotic therapy and prevention of thrombosis. Chest 2012;141:e227S–77S.
19. Braz LG. Perioperative cardiac arrest: a study of 53 718 anaesthetics over 9 yr from a Brazilian teaching hospital. Br J Anaesth 2006;96:569–75.
20. Ferreyra G, Long Y, Ranieri VM. Respiratory complications after major surgery. Curr Opin Crit Care 2009;15:342–8.
21. Smetana GW, Lawrence VA, Cornell JE. Preoperative pulmonary risk stratification for noncardiothoracic surgery: systematic review for the American College of Physicians. Ann Intern Med 2006;144:581.
22. Smetana GW. Preoperative pulmonary evaluation. N Engl J Med 1999;340:937–44.
23. Hedenstierna G. Oxygen and anesthesia: what lung do we deliver to the post-operative ward? Acta Anaesthesiol Scand 2012;56:675–85.
24. Smetana GW, Lawrence VA, Cornell JE. Postoperative pulmonary complications: an update on risk

assessment and reduction. Cleve Clin J Med 2009; 76:S60–5.

25. Turan A, Mascha EJ, Roberman D, et al. Smoking and perioperative outcomes. Anesthesiology 2011; 114:837–46.

26. Valkenet K, van de Port IG, Dronkers JJ, et al. The effects of preoperative exercise therapy on postoperative outcome: a systematic review. Clin Rehabil 2011;25:99–111.

27. Freitas ER, Soares BG, Cardoso JR, et al. Incentive spirometry for preventing pulmonary complications after coronary artery bypass graft. Cochrane Database Syst Rev 2012;9:CD004466.

28. Wong J, Lam DP, Abrishami A, et al. Short-term preoperative smoking cessation and postoperative complications: a systematic review and meta-analysis. Can J Anaesth 2011;59:268–79.

29. Cook TM, Woodall N, Frerk C. Major complications of airway management in the UK: results of the Fourth National Audit Project of the Royal College of Anaesthetists and the Difficult Airway Society. Part 1: anaesthesia. Br J Anaesth 2011; 106:617–31.

30. Kluger MT, Short TG. Aspiration during anaesthesia: a review of 133 cases from the Australian Anaesthetic Incident Monitoring Study (AIMS). Anaesthesia 1999;54:19–26.

31. Westhorpe RN. Crisis management during anaesthesia: bronchospasm. Qual Saf Health Care 2005;14:1–6.

32. Dewachter P, Mouton-Faivre C, Emala CW, et al. Case scenario: bronchospasm during anesthetic induction. Anesthesiology 2011;114:1200–10.

33. Olsson GL. Bronchospasm during anaesthesia. A computer-aided incidence study of 136,929 patients. Acta Anaesthesiol Scand 1987;31: 244–52.

34. Rudolph JL, Schreiber KA, Culley DJ, et al. Measurement of post-operative cognitive dysfunction after cardiac surgery: a systematic review. Acta Anaesthesiol Scand 2010;54:663–77.

35. Evered L, Scott DA, Silbert B, et al. Postoperative cognitive dysfunction is independent of type of surgery and anesthetic. Anesth Analg 2011;12: 1179–85.

36. Rudolph JL, Marcantonio ER. Postoperative delirium. Anesth Analg 2011;112:1202–11.

37. Hudetz AG, Hemmings HC. Anaesthesia awareness: 3 years of progress. Br J Anaesth 2012; 108:180–2.

38. Hardman JG. Awareness during anaesthesia. Cont Educ Anaesth Crit Care Pain 2005;5:183–6.

39. Pandit JJ, Cook TM, Jonker WR, et al. A national survey of anaesthetists (NAP5 Baseline) to estimate an annual incidence of accidental awareness during general anaesthesia in the UK. Anaesthesia 2013;68:343–53.

40. Leslie K, Chan MT, Myles PS, et al. Posttraumatic stress disorder in aware patients from the B-Aware Trial. Anesth Analg 2010;110:823–8.

41. Myles PS, Leslie K, McNeil J, et al. Bispectral index monitoring to prevent awareness during anaesthesia: the B-Aware randomised controlled trial. Lancet 2004;363:1757–63.

42. Avidan MS, Zhang L, Burnside BA, et al. Anesthesia awareness and the bispectral index. N Engl J Med 2008;358:1097–108.

43. Avidan MS, Jacobsohn E, Glick D, et al. Prevention of intraoperative awareness in a high-risk surgical population. N Engl J Med 2011;365:591–600.

44. Mashour GA, Shanks A, Tremper KK, et al. Prevention of intraoperative awareness with explicit recall in an unselected surgical population: a randomized comparative effectiveness trial. Anesthesiology 2012;117:717–25.

45. Sear JW. Kidney dysfunction in the postoperative period. Br J Anaesth 2005;95:20–32.

46. Bellomo R, Ronco C, Kellum JA, et al. Acute renal failure: definition, outcome measures, animal models, fluid therapy and information technology needs: the Second International Consensus Conference of the Acute Dialysis Quality Inititative (ADQI) Group. Crit Care 2004;8:R204–12.

47. Kidney Disease: Improving Global Outcomes (KDIGO) Acute Kidney Injury Work Group. Clinical Practice Guideline for Acute Kidney Injury. Kidney Int Suppl 2012;2:1–141.

48. Calvert S, Shaw A. Perioperative acute kidney injury. Periop Med 2012;1:1–11.

49. Borthwick E, Ferguson A. Perioperative acute kidney injury: risk factors, recognition, management, and outcomes. BMJ 2010;341:c3365.

50. Carmichael P, Carmichael AR. Acute renal failure in the surgical setting. ANZ J Surg 2003;73:144–53.

51. Gentz BA, Malan TP. Renal toxicity with sevoflurane: a storm in a teacup. Drugs 2001;61:2155–62.

52. Wagener G, Brentjens TE. Renal disease: the anesthesiologist's perspective. Anesthesiol Clin 2006; 24:523–47.

53. Webb ST, Allen JS. Perioperative renal protection. Cont Educ Anaesth Crit Care Pain 2008;8:176–80.

54. Gan TJ, Meyer TA, Apfel CC, et al. Society for Ambulatory Anesthesia guidelines for the management of postoperative nausea and vomiting. Anesth Analg 2007;105:1615–28.

55. Apfel CC, Läärä E, Koivuranta M, et al. A simplified risk score for predicting postoperative nausea and vomiting: conclusions from cross-validations between two centers. Anesthesiology 1999;91:693–700.

56. Apfel CC, Philip BK, Cakmakkaya OS, et al. Who is at risk for postdischarge nausea and vomiting after ambulatory surgery? Anesthesiology 2012;117: 475–86.

57. Apfel CC, Korttila K, Abdalla M, et al. A factorial trial of six interventions for the prevention of postoperative nausea and vomiting. N Engl J Med 2004;350:2441–51.

58. Gan TJ. Risk factors for postoperative nausea and vomiting. Anesth Analg 2006;102:1884–98.

59. Chandrakantan A, Glass PS. Multimodal therapies for postoperative nausea and vomiting, and pain. Br J Anaesth 2011;107:i27–40.

60. Higgins PP, Chung F, Mezei G. Postoperative sore throat after ambulatory surgery. Br J Anaesth 2002;88:582–4.

61. McHardy FE, Chung F. Postoperative sore throat: cause, prevention and treatment. Anaesthesia 1999;54:444–53.

62. Stout DM, Bishop MJ, Dwersteg JF, et al. Correlation of endotracheal tube size with sore throat and hoarseness following general anesthesia. Anesthesiology 1987;67:419–21.

63. Scuderi PE. Postoperative sore throat. Anesth Analg 2010;111:831–2.

64. Seet E, Yousaf F, Gupta S, et al. Use of manometry for laryngeal mask airway reduces postoperative pharyngolaryngeal adverse events: a prospective, randomized trial. Anesthesiology 2010;112:652–7.

65. Newland MC, Ellis SJ, Peters KR, et al. Dental injury associated with anesthesia: a report of 161,687 anesthetics given over 14 years. J Clin Anesth 2007;19:339–45.

66. Windsor J, Lockie J. Anaesthesia and dental trauma. Anaesth Int Care Med 2008;9:355–7.

67. Harper NJ, Dixon T, Dugué P, et al. Suspected anaphylactic reactions associated with anaesthesia. Anaesthesia 2009;64:199–211.

68. Dewachter P, Mouton-Faivre C, Emala CW. Anaphylaxis and anesthesia: controversies and new insights. Anesthesiology 2009;111:1141–50.

69. Halsall PJ, Hopkins PM. Malignant hyperthermia. Cont Educ Anaesth Crit Care Pain 2003;3:5–9.

70. Wappler F. Anesthesia for patients with a history of malignant hyperthermia. Curr Opin Anaesthesiol 2010;23:417–22.

71. Appiah-Ankam J, Hunter JM. Pharmacology of neuromuscular blocking drugs. Cont Educ Anaesth Crit Care Pain 2004;4:2–7.

72. Shnaider I, Chung F. Outcomes in day surgery. Curr Opin Anaesthesiol 2006;19:622–9.

73. Awad IT, Chung F. Factors affecting recovery and discharge following ambulatory surgery. Can J Anaesth 2006;53:858–72.

74. Mandal A, Imran D, McKinnell T, et al. Unplanned admissions following ambulatory plastic surgery – a retrospective study. Ann R Coll Surg Engl 2005; 87:466–8.

A Primer on Local Anesthetics for Plastic Surgery

Kevin Armstrong, MD

KEYWORDS

- Local anesthetics • Mechanism • Sodium channel • Tumescent anesthesia • Duration of action
- Complications

KEY POINTS

- Local anesthetics are efficacious for several plastic surgery procedures.
- Amino amides are the most commonly used local anesthetics.
- Potency, onset, and duration are related to lipid solubility and protein binding.
- Different agents have differing duration and onset.
- Local anesthetics block the voltage-gated sodium channel nonselectively.
- The voltage-gated sodium channel offers the potential for selectivity.
- Metabolism of amide local anesthetics depends on liver function.
- The addition of adjuvants can alter efficacy and safety.
- Local anesthetic systemic toxicity is life threatening.
- Bupivacaine in large doses is potentially fatal.
- Levobupivacaine and ropivacaine are safer agents and are suitable substitutes for bupivacaine.
- Where large doses of local anesthetic are used, lipid rescue kits, which can reduce morbidity and mortality, should be available.

INTRODUCTION

Local anesthetics are a major contributor to medical and dental practice throughout the world. No doubt most, if not all readers are aware of the effectiveness of this class of medication through personal experience. Provision and delivery of anesthesia and/or analgesia using local anesthetic can be accomplished in several ways. Local anesthetics have been administered as a field block, injection near minor or major nerves and plexuses, and injection into the epidural or intrathecal space. Other methods include transcutaneous application, tumescent anesthesia, and intravenous delivery.

HISTORY

Since the introduction of cocaine to medical practice in 1884, local anesthetics have been and continue to be a valuable tool in surgical practice.

Since its isolation in 1855, cocaine was first synthesized in 1898. All synthetic local anesthetics are derivatives of cocaine. Many readers will recognize a handful of the 20 or so synthetic agents used historically. Like any pharmaceutical agent, there have been continued attempts to improve the efficacy and safety of this class of medication. Between 1891 and the 1970s several amino-ester (ester) and amino-amide (amide) local anesthetics have been synthesized.[1] Two newer agents have since been developed and introduced, primarily to address improved safety.

BASIC AND CLINICAL SCIENCE OF LOCAL ANESTHETICS
Amides

The most versatile of the group continues to be lidocaine. Lidocaine and the majority of local

Disclosures: None.
Department of Anesthesia and Perioperative Medicine, Schulich School of Medicine and Dentistry, Western University, 1151 Richmond Street, London, ON N6A 3K7, Canada
E-mail address: kevin.armstrong@sjhc.london.on.ca

Clin Plastic Surg 40 (2013) 515–528
http://dx.doi.org/10.1016/j.cps.2013.07.002

anesthetics currently used in surgical practice are amides. First developed in 1943, it is functional, relatively rapid in onset and removed, safe, and its use is extensive. The vast majority of plastic surgeons have a working clinical knowledge of lidocaine use. Perhaps the second most commonly used agent is bupivacaine, first developed in 1957 and released for clinical use in 1963. It is more potent and longer acting than lidocaine, and provides suitable anesthesia and/or postprocedure pain control on the order of 2 to 4 times that of lidocaine. The major drawback to its use is safety. Several fatalities caused by local anesthetic systemic toxicity (LAST) have involved the use of bupivacaine.[1]

Prilocaine was first synthesized in 1953. Its most common usage today is as a component of EMLA (a mixture of lidocaine and prilocaine). Some see this as a useful agent for intravenous regional anesthesia (IVRA). Prilocaine is also known for one of its toxic reactions, methemoglobinemia.

Mepivacaine, first synthesized in 1956, is similar to lidocaine with regard to onset and duration of action. It is thought to have some vasoconstrictive properties, which is a characteristic of few local anesthetics. Mepivacaine is a chiral molecule, and is sold as a racemic mixture of R and S optical isomers.

Articaine (synthesized in 1969) has extensive use in dental anesthesia. A PubMed search results in more than 300 references since the year 2000, most of which are related to dental practice, with some anesthesia studies. Its use in tumescent anesthesia for liposuction has been evaluated.[2] Possible advantages are rapid onset and short duration, attributable to an additional ester group on the lipophilic side chain that is rapidly metabolized.

Esters

Cocaine is still used in medical practice, primarily in nasal surgery. Other agents with fewer side effects are available, but cocaine's vasoconstrictive effects remain the primary reason for its use. Systemic absorption of cocaine can result in hemodynamic alteration in the patient.

Benzocaine, first synthesized in 1890, is not used in the clinical situation but is present in some over-the-counter cough drops.

Tetracaine was synthesized in the 1930s; its primary use is in topical anesthesia (ophthalmology) and in wound anesthesia.

Chlorprocaine, first introduced in 1955, is a rapid-onset, short-acting agent. Like most esters, it is rapidly metabolized by plasma esterases, so it is viewed as being very safe. In those with pseudocholinesterase deficiency, duration may be longer and the safety reduced. Since 2013, its

availability in North America has been limited because of a manufacturing issue.

Newer Agents

For several years the agents listed thus far were the basis of local anesthesia. In response to fatalities involving bupivacaine, a search for a safer alternative was undertaken. Two commercially available amides were the result of this search: ropivacaine and levobupivacaine.

Synthesized in 1993 and introduced in 1996, ropivacaine is a single enantiomer. It has an improved risk profile in comparison with bupivacaine, and a similar duration of action. Ropivacaine does not cause the same degree of vasodilation as many local anesthetics. Use of ropivacaine in plastic surgery is limited,[3] although its use has been evaluated in digital nerve blocks[4] and infiltrative anesthesia.[5]

Similarly, levobupivacaine is the S-enantiomer of bupivacaine. Released in the late 1990s, its safety profile is better than that of racemic bupivacaine. The clinical effect is similar to that of ropivacaine and bupivacaine,[6] but studies do exist demonstrating superiority of one over the other.[7–9] Much of the research regarding comparison with ropivacaine has been in peripheral nerve block and neuraxial anesthesia/analgesia.

The difference between agents is frequently identified as potency. Lack of familiarity, cost, and limited improvement on currently available local anesthetics have hindered the adoption of these 2 agents. However, in situations where large doses of local anesthetic are used, either of these newer agents should be considered.

Mixing of Local Anesthetics

Depending on the intended use of a local anesthetic, a clinician may look at the various properties of a particular anesthetic (speed of onset, duration, dosage, toxicity, and so forth) and "wish" for an improved picture. The mixing of local anesthetics has been evaluated, with varying results.[10,11] Caution should be exercised when mixing agents because the risk of error is possible. The practice of mixing agents is most commonly used in peripheral nerve block.

Structure

Synthetic local anesthetics are all derivatives of cocaine, are small molecules with molecular weights of less than 500, and fall primarily into 2 categories (**Fig. 1**). A lipophilic portion and a hydrophilic portion are linked by either an amino ester or an amide. Modification to either of the side chains can change the physical properties of the agent.

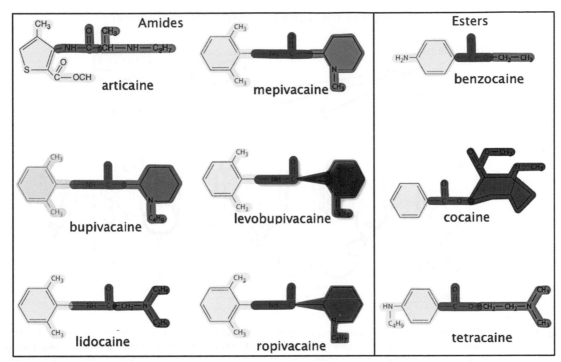

Fig. 1. Amino-amide and amino-ester local anesthetics. The link is represented by red, and yellow represents the lipophilic side chain. Blue indicates the hydrophilic side chain. Mepivacaine, bupivacaine, and ropivacaine exist as optical isomers. Levobupivacaine and ropivacaine are marketed as isolated L-isomers.

For agents with a chiral carbon (ie, mepivacaine and bupivacaine) it is possible to separate racemic mixtures to realize a single optical isomer. The isolated optical isomer is one of the more recent advances to show potential for clinical use.[1]

Mechanism of Action

Many readers will be familiar with the concepts of transmembrane potential and the action potential in excitatory cells. This action potential is the unit of information transfer in the motor, sensory, or autonomic nervous system. Sodium flux across the cellular membrane is a primary contributor to the development and propagation of the action potential. Local anesthetics reduce or stop sodium movement across the membrane by blocking the voltage-gated sodium channel. This blockade of the sodium channel is accepted as the mechanism whereby local anesthetics work. When enough sodium channels are blocked, neural traffic is stopped and anesthesia results. These agents also cause nonselective blockade of potassium and/or calcium channels.[12] These secondary effects contribute to side effects and toxicity.

The Sodium Channel

To a clinical physician, the significance of this molecular-complex voltage-gated sodium may

not be readily apparent. However, the structure and function of these channels is a basis for understanding the mechanisms, complications, and future developments of local anesthetics. The sodium channel is composed of 1 α and 2 β subunits. The α subunit is further divided into 4 domains, and each domain has 6 transmembrane segments (**Fig. 2**). Often represented as a 2-dimensional linear structure across the cell membrane, in vivo its 3-dimensional structure forms a channel. Two of the transmembranal segments (S5 and S6) from each domain contribute to a channel which, when open, allows the sodium ion to traverse the membrane. The regulation of this channel's patency is determined by a voltage-sensitive (charged) portion of a segment from each domain. In a changing electrical field, such as occurs during the action potential, a conformational change in the channel results in closing or opening of that channel.[13] Local anesthetics bind to a segment of the α subunit (segment 6 of domain 4). When this occurs the channel does not open, regardless of voltage change.

The voltage-gated sodium channel exists in 3 conformational states. The "neutral" state can be considered the resting closed state. Transient changes in transmembrane voltage (toward less negative) results in a conformational change to the activated open state. During this time there is

Alpha Subunit of the Voltage Gated Sodium Channel

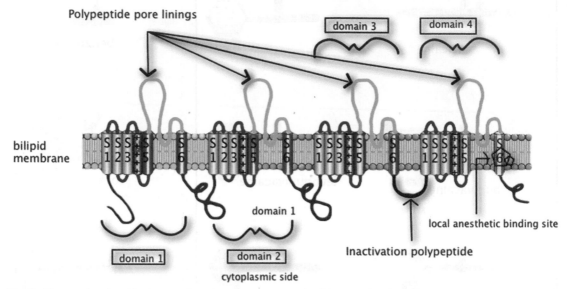

Fig. 2. The α subunit with 4 repeating domains, composed of 6 repeating helical segments. Segment 4 is the voltage sensor, owing to its heavy positive charge. Movement of segment 4, in the changing electric field during an action potential, causes a conformational change (open then closed). The subunit folds to form the channel. Segments 5 and 6 from each domain approximate to form the pore. Several polypeptides contribute to the functioning of the channel. Four peptides that connect S5 and S6 (*green*) fold inward to line the ion pore. The polypeptide joining S6 of domain 3 and S1 of domain 4 is the inactivation gate. Local anesthetics bind to segment 6 from the cytoplasmic side of the membrane and within the pore.

significant ion movement and subsequent regional alteration in the transmembrane potential, which results in nearby voltage-gated channels moving to the activated open state and propagation of the action potential. As the transmembrane potential returns to its baseline state through the movement of primarily potassium ions, the channel changes to an inactivated closed state, by way of a voltage-sensitive mechanism.

Local anesthetics bind to a receptor on the sixth segment of the fourth domain, which causes the channel to become stabilized in the inactivated closed state. Movement of sodium ions is thus halted, regardless of changes in transmembrane potential. The result is failure of the action potential to propagate, and potential sensory and motor information is not transmitted.

For an agent to access the receptor site it must enter the cell. Larger molecules, such as pufferfish toxin, block sodium conduction from the outside of the cell. There is specificity for various sodium channels, and the blockade is probably a physical obstruction rather than the conformational change that results from the action of local anesthetic. To enter the cell requires movement across the bilipid cell membrane. Physical properties, in particular the lipophilicity of a particular local anesthetic,

will determine the amount and speed at which this movement occurs.

Potency of Local Anesthetics

In general terms, local anesthetics have a low affinity for the sodium channel. The relatively large doses account for the effectiveness of the agents. Potency describes the relative activity of 2 medications with the same mechanism of action. A medication is more potent if a lesser "amount" of an agent is required to produce the same effect when compared with the other. Considering the 2 most commonly used agents, lidocaine and bupivacaine, the latter is more potent. A major contributor is lipid solubility (**Table 1**). A related phenomenon is the duration of action. Generally speaking, more potent agents have a longer duration of action (**Table 2**). With respect to bupivacaine, its greater toxicity is related to potency.

Potential Future

The search for ideal medications has been a goal of pharmacology since its beginnings. In the context of local anesthesia, such an agent or agents would block pain sensation only (in many situations). The concept of receptor and

Table 1
Physical properties of local anesthetics

Local Anesthetic	Toxicity	Lipid Solubility	Protein Binding (%)	Potency	pK_a	Onset	Duration of Action Relative	Hours
Cocaine	High	—	98	Low	8.7	Slow	Long	—
2-Chloroprocaine	Low	Low	0	High	9.1	Very rapid	Short	0.5–1
Tetracaine	High	High	76	High	8.4	Slow	Long	2–6
Articaine	Low	High	94	—	7.8	Rapid	Short	1
Bupivacaine	High	High	96	High	8.1	Slow	Long	3–8
Lidocaine	Low	Low	65	Low	7.8	Rapid	Medium	1–3
Levobupivacaine	Intermediate	High	96	High	8.1	Moderate	Long	3–8
Mepivacaine	Intermediate	Low	78	Low	7.7	Moderate	Medium	2–4
Prilocaine	Intermediate	Low	55	Low	8.0	—	Medium	—
Ropivacaine	Intermediate	Intermediate	93	High	8.1	Moderate	Long	3–8

The physical properties of a local anesthetic will affect its onset, duration, and toxicity. The majority of local anesthetics are small molecules, with molecular weights ranging from 246 Da (mepivacaine) to 288 Da (bupivacaine). The pK_a in the setting of the environmental pH will affect lipid solubility. Most agents have a pK_a greater than 7.7. Higher percentage of protein binding tends to lead to longer duration of action. Duration varies according to agent, site of application, and addition of adjuvants for some agents. Potency is reported as high, intermediate, or low, and is relative to other agents.

antagonist is well established in medicine, as are antagonists for those receptors. Common examples include the α, β, opioid, neuromuscular, and cholinergic receptors. The voltage-gated sodium channel has a receptor for low molecular weight local anesthetics. Recent findings have further elucidated the structure of the voltage-gated sodium channel.[14] In 2013 there are 9 distinguishable subtypes of the voltage-gated sodium channel, and the potential for selectivity is possible.[15] Much attention is now directed toward subtype 1.7 (Nav1.7), as this channel is considered to be present in the peripheral nerve system, and is important in the sympathetic nervous system and primary afferent neurons. Pufferfish toxin and other toxins do show selectivity for various ion channels, but the specificity of any agent is limited. Smaller compounds with names such as A-803467 have selectivity for the Nav1.7, and offer promise for more directed therapy.

Onset of Effectiveness

Another consideration regarding local anesthetics is time to onset. Regardless of the agent, time is required for a local anesthetic to become effective. This onset time is usually in the range of minutes (see **Table 1**), and also depends on where or how the agent is administered. Many attempts have been made to reduce the time between injection or application and effect. Such approaches include altering pH; adding opioids, steroids, or

vasoconstrictors; mixing agents; and warming the agent. There are data to suggest that some maneuvers are beneficial, but the improvement may be small. In addition, altering an agent may increase the number of errors.

Lipid Solubility

Lipid solubility is a requirement for local anesthetics to enter the cell, because the receptor is accessed from within.[1] The lipid bilayer is a barrier for hydrophilic molecules, because it is a very lipid-dense environment (see **Fig. 2**). An agent's lipophilicity (see **Table 1**) depends on the hydrophobic side chain and is affected by the electrical state (charged or uncharged).

Most local anesthetics are weak bases and are prepared as hydrochloride salts, frequently expressed as

$$NH_4^- + H^+ \leftrightarrow NH_4H$$

With the exception of prilocaine, all agents have a pH greater than 7.7. The pK_a is the pH at which 50% of a salt is ionized (NH_4^-) and 50% is un-ionized (NH_4H). The Henderson-Hasselbalch equation describes the ratio of these 2 states.

Commercially available local anesthetics have a pH of 3 to 5, depending on the agent and whether epinephrine is in the preparation. A low pH improves agent stability. To promote the un-ionized form of the agent, which in turn promotes transmembranal movement, it would be advantageous

Table 2
A general guideline for safe dosage and expected durations of various local anesthetics for the average adult patient

Local Anesthetic Preparations Concentration in Volume % (mass/mL)	Maximal Single Dosing by Mass or Volume			Expected Duration by Site or Administration Appropriate Dose (hours)		
	mg/kg	Maximal Dose (mg)	Max Volume (mL)	Infiltration (min)	PNB (min)	Epidural (min)
Lidocaine Plain						
0.5% (5mg/mL)	5	200–300	40–60	75–90	90–120	30–45
1% (10 mg/mL)	5	200–300	20–30	75–90	90–120	30–45
Lidocaine plus epinephrine	there is 5 mcg/mL of epinephrine in commercial preparation of lidocaine +epi					
0.5% (5 mg/mL) + epinephrine	7	500	100	90–180	120–240	80–120
1% (10 mg/mL) + epinephrine	7	500	50	90–180	120–240	120–180
Buupivacaine	there is 5 mcg/mL of epinephrine in commercial preparation of bupivacaine + epi					
0.25% (2.5 mg/mL)	2.0	175	70	180–360	360–720	165–225
0.5% (5 mg/mL)	2.0	175	35	180–360	360–720	165–225
0.25% (2.5 mg/mL) + epi	3.0	225	90	200–400	360–720	165–225
Ropivacaine/Levobupivacaine	the addition of epinephrine does not affect maximal dose or duration					
0.5% (5mg/mL)	3.0	225–300	45–60	180–240	360–720	165–225
ropivacaine 0.5% + epi	3.0	225–300	45–60	180–240	360–720	165–225
levobupivacaine 0.5%	3.0	225–300	45–60	NA	360–720	165–225
Tumescent lidocaine with epinephrine	Preparation involves diluting of plain lidocaine with with normal saline and the addition of epinephrine (0.5–1 mcg/mL) and sodium bicabonate to 1000 mLs					
0.05–.1% (0.5–1 mg/mL)	55	3500[a]	3500–7000	480–1200	—	—

The lowest dose to produce the desired effect should be employed.
In situations where there is cardiac, liver or renal disease, dose adjustment should be considered.
Following these guidelines does not guarantee safety.
Tumescent anesthesia.
Doses of lidocaine up to 10 times those which appear in the product monograph have been evaluated and used in Clinical practice for a number of years.
Maximum doses would suggest extensive liposuction involving multiple operative sites.
[a] Based on 50/Kg for a 70 kg patient.

to make the injected local anesthetic, or the environment, basic. The addition of sodium bicarbonate (NaHCO$_3$) can increase the pH of the solution.[16] Excessive HCO$_3$ can decrease aqueous solubility and result in precipitation.[1]

Many readers are familiar with the knowledge or have experienced that local anesthetics are less effective at infected sites. This feature can be explained by the acidic conditions of infected tissue. The low pH drives the balance toward the ionized state, with decreased transmembranal movement and decreased effectiveness.

Duration of Action

Like onset, the duration of action depends on several variables that include the agent itself, the patient's age, the anatomic site of administration, circulatory status, the use of adjuvants, and so forth. This information is not always readily available from published data. In general, more potent agents are considered to be long acting (3–12 hours), whereas less potent agents are thought of as short acting (2–4 hours). Combining short-acting and long-acting agents may result in an intermediate duration.[11] **Table 2** provides some general times for duration of action based on some of these variables. Depending on the goal (eg, duration of surgery and postoperative pain relief), the provider may choose a particular agent.

The recovery from the effects of local anesthetics is a pharmacokinetic phenomenon. There must be sufficient reduction of drug at the site of action, so that blockage of the sodium channels is reduced. This reduction in the amount of local anesthetic occurs as a result of diffusion out of and away from the axon. The deposition of local anesthetic in the vicinity of the axon and intended movement into the axons is driven essentially by a concentration gradient from high to low concentration. There is also movement of the local anesthetic into the vascularity (and other cells/tissues) down a similar concentration gradient. Depending on the area of the body (vascular supply) and state of the cardiovascular system, duration will vary. In areas where metabolism is low and the vascular supply is low (ie, adipose), removal of local anesthetics will similarly be low and a longer duration of action will be apparent. In individuals with a very dynamic circulation (younger vs older individuals), removal of local anesthetic will be increased and, consequently, duration will be shorter.[17]

Metabolism

Metabolism can occur in the tissues, but the majority occurs away from the nerve. The specifics of metabolism depend on the type of local anesthetic. As described previously, these agents are characterized as either esters or amides. Esters are hydrolyzed by esterases such as plasma cholinesterase, whereas amides are metabolized in the liver by the cytochrome P450 system.[1] Small amounts of some local anesthetics may be eliminated without metabolism. Metabolism results in a more water-soluble compound and thus promotes renal elimination. Given that the liver synthesizes esterases and directly metabolizes amides, the level of local anesthetic will be higher in liver disease.[18] However, adjustment of local anesthetic dosing should be considered in those with significant liver disease.[19]

Elimination of Local Anesthetics

Elimination of unaltered local anesthetics does occur. As much as 5% of unaltered drug may be eliminated directly.[1] After metabolism, water-soluble metabolites are eliminated by the kidney. Some metabolites are active, and are metabolized further to reduce the effect before elimination. In addition, some of the dose injected into or absorbed into the vascular system is extracted by the lung.[13]

ADJUVANTS TO LOCAL ANESTHETICS

Many attempts have been made to improve the clinical profile of local anesthetics. Some of the goals include reducing the pain on injection, reducing the onset time, prolonging the duration of action, reducing toxicity, and improving efficacy. The addition of adjuvants may be of benefit.

Epinephrine

Epinephrine and phenylephrine have a vasoconstrictive effect, and have been used to improve infiltrative[20] and peripheral nerve block anesthesia.[1,13] In the case of commercially available local anesthetics, epinephrine containing solutions of both bupivacaine and lidocaine are available. Both local anesthetics are considered to have vasodilating effects, and vasoconstriction would produce a desirable effect. The primary goal is to prolong the duration of action by reducing systemic uptake, increase the amount of drug at the neuron, and increasing the time available for neural uptake. Epinephrine has also been used as a marker for intravascular injection. Fifteen micrograms (3 mL of a 1:200,000 solution) will produce signs (increased heart rate, blood pressure) and symptoms consistent with epinephrine. The symptoms (eg, palpitations, anxiety, headache, shortness of breath) may be reported as an allergic reaction. Infiltration at sites with limited arterial supply is a concern for some, but there is evidence that this may not be the case in patients with vascular compromise.[21] Epinephrine is sometimes added to bupivacaine, and to lidocaine for peripheral nerve blockade, because each has vasodilating effects. As identified previously, commercially prepared epinephrine-containing solutions may affect onset related to solution pH.

Bicarbonate

Alteration of pH can be achieved by adding $NaHCO_3$. As described earlier, increasing the pH toward the pK_a of the agent can result in faster onset.[16,22] This approach is generally practiced when using bupivacaine. Excessive sodium bicarbonate can result in precipitation out of solution. One milliliter of 8.4% $NaHCO_3$ is generally the volume that will be added to 20 mL of 0.5% bupivacaine to promote onset.[22] A higher pH has been identified as a means to reduce pain on infiltration.[23]

Opioids

The addition of opioids to local anesthetics is practiced in neuraxial and infiltrative anesthesia.[20,24] Its use in peripheral nerve blockade is less clear.[24,25] The mechanism is believed to be via peripheral opioid receptors in the infiltrative application, and spinal cord opioids in neuraxial anesthesia.

Nonsteroidal Anti-Inflammatory Agents

Parenteral preparations of nonsteroidal anti-inflammatory agents such as ketorolac and paracetamol have been combined with local anesthetics and opioids. Referred to as local infiltration analgesia, the most accepted use is in periarticular injection following knee arthroplasty[20] and IVRA.[26] The mechanism is believed to be a local anti-inflammatory effect.

Steroids

The addition of steroids to local anesthetics for peripheral nerve block may potentially prolong the analgesic effect.[27,28]

Temperature

Pain on injection of local anesthetics is a well-known phenomenon. The most effective measure is the warming of local anesthetics to body temperature,[29] which may be accomplished by various commercially available warmers.

CHOICE OF ANESTHETIC

Choice of an anesthetic is based on efficacy, duration of action, safety, familiarity, and the test of time. In North America, lidocaine and bupivacaine are commonly used. Depending on the situation and amount of drug used, either of these agents can achieve an effective, safe, and appropriate duration of action. Because all local anesthetics are no longer under patent, they are relatively inexpensive. The long-acting drugs levobupivacaine and ropivacaine have been shown to have better cardiac safety when compared with bupivacaine.[12,30] The impact of cost on choice of local anesthetic is an important consideration in the current fiscal environment. However, safety must also be considered when using large volumes of local anesthetics.

ADMINISTRATION OF ANESTHETIC

A common method for delivery of local anesthetics is local infiltration. For many procedures involving cutaneous and soft-tissue procedures, this is very effective. Limitations may include the extent of work to be done, the extent of work on deeper structures, and the volume of local anesthetic required. The accepted safe volumes for infiltration for average sized adults are listed in **Table 2**.

Transcutaneous Delivery

Topical and transcutaneous administration of local anesthetics has a particular niche in pediatric medicine. Perhaps the most well known is EMLA, a eutectic mixture of lidocaine and prilocaine that exists as a cream. When mixed together the melting point is lower than that of each agent by itself, which allows anesthesia to occur through intact skin. Its primary use is for intravenous starts. Others have used this product for debridement of leg ulcers,[31] skin grafting,[32] and after breast surgery for cancer,[33] among other applications. One of its limitations is that it requires 45 to 60 minutes before effectiveness. However, there can be complications secondary to its use, such as seizures and methemoglobinemia.[34]

In pediatric emergency rooms, a mixture of local anesthetics has been used to anesthetize lacerations in children before cleaning and suturing. Lidocaine (4%), epinephrine (0.05%) and tetracaine (0.5%) (LET) has replaced a mixture of tetracaine (1%), adrenalin (1:4000), and cocaine (4%) (TAC).[35]

Extended-release preparations (liposomes and polymers) are a potentially new means for drug delivery. Encapsulated local anesthetics have been evaluated as a delivery method, with some success.[36,37] Other transcutaneous delivery systems, such as iontophoresis, have been studied, but adoption into clinical practice has been limited. Transcutaneous patches for many medications including lidocaine do exist. However, the delivery rate would not produce anesthesia. These new developments show promise, but also require caution.

Tumescent Anesthesia

Traditionally tumescent anesthesia involves the use of large volumes of dilute local anesthetics for liposuction. Clinicians now find utility of this technique for other surgeries. The term tumescent refers to the physical appearance of tissues after the instillation of large volumes. The primary agent used, is very low concentration (0.05-0.1%) of lidocaine, mixed with epinephrine. More common preparations involve the dilution of 500 to 1000 mg to 1000 mL with normal saline. Epinephrine (0.5 mg to 1 mg), and sodium bicarbonate are also added to the preparation. Doses in the range of 35 mg/kg and, more recently, 55 mg/kg have been demonstrated as safe.[38] Such large doses would indicate extensive sites of treatment and duration of liposuction. Maximal dose would mean that approximately 7 litres of the 0.05% solution is used in the 70 Kg patient.

Mixed lidocaine and bupivacaine has also been evaluated.[39] It is recognized that the peak level of local anesthetic occurs 8 to 12 hours after the procedure,[40] meaning that this may occur beyond the bounds of a health care facility. Occasionally the death of a young person will occur in this setting, although the etiology of such mortality has not been fully established. Recently it has been suggested that fat emboli may be a major contributor.[41] The specific technique of tumescent anesthesia is beyond the scope of this chapter.

The apparent safety of this practice is illustrative of a concept described earlier where systemic absorption of local anesthetics is dependent to some degree on the vascularity of the tissue. A recurrent theme regarding the safe use of local anesthetics is that caution is to be exercised and that the lowest dose to produce the desired effect should be employed.

Intravenous Regional Anesthesia

IVRA, sometimes referred to as a Bier block, is an anesthetic technique used for procedures involving upper limbs, and less so for lower limbs. IVRA is fairly effective and requires common skills of practitioners, although there are some precautions to be observed. Such precautions are necessary because if a large dose of local anesthetic is delivered directly to the vascular system over a short period (ie, cuff failure), toxicity is likely. Depending on the agent, this may be fatal. For this reason lidocaine and prilocaine are the agents of choice, but mepivacaine and ropivacaine[42] have also been evaluated. Diligent monitoring of the patient is required, as well as specialized equipment and personnel. At the time of tourniquet deflation, if the procedure is shorter than 40 minutes many recommend monitoring for signs of systemic toxicity with intermittent cuff deflation. Offset of IVRA is rapid. When this form of anesthesia is chosen, postoperative pain management should be considered.

Nerve Blockade

Minor nerve blockade is a skill familiar to most plastic surgeons. The delivery of effective local anesthetic safely to the desired nerve(s) is beyond the scope of this article. The amount of local anesthetic generally accepted to be safe is presented in **Table 2**. Provision of anesthesia by major peripheral and plexus block as well as neuraxial blockade is addressed in the articles by Huq and Ahmed and by Offierski elsewhere in this publication.

Liposomal Encapsulated Local Anesthetics

One of the limitations of local anesthetics is the duration of effect for postoperative analgesia. Liposomal delivery systems may provide a solution.[36,37]

Some challenges to be overcome are stability of the liposomes once injected and the consistency of delivery. An unexpected release of large doses of local anesthetic may produce toxicity. In addition, long exposure of tissue to local anesthetics may cause local myotoxicity.[43,44]

COMPLICATIONS AND REACTIONS
Failure

Failure to complete a procedure to the satisfaction of the patient, surgeon, and anesthesiologist can occur when local anesthetics are used. The reason for this failure is sometimes difficult to ascertain. Possible causes include insufficient dose, insufficient time, inaccurate delivery, individual variation in response to local anesthetic, and variation in anatomy. Of these, inaccurate delivery and insufficient time are perhaps the most common. The consistency with which local anesthetics block sodium currents and thus propagate the action potential is sound, but efficacy can be unpredictable at times.

Esters Versus Amides Versus Preservative

Reactions to local anesthetics are reported with some frequency. Allergy is one of these possibilities, which can and does occur. The most common agents implicated in allergy are the esters. The hydrolysis of an ester results in the potential allergen, *para*-aminobenzoic acid (PABA).[1,45] True allergy to amides is less likely. The preservative methylparaben may be present in some formulations of local anesthetics and is similar to PABA, which can trigger an allergic response.[45]

Epinephrine

Other reactions may secondarily be due to the use of adjuvants, the most common of which is epinephrine. Tachycardia, hypertension, tremor, and a sense of "impending doom" may occur if epinephrine is injected intravascularly. The occurrence of such can be reduced if the physician:

1. Is aware of the possibility
2. Injects slowly
3. Aspirates intermittently
4. Visualizes local anesthetic on ultrasonography
5. Maintains contact with the patient

Systemic absorption can result in similar symptoms, but usually over a longer time frame.

Methemoglobinemia

Excessive vascular levels of prilocaine and benzocaine can result in methemoglobinemia.[1] This condition can occur when enough *O*-toluidine is generated from hepatic metabolism and oxidizes hemoglobin to methemoglobin. The patient can appear blue, and the ability to transport oxygen can be reduced. Methemoglobinemia is limited to prilocaine and benzocaine use. There are case reports in the pediatric literature of this complication secondary to ELMA.[34]

Tissue Injury

Local anesthetics can be injurious to some tissues, the most notable of which is the chondrocyte. In the 1990s, the use of intra-articular injection of bupivacaine resulted in chondrolysis.[46] Though not a usual practice by plastic surgeons, this illustrates that some tissues may be susceptible to injury. As highlighted earlier, there may be potential for local myotoxicity.[43,44]

Neurotoxicity

The concentration of currently available local anesthetics is unlikely to cause nerve injury. Nerve dysfunction and injury following the use of local anesthetics probably involves multiple mechanisms. The agent itself may play some role, but this is rare, and incompletely understood. The use of epinephrine may be contributory, because ischemia is an injury-producing event.

Limitations

The use of local anesthetics can provide an alternative to a general anesthetic. Anesthesia can be accomplished in several ways. Local infiltration, IVRA, distal or proximal peripheral nerve blockade, and neuraxial blockade are some of the choices. In addition, local anesthetics can be used for post-procedure pain management. However, preference of the patient, surgeon, or anesthesiologist can limit its suitability. Other limitations include duration of the procedure, duration of action, fear, unrealistic expectations, and impatience.

LOCAL ANESTHETIC SYSTEMIC TOXICITY

A common question is: what is the maximum dosage of a local anesthetic? Arriving at such an answer is challenging because the data available is difficult to interpret. As with most characteristics of local anesthetics, several variables are not applicable to all situations. The agent (ie. bupivacaine vs ropivacaine), dose, method of delivery (tumescent vs infiltration vs peripheral nerve block), site (intravascular vs tissue), rate of delivery, and use of adjuvants are some of the variables to consider. An appropriate starting point is the agent itself. There are general guidelines for dosages based on body weight. Examples of commonly accepted,

single time, maximum dosages for the average sized adult are presented in **Table 2**. However, very small amounts of drug can produce central nervous system toxicity if injected into the carotid or vertebral artery. To reduce the risk of systemic toxicity in the context of maximal doses a few strategies are to be considered: The lowest dose to produce the desired effect should be employed. Where maximal doses are used, caution is imperative. In situations where there is cardiac, liver or renal disease, dose adjustment should be considered. Finally it is important to understand that following these guidelines does not ensure that toxicity will not occur safety.

Higher Allowable Doses

Adding further confusion to the situation for the generalist is the use of tumescent anesthesia, for which extremely large doses of lidocaine have been approved for use.[38] Initially 35 mg/kg, the latest approved dose is 55 mg/kg (1997 onward), with no apparent toxicity issues. This circumstance perhaps illustrates a concept discussed earlier, namely that the site and circulatory condition of the tissue is a major contributor to systemic uptake. IVRA potentially exposes patients to systemic toxicity. A large dose of anesthetic can be delivered directly into the vascular system if precautions (ie, choice of agent, and availability of specialized equipment and personnel) are not taken.

Signs and Symptoms of Toxicity

The most serious consequence of LAST is death, which has occurred in several settings.[1] The progress of the signs and symptoms are traditionally described as mild to severe, and affect the central nervous system and cardiovascular system.

Initial signs and symptoms are excitatory:

- Ringing in the ears
- Metallic taste in the mouth
- Agitation
- Tachycardia
- Seizure

Later symptoms and signs are depressant:

- Unconsciousness
- Respiratory arrest
- Bradycardia
- Hypotension
- Cardiovascular arrest[47]

The agent and dose of medication will also affect the outcome. Understandably, this is of significant concern because serious morbidity and/or mortality can result. In the vast majority of cases, death has been associated with bupivacaine. Patients experiencing LAST secondary to bupivacaine have been very difficult to treat.

The most effective treatment of LAST is avoidance. A relatively new development in the treatment of LAST is lipid rescue.[47-49] Before the advent of this mode of treatment, local anesthetic toxicity involving bupivacaine in clinical and laboratory settings was refractory to any treatment and frequently fatal. The proposed mechanism of action is discussed in the next section.

Physiology of Toxicity

As outlined earlier, the mechanism of local anesthetics action is blockade of the sodium channel. In addition to voltage-gated sodium channels, there are potassium and calcium voltage-gated channels, each with a role to play in the electrical functioning of excitatory tissue. There are also subspecies of any of the voltage-gated channels. Each or any of these are blocked to some degree by local anesthetics in a nonspecific way, depending on the agent.[15,50,51] In the context of systemic delivery or absorption, the excitable tissues of the central nervous and cardiac system, when exposed to toxic levels, result in the previously described signs and symptoms. Normal functioning of the central nervous system involves both excitatory and inhibitory neurons. As LAST progresses, the inhibitory neurons are blocked first. This lack of inhibition on the excitatory neuron is thought to be the mechanism of the observed seizure. The functioning of the heart depends on a mechanism similar to that of the neuron. As predicted, blockade of the ion channels will affect initiation of contraction, propagation of the contraction, and repolarization. A toxic level of local anesthetic results in decreased contractility and several arrhythmias, the first of which to occur is perhaps bradycardia. Ventricular fibrillation is the most serious of the dysrhythmias. The mechanism seems intuitive, given the voltage-gated channel blocking effect of this class of medication.[1] It would be expected that patients with cardiovascular disease are more likely to be affected.

With respect to the extent of compromise, the agent itself plays a role. Shorter-acting lidocaine is less cardiotoxic than the longer-acting and more potent bupivacaine. Most reported deaths related to LAST involve bupivacaine.[1] The difference between short-acting and longer-acting agents may be related to their physical properties. The more potent agents are more lipid soluble and protein bound. As such, the duration of blockade of any voltage-gated channel is probably longer and thus the recovery is delayed. The newer agents ropivacaine and levobupivacaine were developed to address this issue of cardiotoxicity.[6,8,12,30,52] It appears that the L-enantiomer behaves differently in the blockade of these channels, and there seems to be selectivity for the voltage-gated channel.[15] These agents are accepted as safer; however, care should be taken when using large doses of any local anesthetic.[15]

Sedation and Toxicity

Benzodiazepines are frequently used in the setting of local anesthetic administration. In the setting of LAST, early neurologic signs and symptoms may be less apparent, and result in a narrowing between the neurologic signs and cardiovascular collapse. In addition, the respiratory depressant effects of benzodiazepines can result in higher CO_2 levels and acidosis, which may worsen toxicity through ion trapping and other electrolyte alteration.[53]

Supportive Treatment

When LAST is suspected, the first form of management is supportive. Calling for help and determining if the patient (1) is conscious and breathing, (2) has a patent airway, (3) has cardiac output (by pulse, blood pressure, or saturation probe), and (4) has intravenous access and supplemental oxygen is warranted. The knowledge that this may progress to seizure or cardiovascular collapse should initiate preparation for full resuscitation, including lipid rescue.[53]

Lipid Rescue

Lipid rescue is perhaps one of the greater advancements in the treatment of LAST, especially with the higher-potency agent bupivacaine. What was once a situation with limited options now offers some promise. Although the exact mechanism is unknown, the most popular mechanism proposed is that intravascular lipid acts as a "sink"[47,54-57] for excess local anesthetic in the circulatory system and reduces the drug available to produce toxicity. The Web site www.lipidrescue.org is dedicated to the topic. Information on overview, treatment, case reports, laboratory investigation, and so forth are presented. Major organizations such as the Association of Anaesthetists of Great Britain and Ireland and the American Society of Regional Anesthesia suggest that lipid rescue kits be available in cases where large doses of local anesthetics are used,[47,53] and also offer advice for developing and maintaining a lipid rescue kit. When LAST does occur, there are suggested alterations to advanced cardiac life support, including the avoidance of vasopressin, calcium-channel blockers, β-blockers, and local anesthetics. The dose of epinephrine is reduced to less than 1 μg/kg. The administration of 20% lipid emulsion in the amounts of 1.5 mL/kg as a bolus and an infusion of 0.25 mL/kg/min is used. There are recommendations for repeat boluses and an increase in infusion rates, all to a maximum of 10 to 12 mg/kg.

SUMMARY

Local anesthetics have a long history in the management of the surgical patient. There are some newer and safer anesthetics available that have not gained much headway in plastic surgery practice. A deeper understanding of the basics of local anesthetics can improve the experience of the user. The issue of safety has changed over the past few years, and caution is to be exercised when large doses of local anesthetics are used. In areas where large doses of local anesthetics are used, a lipid rescue kit should be developed and made available.

REFERENCES

1. Berde CB, Strichartz GR. Local anesthetics. Chapter 30. In: Miller RD, editor. Miller's anesthesia. 7th edition. Philadelphia: Churchill Livingstone; 2009.
2. Grossmann M, Sattler G, Pistner H, et al. Pharmacokinetics of articaine hydrochloride in tumescent local anesthesia for liposuction. J Clin Pharmacol 2004;44(11):1282–9.
3. Koeppe T, Constantinescu MA, Schneider J, et al. Current trends in local anesthesia in cosmetic plastic surgery of the head and neck: results of a German national survey and observations on the use of ropivacaine. Plast Reconstr Surg 2005;115(6):1723–30.
4. Keramidas EG, Rodopoulou SG. Ropivacaine versus lidocaine in digital nerve blocks: a prospective study. Plast Reconstr Surg 2007;119(7):2148–52.
5. Kakagia D, Fotiadis S, Tripsiannis G. Comparative efficacy of ropivacaine and bupivacaine infiltrative analgesia in otoplasty. Ann Plast Surg 2005;54(4):409–11.
6. Leone S, Di Cianni S, Casati A, et al. Pharmacology, toxicology, and clinical use of new long acting local anesthetics, ropivacaine and levobupivacaine. Acta Biomed 2008;79(2):92–105.
7. Kakagia D, Fotiadis S, Tripsiannis G. Levobupivacaine versus ropivacaine infiltration analgesia for mastopexy: a comparative study of 2 long-acting anesthetic drugs in infiltrative anesthesia for mastopexy. Ann Plast Surg 2005;55(3):258–61.
8. Zink W, Graf BM. The toxicity of local anesthetics: the place of ropivacaine and levobupivacaine. Curr Opin Anaesthesiol 2008;21(5):645–50.
9. Kakagia DD, Fotiadis S, Tripsiannis G, et al. Postoperative analgesic effect of locally infiltrated levobupivacaine in Fleur-de-Lys abdominoplasty. Aesthetic Plast Surg 2007;31(2):128–32.
10. Laur JJ, Bayman EO, Foldes PJ, et al. Triple-blind randomized clinical trial of time until sensory change using 1.5% mepivacaine with epinephrine, 0.5% bupivacaine, or an equal mixture of both for infraclavicular block. Reg Anesth Pain Med 2012;37(1):28–33.
11. Gadsden J, Hadzic A, Gandhi K, et al. The effect of mixing 1.5% mepivacaine and 0.5% bupivacaine on duration of analgesia and latency of block onset in ultrasound-guided interscalene block. Anesth Analg 2011;112(2):471–6.
12. Gristwood RW. Cardiac and CNS toxicity of levobupivacaine: strengths of evidence for advantage over bupivacaine. Drug Saf 2002;25(3):153–63.
13. Raj PP. Local anesthetics. Chapter 13. In: Raj PP, editor. Textbook of regional anesthesia. 1st edition. Churchill Livingstone; 2002.
14. Payandeh J, Scheuer T, Zheng N, et al. The crystal structure of a voltage-gated sodium channel. Nature 2011;475:353–8.
15. England S, de Groot MJ. Subtype-selective targeting of voltage-gated sodium channels. Br J Pharmacol 2009;158(6):1413–25.
16. Milner QJ, Guard BC, Allen JG. Alkalinization of amide local anaesthetics by addition of 1% sodium bicarbonate solution. Eur J Anaesthesiol 2000;17(1):38–42.
17. Leeson S, Strichartz G. Kinetics of uptake and washout of lidocaine in rat sciatic nerve in vitro. Anesth Analg 2013;116(3):694–702.
18. Lauprecht AE, Wenger FA, El Fadil O, et al. Levobupivacaine plasma concentrations following major liver resection. J Anesth 2011;25(3):369–75.
19. Rosenberg PH, Veering BT, Urmey WF. Maximum recommended doses of local anesthetics: a multifactorial concept. Reg Anesth Pain Med 2004;29(6):564–75 [discussion: 524].
20. Essving P, Axelsson K, Åberg E, et al. Local infiltration analgesia versus intrathecal morphine for postoperative pain management after total knee arthroplasty: a randomized controlled trial. Anesth Analg 2011;113(4):926–33.
21. Chowdhry S, Seidenstricker L, Cooney DS, et al. Epinephrine and hand surgery. J Hand Surg Am 2012;37(6):1254–6.
22. Patel M, Craig R, Laishley R, et al. A comparison between epidural anaesthesia using alkalinized

solution and spinal (combined spinal/epidural) anaesthesia for elective caesarean section. Int J Obstet Anesth 1996;5(4):236–9.

23. Cepeda MS, Tzortzopoulou A, Thackrey M, et al. Adjusting the pH of lidocaine for reducing pain on injection. Cochrane Database Syst Rev 2010;(12):CD006581.

24. Axelsson K, Gupta A. Local anaesthetic adjuvants: neuraxial versus peripheral nerve block. Curr Opin Anaesthesiol 2009;22(5):649–54.

25. Murphy DB, McCartney CJ, Chan VW. Novel analgesic adjuncts for brachial plexus block: a systematic review. Anesth Analg 2000;90(5):1122–8.

26. Sen H, Kulahci Y, Bicerer E, et al. The analgesic effect of paracetamol when added to lidocaine for intravenous regional anesthesia. Anesth Analg 2009;109(4):1327–30.

27. Parrington SJ, O'Donnell D, Chan VW, et al. Dexamethasone added to mepivacaine prolongs the duration of analgesia after supraclavicular brachial plexus blockade. Reg Anesth Pain Med 2010; 35(5):422–6.

28. Vieira PA, Pulai I, Tsao GC, et al. Dexamethasone with bupivacaine increases duration of analgesia in ultrasound-guided interscalene brachial plexus blockade. Eur J Anaesthesiol 2010;27(3):285–8.

29. Jones JS, Plzak C, Wynn BN, et al. Effect of temperature and pH adjustment of bupivacaine for intradermal anesthesia. pain and temperature. Am J Emerg Med 1998;16(2):117–20.

30. Graf BM. The cardiotoxicity of local anesthetics: the place of ropivacaine. Curr Top Med Chem 2001; 1(3):207–14.

31. Briggs M, Nelson EA, Martyn-St James M. Topical agents or dressings for pain in venous leg ulcers. Cochrane Database Syst Rev 2010;(11):CD001177.

32. Wahlgren CF, Lillieborg S. Split-skin grafting with lidocaine-prilocaine cream: a meta-analysis of efficacy and safety in geriatric versus nongeriatric patients. Plast Reconstr Surg 2001;107(3): 750–6.

33. Fassoulaki A, Sarantopoulos C, Melemeni A, et al. EMLA reduces acute and chronic pain after breast surgery for cancer. Reg Anesth Pain Med 2000; 25(4):350–5.

34. Larson A, Stidham T, Banerji S, et al. Seizures and methemoglobinemia in an infant after excessive EMLA application. Pediatr Emerg Care 2013; 29(3):377–9.

35. Schilling CG, Bank DE, Borchert BA, et al. Tetracaine, epinephrine (adrenalin), and cocaine (TAC) versus lidocaine, epinephrine, and tetracaine (LET) for anesthesia of lacerations in children. Ann Emerg Med 1995;25(2):203–8.

36. Weiniger CF, Golovanevski L, Domb AJ, et al. Extended release formulations for local anaesthetic agents. Anaesthesia 2012;67(8):906–16.

37. Cohen R, Kanaan H, Grant GJ, et al. Prolonged analgesia from Bupisome and Bupigel formulations: from design and fabrication to improved stability. J Control Release 2012;160(2):346–52.

38. Ostad A, Kageyama N, Moy RL. Tumescent anesthesia with a lidocaine dose of 55 mg/kg is safe for liposuction. Dermatol Surg 1996;22(11): 921–7.

39. Swanson E. Prospective study of lidocaine, bupivacaine, and epinephrine levels and blood loss in patients undergoing liposuction and abdominoplasty. Plast Reconstr Surg 2012;130(3): 702–22.

40. Klein JA. The tumescent technique. Anesthesia and modified liposuction technique. Dermatol Clin 1990;8(3):425–37.

41. Senen D, Atakul D, Erten G, et al. Evaluation of the risk of systemic fat mobilization and fat embolus following liposuction with dry and tumescent technique: an experimental study on rats. Aesthetic Plast Surg 2009;33(5):730–7.

42. Asik I, Kocum AI, Goktug A, et al. Comparison of ropivacaine 0.2% and 0.25% with lidocaine 0.5% for intravenous regional anesthesia. J Clin Anesth 2009;21(6):401–7.

43. Padera R, Bellas E, Tse JY, et al. Local myotoxicity from sustained release of bupivacaine from microparticles. Anesthesiology 2008;108(5):921–8.

44. McAlvin JB, Reznor G, Shankarappa SA, et al. Local toxicity from local anesthetic polymeric microparticles. Anesth Analg 2013;116(4):794–803.

45. Eggleston ST, Lush LW. Understanding allergic reactions to local anesthetics. Ann Pharmacother 1996;30(7–8):851–7.

46. Noyes FR, Fleckenstein CM, Barber-Westin SD. The development of postoperative knee chondrolysis after intra-articular pain pump infusion of an anesthetic medication: a series of twenty-one cases. J Bone Joint Surg Am 2012;94(16):1448–57.

47. Bern S, Akpa BS, Kuo I, et al. Lipid resuscitation: a life-saving antidote for local anesthetic toxicity. Curr Pharm Biotechnol 2011;12(2):313–9.

48. Weinberg GL. Treatment of local anesthetic systemic toxicity (LAST). Reg Anesth Pain Med 2010; 35(2):188–93.

49. Dillane D, Finucane BT. Local anesthetic systemic toxicity. Can J Anaesth 2010;57(4):368–80.

50. Wolfe JW, Butterworth JF. Local anesthetic systemic toxicity: update on mechanisms and treatment. Curr Opin Anaesthesiol 2011;24(5):561–6.

51. Lönnqvist PA. Toxicity of local anesthetic drugs: a pediatric perspective. Paediatr Anaesth 2012; 22(1):39–43.

52. Ohmura S, Kawada M, Ohta T, et al. Systemic toxicity and resuscitation in bupivacaine-, levobupivacaine-, or ropivacaine-infused rats. Anesth Analg 2001;93(3):743–8.

53. Neal JM, Mulroy MF, Weinberg GL. American Society of Regional Anesthesia and Pain Medicine checklist for managing local anesthetic systemic toxicity: 2012 version. Reg Anesth Pain Med 2012;37(1):16–8.
54. Cave G, Harvey M, Graudins A. Intravenous lipid emulsion as antidote: a summary of published human experience. Emerg Med Australas 2011; 23(2):123–41.
55. Kuo I, Akpa BS. Validity of the lipid sink as a mechanism for the reversal of local anesthetic systemic toxicity: a physiologically-based pharmacokinetic model study. Anesthesiology 2013; 118(6):1350–61.
56. Shi K, Xia Y, Wang Q, et al. The effect of lipid emulsion on pharmacokinetics and tissue distribution of bupivacaine in rats. Anesth Analg 2013;116(4): 804–9.
57. Picard J, Ward SC, Zumpe R, et al. Guidelines and the adoption of 'lipid rescue' therapy for local anaesthetic toxicity. Anaesthesia 2009; 64(2):122–5.

Costs of Regional and General Anesthesia
What the Plastic Surgeon Needs to Know

Douglas R. McKay, MD, MBA, FRCSC

KEYWORDS

- Local anesthesia • Regional anesthesia • General anesthesia • Anesthesiology • Plastic surgery
- Health care costs

KEY POINTS

- The standard 4 cost analyses used in health care are:
  - Cost analysis
  - Cost-benefit analysis
  - Cost-effectiveness analysis
  - Cost-utility analysis
- Indirect costing is far more complicated than direct costing and at times seemingly arbitrary, but the indirect costs of the procedure ultimately determine its value, particularly when the patient's perception of quality is included in the analysis.
- Time intervals related to scheduling and monitoring procedures that are of chief concern are anesthesia-controlled time, turnover time, and case duration.
- Research protocols require that the surgeon and anesthesiologist be amenable to using either regional or general anesthesia, and that both techniques are suitable for the intervention at hand but still allow the patient to choose between modalities.

INTRODUCTION

Surgery costs a great deal of money. Cost should be easy to quantify as it appears to be objective, but determining the exact cost of a procedure is very difficult and almost always subjective. Direct and indirect costs must be considered from the perspective of all parties: the patient, the health care system, the provider, society, and so forth. Analyses cannot be limited to per-case costing from only the purveyor's perspective. Social costing and the qualitative outcomes of the intervention are critical variables to consider when calculating and comparing cost.

A significant amount of money spent on health care is driven and controlled by anesthesiology. An estimated 3% to 5% per annum comes under the auspices of anesthesia providers through their control of the operating and recovery rooms, and through the supplies and services they consume preparing patients for a procedure, and tending to their aftercare.[1] There are significant cost savings to be had by choosing a regional or local anesthesia technique for plastic surgery procedures, but research to this end is limited. Many advantages with respect to cost are assumed, but lack validation through rigorous evaluation.[2]

Many plastic surgery procedures can be performed under local anesthesia. In fact so commonplace is the use of local anesthesia that practitioners execute a many procedures under local anesthesia without much thought to the implications of the anesthetic technique on outcomes and cost. What constitutes a local anesthetic

Departments of Surgery and Oncology, Hotel Dieu Hospital, Queens University, 166 Brock Street, Kingston, Ontario K7L 5G2, Canada
E-mail address: mckayd1@KGH.KARI.NET

Clin Plastic Surg 40 (2013) 529–535
http://dx.doi.org/10.1016/j.cps.2013.07.003
0094-1298/13/$ – see front matter © 2013 Elsevier Inc. All rights reserved.

procedure is subject to debate: Plastic surgery can be performed using direct infiltration, field blocks, nerve blocks, plexus blocks, intravenous regional anesthesia (IVRA), and spinal blocks, and all of these techniques can be supplemented with adjuvant conscious sedation or monitored anesthesia care (MAC). Caution must be exercised when assumptions about cost are made across this variety of techniques.

Plastic surgeons tend to concern themselves less with the cost of an intervention, focusing, rightly so, on outcomes. The literature echoes this sentiment. The percentage of gross domestic product spent on health care is more than 10% for the top 10 spenders worldwide.[3] In the United States this amounts to some US$2.6 trillion per year and about CAN$200 billion per year.[4,5] In the province of Ontario, Canada's most populous province, 50% of the provincial budget is allocated to health care and, if unchecked, is projected to increase to 80% of the budget by 2030.[6] Escalation should be expected, based on the technology-driven nature of health care.[7] Every health care provider should be concerned with cost. Resources are not limitless. The implication of the anesthesia technique used on plastic surgery procedural costing is explored in this article, as are future avenues for research planning to this end.

ARE THE OUTCOMES EQUIVALENT?

Implicit in the comparison of different techniques is the assumption that outcomes are equivalent. General anesthesia (GA) carries the risk of death as well as other major medical complications.[8] There is a wealth of research demonstrating a decrease in postoperative symptoms and complications when local anesthetic techniques are used; similarly, there is a body of literature showing no untoward or obvious increase in surgical complications as a result. However, as risks such as respiratory complications decrease as a result of avoiding GA, the risks directly attributable to the local anesthetic technique must increase. The cost of the treatment of complications incurred, and the savings realized through the avoidance of others, must be factored into the costing equation, thus complicating the problem of accurate allocation.

Lalonde has prolifically published on the use of local anesthesia for plastic surgery procedures.[9] His work also serves as an excellent example of what is required to demonstrate equivalence.[10,11] In lieu of publishing a case series with no untoward complications, he first demonstrates equivalence in outcomes when different anesthesia techniques are used, and then demonstrates favorable cost and efficiency metrics. This first step of demonstrating outcome equivalence is essential before undertaking cost comparisons.

COSTS BEYOND MERE DOLLARS AND CENTS

Many allude to cost without understanding the difference between the modalities of cost analysis commonly used in health care. The standard 4 analyses are[12]:

1. Cost analysis
2. Cost-benefit analysis
3. Cost-effectiveness analysis
4. Cost-utility analysis

The differences must be appreciated in order to interpret research and apply conclusions to clinical practice. The differences are also integral to research design if an economic analytical component is to be included.

- Cost-analysis sums dollars spent
- Cost-benefit analysis assigns dollar values to health care output
- Cost-effectiveness calculates the cost of a specific health care end point
- Cost-utility analysis determines the value of an intervention in terms of its qualitative outcome[13]

A common plastic surgery procedure, the flexor tendon repair, can be used to illustrate these differences. A cost analysis would determine the average amount spent on the surgical repair regardless of outcome; a cost-benefit analysis would calculate the cost of a successful repair; cost-effectiveness analysis would calculate the cost of a return to function or any other given end point; and a cost-utility analysis would determine quality-of-life years (QALY) gained through the intervention, allowing the investigator to ascribe a dollar value to each year gained. The utility analysis is the only type of cost analysis that includes the patient's perception of value in the calculation while allowing for cross-comparison between disciplines. This type of analysis advantageously allows an institution or individual to compare the value of a dollar spent on different treatments. A provider could compare the value of money spent on flexor tendon repairs with the value of dollars spent on breast reduction, and allocate funding to optimize outcomes in terms of QALY.

COMPARE APPLES WITH APPLES AND ORANGES WITH ORANGES

The significant differences between the modalities of cost analyses highlight the pitfalls of making conclusions and business decisions based on the cost research without understanding the calculations that lead to the conclusions. Unfortunately, very few articles in the plastic surgery literature include some form of economic analysis.[14] The same is true of the anesthesia literature, and most research fails to adequately explain the assumptions used that lead to indirect cost allocation. When one reviews articles comparing anesthesia techniques in plastic surgery procedures looking for cost analysis, the search proves thoroughly unsatisfying.

Many plastic surgeons look to the literature to find support endorsing the safety of performing a particular procedure under local anesthesia. Many do so because it is intuitively less expensive or more profitable, they believe it is safer, or they believe that it expedites time to resolution by avoiding the main operating room, while advantageously increasing throughput and profit.

The ability to perform a procedure using a local anesthesia technique advantageously increases the number of available venues for its execution. Procedures classically executed in hospital operating rooms may be performed in an ambulatory minor procedure suite, an operating room, or an examining room. Based on the law of supply and demand, access to multiple venues for procedural execution will ultimately drive down cost in the long run through supply surplus and the commodification of procedural execution.

Caution must be exercised when equating procedures performed in different venues with respect to both outcomes and cost. It may not be possible to equate sterility, lighting, and instrument availability between the office setting and an operating room; it is easier to do so between a dedicated procedure facility or minor procedure suite and an operating room, but the construction of such a venue must be factored into costing, as must the opportunity cost of the lost real estate to the institution or individual. Procedures performed at different venues cannot be assumed as equivalent entities with respect to cost. While some cost allocations will be the same (cost of equipment, drugs, and so forth) many will vary, and this holds particularly true with respect to indirect allocations. The cost of sterilizing instruments, nurse staffing of the recovery room, even utility consumption, will be drastically different when comparing an office procedure with one performed in a tertiary care center. One might intuit that costs are less for office procedures, but a rigorous cost analysis may prove otherwise; a well-run public hospital may have a lower indirect per-case cost allocation than may a high-end private hospital or aesthetic institute. This pitfall limits blanket recommendations based on presumptions as opposed to rigorous analysis.

DIRECT AND INDIRECT COSTS

Direct costs are generally easy to allocate. One simply sums the cost of the drugs and equipment used and the fees applied for a given intervention. Chilvers and colleagues[15] and others show that the cost of drugs and equipment required are less when regional anesthesia (RA) or local option is used.[2]

Indirect costing is far more complicated and at times seemingly arbitrary. However, the indirect costs of the procedure will ultimately determine its value, particularly when the patient's perception of quality is included in the analysis. Indirect costs to the institution include unplanned admissions and long stays in the recovery room. Indirect costs from the patient's perspective include time off work, caregiver requirements, and perceived sacrifices of quality of life, among others, and have a major impact on the economy as a whole. However, as these costs are borne by the patient or their employers, they are largely ignored. The patient's perspective is rarely included in cost analysis, resulting in the underreporting of indirect costs.[12]

Some have suggested that anesthetic modalities should be evaluated using either cost-benefit or cost-effectiveness analyses.[1] Thoma and colleagues[16] convincingly argue that cost-utility analyses—those that take into account the patient's notion of qualitative outcomes—must be the modality of analysis used moving forward. Thoma also points to a dearth of qualitative analysis in the plastic surgery literature, threatening the discipline's viability in tight economic times and in the future.

Given that each individual's notion of quality varies, accurate costing becomes challenging. One could argue that local anesthesia procedures can generally be accommodated in a more timely fashion. Surgeons have greater access to their offices than to operating rooms. For example, a flexor tendon procedure may be performed under local anesthetic in the office on the day of presentation rather than on the next available operating-room day. From a utility perspective one could assume that this "1-stop shop" would favorably affect costing through a shorter time to resolution. However, this presumption would need to be tempered by the fact that some patients will find a local procedure and block traumatizing.

TOTAL SOCIAL COSTING

A cost analysis cannot be considered complete unless the patient's perspective and costs are analyzed. It is interesting that studies aimed at quantifying cost differences between anesthesia techniques include the patient's preference as the deciding factor when choosing a modality. The research protocols require that the surgeon and anesthesiologist be amenable to using either technique, and that both techniques are suitable for the intervention at hand but still allow the patient to choose between modalities. The investigators realize an adequate sample size for each modality, allowing them to perform statistical analysis; this suggests that patients ascribe value to one modality over another. If one technique is imposed over another based on savings to the provider while the patient's perception of quality of care is sacrificed, the dollar value of QALY will increase. Whereas one patient may chose the lower postoperative-symptom profile of an RA, the needle-phobic patient would ascribe significantly more value to the oblivion and amnesia of a general anesthetic. The patient's perception of quality must be further explored and integrated into cost analysis to avoid pedantic practice.

COSTING LOCAL ANESTHESIA PROCEDURES AND PLASTIC SURGERY

Research of this nature is more prolific in the orthopedic literature using a limb-procedure model. At times cost conclusions relevant to plastic surgery can be made with caution, and at times not. Conclusions made about breast surgery using an anterior cruciate ligament (ACL) repair model may lead to incorrect assumptions. Investigators must study the anesthesia technique used in the context of the procedure before evaluating the cost.[17]

ANESTHESIA-RELATED METRICS

A primer on anesthesia-related descriptive metrics is required; these metrics will determine a great deal of the easily indirect costing amenable to allocation. The time intervals related to scheduling and monitoring procedures are objectively defined.[18] Those of chief concern are anesthesia-controlled time (ACT), turnover time (TOT), and case duration.[19]

ACT covers the period from entry to the operating room until the beginning of positioning and preparation, whereas the postoperative ACT spans the time from procedural completion to the operating-room exit. The TOT is the time from one patient's operating-room exit to the next patient's entry time for a sequentially scheduled case. Any research aimed at delineating cost differences must begin with the evaluation of these parameters.

FAVORABLE AND UNFAVORABLE COSTING IMPLICATIONS FOR PROCEDURE TIME

One can compare and contrast 2 limb surgery research models from the literature to demonstrate the complexity of drawing conclusions about indirect costing from varied sources. Williams and colleagues[20] demonstrate significant cost savings when RA rather than GA is used for ACL repair. Cost savings are attributed to decreased ACT as a result of shorter induction times when RA is compared with GA. The procedures in this case are performed in the main operating room, and ACT equates to expensive operating-room time and a drop in indirectly cost-allocated operating-room time.

Contrast this to a hand surgery costing study by Chan and colleagues,[21] who compared GA, IVRA, and RA. In this case the RA used was a brachial plexus block (BPB). ACT increased when RA was used. In this study ACT was greatest when the BPB was used and was equivalent when either an IVRA or GA was used. Although the RA was directly cost-allocated as less, if the BPB was done in the operating room, more expensive operating-room time was used, increasing indirect costing. To complicate matters, operating-room time costs vary depending on who is using that time: time controlled by anesthesia costs less than the portion of the case controlled by the surgeon, and each carries opportunity costs of the other.

These contradictory findings are intuitive. The complexity of the modality used—spinal anesthesia versus a BPB—will confound cost analysis. Plastic surgeons must exercise caution when drawing conclusions, which would come as no surprise to a surgeon who has waited for a BPB to be performed in the operating room.

Surgeon operating-room time costs more than ACT operating-room time, but ACT is not free. The use of an induction room can help to decrease the cost of ACT and increase the availability of procedural time, but the construction of multiple induction rooms requires foresight, costs money, and carries an opportunity cost.

FAVORABLE IMPLICATIONS ON AFTERCARE AND MANAGEMENT COSTS

One must look beyond the duration of the procedure to find the true cost advantages of RA techniques. Aftercare appears to be universally cheaper as a result of the postoperative symptom profile for the RA patient. Moreover, it seems safe to apply this conclusion across disciplines and a variety of procedures.

Again, one is drawn to the work of Williams and colleagues[19] and Chan and colleagues.[21] Williams demonstrates unequivocally that RA use decreases the incidence of postoperative nausea and vomiting (PONV), reduces or eliminates acute postoperative pain, decreases the need for mandatory recovery room or PACU stays, and decreases the incidence of unplanned admissions and related costs.[19] Here Chan's group agrees.[21] Decreased PONV and acute postoperative pain decreases the amount of medication required following a procedure. Chilvers and colleagues[15] confirm these direct cost savings in their analysis of the pharmacoeconomic study of IVRA and GA for outpatient hand surgery. The reality is that most anesthesia drugs are relatively cheap when compared with the cost of running an operating or recovery room. The symptoms these medications counteract and the side-effect profile they carry is the hidden source of cost in aftercare; both can prolong a patient's duration of stay in the postanesthesia care unit (PACU), increasing direct and indirect costs.

The failure to control the postoperative symptoms of pain and PONV when a GA is used may result in unplanned admissions. Similarly, adequate symptom control may require large doses of antiemetics or opioid analgesics, both of which carry sedating side-effect profiles that can result in unplanned admissions. Unplanned admissions are costly and unpredictable. Unpredictable events require contingency plans; contingencies require resource allocation. These unlikely events dramatically increase costs either through overallocation of expensive resources and their ineffective use (ie, nurse staffing to ensure the system can accommodate the event whereby the nurse is idle if the event does not occur) or through expensive last-minute accommodations (ie, emergency staffing at overtime rates), and can drastically increase yearly per-case costs through system inefficiencies.

When the opportunity exists to use a local or RA technique, the per-case aftercare costs appear to decrease, with few exceptions. These savings are both direct and indirect in nature, and are intuitive and universal.

THE PLASTIC SURGEON AS ANESTHESIOLOGIST, AND OPPORTUNITY COSTING

A thorough economic analysis necessitates the inclusion of opportunity costs. An opportunity cost is the revenue gained or lost as a result of a path not taken. Imagine a decision tree in which 2 options are available to the decision maker; each

having the potential to generate revenue. The decision maker can only choose one path or the other. Path A generates revenue at the expense of the revenue generated by path B. An economist will account for this "lost" revenue by subtracting it from the revenue gained as the result of the path taken, and label this loss as an opportunity cost.

The use of a local anesthetic can favorably or negatively affect ACT. This impact on the plastic surgeon can be minimized through the use of a block room. Nevertheless, many plastic surgery procedures use local anesthesia techniques administered by the surgeon at a significant opportunity cost. The surgeon cannot operate when he or she is administering anesthesia, and loses the opportunity to generate revenue through procedures. A variation on the induction-room concept can be annexed but this requires access to multiple-procedure room, which again increases costs. Moreover, if the patient is in the procedure room while awaiting the onset of anesthesia, the procedure room is underoptimized as a resource.

Another concept fundamental to organizational optimization is the notion of core competency. In general terms a system is optimized when an individual or an organization remain true to their core competencies. CEOs do not do their own faxing because their efforts are best put toward running the organization, and they are likely less efficient than their administrative assistants at faxing. To this end, one could argue that surgeons should operate and anesthesiologists should anesthetize. In reality, one compares the revenues lost and gained. If the time lost to the surgeon through induction is still offset by an increase in surgical volume (ie, the local anesthetic procedure minimizes the need for operating-room time, or decreases the cost of administering the procedure and increases revenue), then the modality should be embraced. Plastic surgeons are now taking on the role of the anesthesiologist,[22] one which they may not be trained to assume. Although some literature exists to assist their mastery of these techniques, the learning curve front-loads the cost of the skill acquisition.[9]

THE UNKNOWN COSTS OF MEDICOLEGAL SETTLEMENTS

The literature shows that RA is more likely to be associated with litigation.[23] Combined with the fact that plastic surgeons are performing tasks beyond the scope of their training, this is potentially concerning. Accurate costing must to some end factor the cost of time lost for defense as well as revenue lost to successful litigation.

SYSTEMS IMPLICATIONS

Health care is delivered within a system. One cannot isolate one element within the system and change it without implications for the system as a whole. Chan and colleagues[21] make a sage point in the conclusions of their costing study with regard to the impact of the intervention in the context of the system. In their study they demonstrated that local anesthesia procedures decreased the overall time required to complete this procedure and assumed this would decrease the overall cost to the hospital, but were surprised to find no impact. The root cause turned out to system based; PACU costs were tied to peak volumes, and unless the intervention favorably affected recovery-room peak volume, there was no overall cost saving despite favorable improvements in anesthesia-related metrics. In fact, an increase in efficiency could theoretically increase recovery-room peak volumes and ultimately increase total cost. In other words, simply changing the anesthetic modality without relevant or compensatory changes in the system may be of no benefit. These investigators propose PACU streamlining to tailor the system to the change, and optimize the return on the intervention.

Dexter and colleagues[24] came to a very important similar conclusion when attempting to quantify the global impact of RA versus GA on the operating room as a system. Although they were able to demonstrate that RA decreased ACT and TOT, the time savings were not large enough to allow them to complete another case each day.

Williams followed this work with RA interventions but reinforced these with compensatory system changes, namely PACU bypass and same-day discharge, to realize cost savings for the institution. Cost savings must be considered when building a system from the ground up so that appropriate resources exist to realize the advantages gleaned through cost-saving interventions.

MANIPULATING OTHER INTANGIBLES THROUGH ANESTHESIA TECHNIQUE USED: ADVANTAGES OF THE OFFICE OVER THE HOSPITAL

Beyond mere dollars and cents, there are advantages to using a local anesthesia technique to take the procedure out of the hospital setting, although they are difficult to quantify. There may even be a cost increase: a surgeon's direct and indirect costs could increase disproportionately to an increase in income by adapting the office setting to accommodate local anesthetic procedures typically performed at the hospital. Both secretarial and nursing human resource costs increase when acquiring staff with skills to facilitate execution of procedures, as do several other previously discussed direct and indirect costs.

However, the capability to execute procedures beyond the walls of the hospital can also alleviate many frustrations surgeons feel when working in a hospital where they have little control over the execution environment. Control of the operating room avoids the common pitfalls that plague many health care institutions: operating-room cancellations for a myriad of reasons including bed space and aftercare limitations, and cases bumped or postponed to accommodate emergencies of greater acuity.

Teamwork and cooperation is easier to engender when the team answers to the operating surgeon. There is an ease to scheduling cases and accommodating additional work in the office, which is to say that doing more work, or more work after hours, is not a fight when the operating surgeon controls all aspects of the execution environment and is not competing with others or fighting for resources. Finally, the surgeon can control the atmosphere and pace in the operating room as the employer, tailoring the workday to his or her style of execution. Although one cannot quantify this in terms of dollars and cents it is of significant advantage, and likely increases productivity over the long term. Even if there were no productivity or cost advantage, some would argue that this improvement in quality is invaluable.

SUMMARY

In general terms RA techniques seem to expand the opportunity for cost savings when executing plastic surgery procedures, but cost allocation is not a simple business. Equivalence must first be demonstrated, and the patient's perception is integral to assigning value to an intervention. Opportunity costs cannot be ignored when the plastic surgeon assumes the role of the anesthesiologist. Most importantly, the system must be modified to optimize the cost savings realized through the intervention.

REFERENCES

1. Johnstone RE, Martinec CL. Costs of anesthesia. Anesth Analg 1993;76:840–8.
2. Greenberg CP. Practical cost-effective regional anesthesia for ambulatory surgery. J Clin Anesth 1995;7:614–21.
3. Available at: http://data.worldbank.org/indicator/SH.XPD.TOTL.ZS. Accessed May 19, 2013.

4. Centers for Medicare and Medicaid Services, Office of the Actuary, National Health Statistics Group. National Health Care Expenditures Data, January 2012.

5. Available at: http://www.cihi.ca/cihi-ext-portal/internet/en/document/spending+and+health+workforce/spending/release_03nov11. Accessed May 20, 2013.

6. Available at: http://occ.on.ca/advocacy/issues/health-care/. Accessed May 20, 2013.

7. Barbash GI, Glied SA. New technology and health care costs—the case of robot-assisted surgery. N Engl J Med 2010;363(8):701–4.

8. Keyes GR, Singer R, Iverson RE, et al. Mortality in outpatient surgery. Plast Reconstr Surg 2008;122: 245–50 [discussion: 251–3].

9. Mustoe TA, Buck DW 2nd, Lalonde DH. The safe management of anesthesia, sedation, and pain in plastic surgery. Plast Reconstr Surg 2010;126(5): 1642–4.

10. Leblanc MR, Lalonde J, Lalonde DH. A detailed cost and efficiency analysis of performing carpal tunnel surgery in the main operating room versus the ambulatory setting in Canada. Hand (N Y) 2007; 2(4):173–8.

11. Lalonde DH. Wide-awake flexor tendon repair. Plast Reconstr Surg 2009;123(2):623–5.

12. Drummond MF, Sculpher MJ, Torrance GW, et al. Methods for the economic evaluation of health care programmes. 3rd edition. New York: Oxford University Press; 2005.

13. Venney JE, Kaluzny AD. Evaluation and decision making for health services. Ann Arbor (MI): Health Administration Press; 1991.

14. Ziolkowski N, Voineskos S, Ignacy T, et al. Systematic review of economic evaluation in plastic surgery. Presented at the 66th Annual Meeting of the Canadian Society of Plastic Surgeons. Toronto, June 5–9, 2012.

15. Chilvers CR, Kinahan A, Vaghadia H, et al. Pharmacoeconomics of intravenous regional anesthesia versus general anesthesia for outpatient hand surgery. Can J Anaesth 1997;44(11):1152–6.

16. Thoma A, Ignacy TA, Ziolkowski N, et al. The performance and publication of cost utility analysis in plastic surgery; making our specialty relevant. Can J Plast Surg 2012;20(3):187–93.

17. Chung KJ, Cha KH, Lee JH, et al. Usefulness of intravenous anesthesia using a target-controlled infusion system with local anesthesia in sub muscular breast augmentation surgery. Arch Plast Surg 2012;39(5):540–5.

18. Donham RT, Maxxei WJ, Jone RL. Association of anesthesia clinical directors' procedure times glossary. Glossary of times used for scheduling and monitoring of diagnostic and therapeutic procedures. Am J Anesthesiol 1996;23:3–12.

19. Williams BA, Motolenich P, Kentor ML. Hospital facilities and resource management: economic impact of a high volume regional anesthesia program for outpatients. Int Anesthesiol Clin 2005; 43(3):43–51.

20. Williams BA, Kentor ML, Williams JP, et al. Process analysis in outpatient knee surgery: effects of regional and general anesthesia on anesthesia-controlled time. Anesthesiology 2000;93:529–38.

21. Chan VW, Peng PW, Kaszas Z, et al. A comparative study of general anesthesia, intravenous regional anesthesia, and axillary block for outpatient hand surgery: clinical outcome and cost analysis. Anesth Analg 2001;93:1181–4.

22. Shapiro FE. Anesthesia for outpatient cosmetic surgery. Curr Opin Anaesthesiol 2008;21:704.

23. Kroll DA, Caplan RA, Posner K, et al. Nerve injury associated with anesthesia. Anesthesiology 1990; 73:202–7.

24. Dexter F, Coffin S, Tinker JH. Decreases in anesthesia controlled time cannot permit one additional surgical operation to be reliably scheduled during the workday. Anesth Analg 1995;81:1263–8.

Local Anesthetics for Skin Grafting and Local Flaps

Hana Farhangkhoee, MD, MSc[a], Eric Yu Kit Li, MD[a],
Achilleas Thoma, MD, MSc, FRCS (C)[a,b,*]

KEYWORDS

- Health care cost • Local anesthetics • Local skin flaps • Skin flaps

KEY POINTS

- Health care resources are limited, and surgeons must adopt evidence-based and efficient practices for improved patient outcomes.
- Use of local anesthesia for skin grafts and local flaps can be an excellent alternative to general anesthetics.
- Appropriate patient selection for the use of local anesthetics is imperative to maintain safety and the standard of care.
- Many factors influence the success of local anesthesia, including method of injection, type and volume of solution, needle characteristics, and how the local anesthetic is injected.

INTRODUCTION

In Canada, as in other jurisdictions, expenditures in health care are coming under scrutiny because of their tremendous burden on the system. For instance, in Ontario, Canada's largest province, health care consumes about 40% of the provincial budget.[1] Over the last 30 years it has been recognized that significant waste occurs in the delivery of health care, estimated to be about 50% in the United States,[2] 25% in Canada,[3] and 20% to 40% on a global basis.[4] The cost and waste in health care continues to increase despite finite resources. This predicament has required all stakeholders in the health care team, including surgeons, to take innovative and prudent steps to manage resources and reduce costs while allowing for long-term competitive advantage. One of the most sought-after and cost-consuming resources in a hospital setting is the operating room. As surgeons we assume the role of not only being the gatekeepers of operating room but also the managers, responsible for its most efficient use. Expectations to reduce surgical waiting times have challenged us to reevaluate the decision to perform most procedures in the main operating room (MOR).

In plastic surgery, many common procedures such as skin grafts and local flaps can be performed safely and easily in the ambulatory setting under local anesthetic (LA). In the authors' geographic region, the notion of performing "complex" procedures in the ambulatory minor procedure room (MPR) began with carpal tunnel release (CTR) more than 30 years ago. At that time, the senior author (A.T.) was faced with the same dilemma: long waiting times arising from limited space in the MOR, or performing the CTR in a less formal environment, namely the MPR. Subsequently, as no significant issues were identified in the latter, this gradually became the standard of care. The procedure can be completed

Funding Sources: Nil.
Conflicts of Interest: Nil.
[a] Division of Plastic Surgery, Department of Surgery, Faculty of Medicine, McMaster University, 1200 Main Street West, Hamilton, Ontario L8S 4L8, Canada; [b] Department of Clinical Epidemiology and Biostatistics, McMaster University, 1200 Main Street West, Hamilton, Ontario L8S 4L8, Canada
* Corresponding author. 206 James Street South, Suite 101, Hamilton, Ontario L8P 3A9, Canada.
E-mail address: athoma@mcmaster.ca

Clin Plastic Surg 40 (2013) 537–549
http://dx.doi.org/10.1016/j.cps.2013.07.004
0094-1298/13/$ – see front matter © 2013 Elsevier Inc. All rights reserved.

with only one attendant nurse without requiring blood work or intravenous infusion. Furthermore, on completion of the procedure the patients are discharged home within minutes, substantially reducing the amount of time spent in the recovery room. This approach bypasses the unnecessary and sometimes adverse complications associated with general anesthesia, such as nausea and vomiting. A recent cost-effectiveness analysis showed that, if performed in the ambulatory setting, CTR would be 4 times cheaper and 2 times faster than if completed in the MOR.[5]

An increasing demand for cost-effective and efficient health care services continues to challenge surgeons to deliver the same quality of care, but more efficiently. For instance, the concept of using LA for minor procedures can be broadened to include skin grafting and local flaps, a practice that in the authors' institution is more commonly performed in the MPR than the MOR. Skin grafts and local flaps are often required after excision of lesions such as basal cell carcinoma (BCC), squamous cell carcinoma (SCC), and malignant melanoma (MM). The purpose of this article is to outline the surgical approach to skin grafts and local flaps using LA.

Although the goal of this issue of *Clinics* is to encourage clinicians to consider the use of LA alone in a minor-procedure setting, it behooves us all to be reminded that many of the patients who require skin grafts and flaps are elderly. The elderly population is not only increasing as a percentage of the whole population but also has higher number of comorbidities that need attention, for example, end-stage renal failure, congestive heart failure, and aortic stenosis. This group of patients is better served in the MOR with anesthesia standby (**Box 1**).

TREATMENT GOALS AND PLANNED OUTCOMES

The treatment goals of using LA for skin grafts and flaps can be divided into surgeon-oriented and patient-oriented goals (**Box 2**).

Patient Selection

The primary surgical objectives are to ensure patient safety and maintain the standard of care. A foremost important safety measure is to identify patients who are suitable for procedures with LA, whether in the MPR or MOR setting (see **Box 1**). Patients who benefit from having their procedures done in the MOR are those with multiple comorbidities, and carry a higher perioperative risk. These patients often require the assistance of an anesthesiologist to help monitor their status during

---

Box 1
Patients suitable for procedures in the main operating room

Candidate for Main Operating Room

Multiple comorbidities requiring anesthesia support

Needle phobias

Psychiatric population

Pediatric population

High anxiety

Inability to tolerate lengthy procedure

---

the procedure. Although LA can still be used, the MOR setting is safer because it allows anesthesia staff to be on standby in case of emergencies. Another cohort for which the MOR would be more appropriate is patients with needle phobia and certain psychiatric conditions. The assumption is that they cannot tolerate the length of the procedure and would generally benefit from light sedation or general anesthesia in the MOR. Pediatric patients, in particular, may have high levels of anxiety during procedures done using LA. It is well known that most young children do not even tolerate a simple dressing change without sedation. Hence, it is imperative to understand that pediatric patients will require sedation or general anesthesia for most procedures. By being able to recognize which patients are suitable for the MPR or MOR, the surgeon appropriately triages patients and maintains the standard of care.

Box 2
Surgical and patient-oriented goals

Surgical Goals

Optimize patient safety

Maintain standard of care

Strengthen physician medical competencies

Minimize operative time

Reduce surgical wait times

Patient Goals

Patient education

Avoid complications associated with general anesthetics

Shorten hospital stay

Mitigate anxiety

Screen for needle phobia

Surgeon-Oriented Goals

Another surgical goal is to strengthen the surgeon's medical competencies, particularly the managerial role. In 1996, the Royal College of Physicians and Surgeons of Canada adopted the CanMeds roles: medical expert, communicator, collaborator, manager, health advocate, scholar, and professional.[6] These roles were implemented to allow the specialist to develop the skills and abilities for better patient outcomes. By using LA, in the MPR the need for sedation or general anesthesia is eliminated. Effectively reducing MOR requirements, this translates into more cases being completed in a specified time frame and a reduction in the surgical wait times. In addition, as most of these cases can be done in the MPR, the surgeons can allocate operating-room resources for patients requiring more extensive procedures. Placing the surgeon in control of the operating room (a finite resource) will foster important managerial skills targeted at improving patient outcomes.

Patient-Oriented Goals

In addition to surgeon-oriented goals there are patient-oriented goals. The main objective for the patient is centered on education, emphasizing the advantages of LA over sedation or general anesthesia. The one major benefit for patients is the avoidance of possible complications such as those related to intravenous insertion (eg, extravasations) or reactions to the general anesthetic (eg, intubation-related adverse events or postoperative nausea and vomiting). The other advantage of using LA is that it gives patients the opportunity to enter and leave the hospital without altering their level of consciousness. The patients resume their usual activities as soon as possible. If sedation or general anesthesia is required; however, they will need to spend more time recovering and possibly be admitted for observation. For instance, after general anesthesia, patients with moderate to severe forms of obstructive sleep apnea are usually admitted overnight to monitor oxygen saturation. The premise is that the effects of the general anesthetic may prevent them from being able to protect their airway during sleep time. By educating the patient on the numerous benefits of LA, the treatment is aimed at reducing any unwarranted anxiety about being awake. It should be noted that patients should be initially screened for uncontrolled anxiety or needle phobia by asking them how they react to the needle from the dentist. If a true phobia exists, consideration can be given to intervention in the MOR under LA with an anesthetist on standby.

PREOPERATIVE PLANNING AND PREPARATION

The preoperative planning should focus on preparing the patient and the ambulatory setting for the intervention. In the case of skin grafts and skin flaps, this includes obtaining informed consent and explaining the risk and benefits of the procedure. The patient's weight and any known allergies should be noted. To guarantee proper organization of the ambulatory setting, a MPR equipped with an operating-room table or equivalent and lighting is required. A nursing staff member is needed to help during the procedure and with patient monitoring. Equipment required includes, but is not limited to: oxygen saturation monitor and blood-pressure cuff; sterile surgical equipment; cautery and silver dermatome for small skin grafts, or a Zimmer dermatome for larger ones. If the surgery is planned in the MOR with an anesthetist on standby because of a patient's significant medical conditions (eg, congestive heart failure or end-stage renal failure), similar equipment is required; however, the surgeon will have the assistance of additional staff members.

PATIENT POSITIONING

For most procedures the patient can be in supine, lateral decubitus, or prone position. It is imperative to apply an oxygen saturation monitor and blood-pressure cuff. The operative site is prepped and draped in the usual standard fashion. For split-thickness skin grafts (STSG), the ipsilateral thigh is generally chosen as the donor site. If needed, hairs from the thigh may be clipped before the procedure. For full-thickness skin grafts (FTSG), donor sites such as the groin, neck, or proximal forearm are chosen based on recipient-site characteristics.

PROCEDURAL APPROACH
Major Steps for Injecting Local Anesthetics

Choice of local anesthetic
The first step is to choose an LA. Several factors influence this decision, including:

- Desired onset of action
- Anticipated length of procedure
- Volumes necessary for adequate anesthesia

Lidocaine has faster onset (within seconds) but shorter duration of action (1.5–2 hours).[7,8] Conversely, bupivacaine has slower onset (within minutes) but longer duration of action (3–6 hours).[7,8]

In certain situations it may be advantageous to use a mix of both fast-acting and long-lasting LA. When only small volumes of LA (eg, grafts and flaps on finger tips) are required, the use of 2% lidocaine, rather than the commonly used 1% concentration, may also be used for faster onset of action.

Lastly, additives to the LA should be considered. Epinephrine, a common premixed additive, has vasoconstrictive effects that provide local hemostasis and restrict vascular absorption.[9] Bicarbonate, which can also be added to preparations, increases the pH of LA and helps to reduce tissue irritation with injection.[7,10]

Safe volumes

The maximum dosage of LA should be calculated before administration. This dosage differs based on the LA, its concentration, and the patient's weight (**Table 1**). For example, for a healthy adult patient who weighs 60 kg, the maximum allowable dosage of lidocaine without epinephrine is 60 kg × 4 mg/kg = 240 mg. If 1% lidocaine is used, it contains 1 g of lidocaine per 100 mL of solution, and therefore 24 mL of this solution can be safely administered. If the operative site is larger and a greater amount of volume is required to achieve anesthetic effect, the solution may be diluted to meet requirements or alternative techniques other than infiltrative anesthesia may be considered (see later discussion). Either sterile normal saline or water can be used to dilute standard concentrations in a syringe or small intravenous bag.[11] Dilute solutions are particularly useful for local anesthesia of large skin graft donor sites.

Epinephrine is often premixed into solutions to avoid medical error. Although this may obviate calculations of maximum dosage, it is important to be aware that the standard premixed concentration is 1:100,000,[9] which corresponds to 1 g of epinephrine per 100,000 mL of solution. If bicarbonate is used, common recommendations include adding

1 mL of sodium bicarbonate 8.4% solution to each 10 mL of lidocaine and or 0.1 mL to each 10 mL of bupivacaine.[8,12] Addition of bicarbonate solution beyond these amounts may lead to precipitation of the LA.

Other patient factors, including age, comorbidities, and medications can affect the maximum safe dosage of LA, and warrant special consideration (**Table 2**).[13]

Type of syringes and needles

The selection of appropriate syringes and needles is often overlooked. Whereas larger syringes may be more convenient, smaller ones confer greater control on the amount and rate of injection.[9] Although smaller-gauge needles (27–30 gauge) are less painful, larger ones may be necessary for areas with thicker skin or increased skin tension (eg, scalp, back, soles).[9] Whereas shorter needles may be appropriate for smaller operative sites (eg, digits), longer needles may facilitate infiltration of larger areas (eg, thigh), because they allow for a greater area of infiltration per skin puncture, thus reducing patient discomfort.[12]

The use of topical anesthetic as an adjunct before LA administration may be considered in select

Table 1 Maximum recommended dosing of local anesthetics and their additives	
Local Anesthetic	**Maximum Dosing**
Lidocaine	4.0 mg/kg up to 300 mg[12,13]
Lidocaine with epinephrine	7.0 mg/kg up to 500 mg[12,13]
Bupivacaine	2.0 mg/kg up to 175 mg[12,13]
Bupivacaine with epinephrine	2.5 mg/kg up to 225 mg[12,13]
Sodium bicarbonate	1 mL of 8.4% solution to each 10 mL of lidocaine[8,12] 0.1 mL of 8.4% solution to each 10 mL of bupivacaine[8]

Table 2 Maximum recommended dosing of local anesthetics based on patient factors	
Factor	**General Recommendations**
Infants	Reduce maximum dosage by 15%
Elderly >70 y	Reduce maximum dosage by 20%
Renal disease	Lidocaine: no dose adjustment necessary Bupivacaine: reduce maximum dosage by 20%
Hepatic disease	Reduce maximum dosage up to 50% based on severity of disease
Cardiac disease	Reduce maximum dosage up to 20% based on severity of disease Use of epinephrine safe in patients with cardiovascular disease[22]
Medications	Caution with drugs affecting the cytochrome P450 enzyme system

Data from Harmatz A. Local anesthetics: uses and toxicities. Surg Clin North Am 2009;89:587–98; and Rosenberg PH, Veering BT, Urmey WF. Maximum recommended doses of local anesthetics: a multifactorial concept. Reg Anesth Pain Med 2004;29:564–75. [discussion: 524].

patients, such as children or needle-phobic patients. Preparations such as EMLA and AMETOP may be used to desensitize the skin before needle injection, and should be applied 30 minutes prior for maximum effectiveness.[12,14]

ADMINISTRATION OF THE LOCAL ANESTHETIC

Injection of LA can proceed before or after standard prepping and draping. Regardless of the approach, the operative site should be cleansed with antiseptic solution before injection to minimize the risk of infection,[8] and stabilized during injection to ensure accuracy of technique; proper precautions should be taken to avoid accidental intravascular injection or injury to peripheral nerves.[13]

Different techniques or combinations of these techniques can be used, including infiltrative anesthesia, field blocks or peripheral nerve blocks, and tumescent anesthesia.

Infiltrative Anesthesia

With infiltrative anesthesia,[9,15] LA is injected along planned incision lines and in the intended operative site, and may be done in an intradermal or subcutaneous fashion, with the former achieving the anesthetic effect more rapidly but with more pain than the latter.[12] The needle is passed along the desired axis, with intermittent aspiration, while asking the patient to report any sensations of paresthesia. If paresthesias are reported, the needle should be slightly retracted and its axis adjusted before repeat advancement. Whenever possible, injections should proceed in a stepwise fashion such that further injections are in a previously anesthetized area for patient comfort. The needle should also be aspirated gently before exiting the skin to avoid unnecessary spillage of LA onto the operative site, which may cause loss of preoperative markings. The advantage of the infiltrative technique is that nerve endings and blood vessels supplying the operative site are directly affected by the anesthetic, which is particularly useful if epinephrine is used for local hemostatic effect. The disadvantage, however, is that the infiltrate may distort the surrounding tissues and anatomic landmarks. Although increased skin tension can assist in harvesting skin grafts, it may pose as a challenge when elevating local flaps.

Field Blocks or Peripheral Nerve Blocks

Field blocks or peripheral nerve blocks[9,15] are techniques that can prevent distortion of the operative site, reduce the amount of LA required, or serve as adjuncts to infiltrative anesthesia. In field blocks, LA is injected in a circumferential pattern around the operative site. This approach is particularly useful when it is difficult or extremely painful to inject in the operative site (eg, ears, penis). In peripheral nerve blocks, small amounts of LA are injected at targeted anatomic sites where peripheral nerves lie, to provide the anesthetic effect in the operative area. The latter technique, however, requires a detailed understanding of anatomy and expert skill to avoid unintentional nerve injury. Multiple blocks may also be required in areas innervated by multiple nerves. Region-specific field or peripheral nerve blocks are covered in articles elsewhere in this issue by Dr Bain.

Tumescent Anesthesia

Tumescent anesthesia[9,15] involves infiltration of LA in subcutaneous adipose tissue via an infusion cannula. Dilute amounts of LA are used in large operative areas to provide both anesthetic and hemostatic effects. Variations exist, but tumescent is generally a combination of 1 L intravenous fluid, 100 mL 1% lidocaine (1 g lidocaine), and a 1-mL ampoule of 1:1000 epinephrine (1 mg of epinephrine).[16] Although this technique is often used to prepare skin graft donor sites in the MOR setting, it may be less ideal in the MPR. The patient may not be able to tolerate the discomfort associated with tumescent dissection and distension, and infusion equipment may also not be readily available for use.

AFTER ADMINISTRATION OF THE LOCAL ANESTHETIC

The total amount of administered anesthetic should be calculated. This action helps keep a tally in the event that additional LA is used intraoperatively, and prevents dosage higher than recommended guidelines. All associated sharps should be disposed of or stored safely, and adequate time should be given to allow for the anesthetic to work. Of note, a recent pilot randomized controlled trial suggested 25 minutes as the most ideal time to wait before incision for maximal hemostatic effect of epinephrine.[17]

Depending on institutional policies as well as nursing and minor room availabilities, it may be possible to administer LA in one room and then attend to a second patient in a different room. In this favorable situation, appropriate time is allowed for the LA to achieve maximum effectiveness without compromising the length of the overall procedure. Unnecessary doses of LA may also be avoided, as they are in fact often administered when insufficient time has been given for the LA to work.

CASE REPRESENTATIONS

Case: Split-Thickness Skin Graft for Basal Cell Carcinoma of Distal Tibia

The first case illustrates the major steps for application of an STSG for excision of a BCC of the distal tibia in a 75-year-old woman (**Fig. 1**). The operation was performed under local anesthesia in the MOR with the anesthesiologists on standby because of significant medical comorbidities. Ten milliliters of 1% lidocaine and epinephrine diluted with 10 mL of normal saline was used to infiltrate the donor and recipient sites. The lesion was excised down to the fascia. An STSG of at least 3 × 3 cm was required. Before harvesting the graft, mineral oil was applied to the thigh and the skin was pulled taut. The STSG was harvested using a Zimmer Dermatome (0.010–0.012 inch [0.254–0.305 mm] deep). The skin graft was then applied to the recipient site and fenestrated with multiple drain holes to avoid seroma collection. The edges of the graft were trimmed to ensure a good fit, and secured into position with plain gut and then a tie-over bolster dressing with 5-0 nylon sutures. The donor site was covered with Tegaderm absorbent.

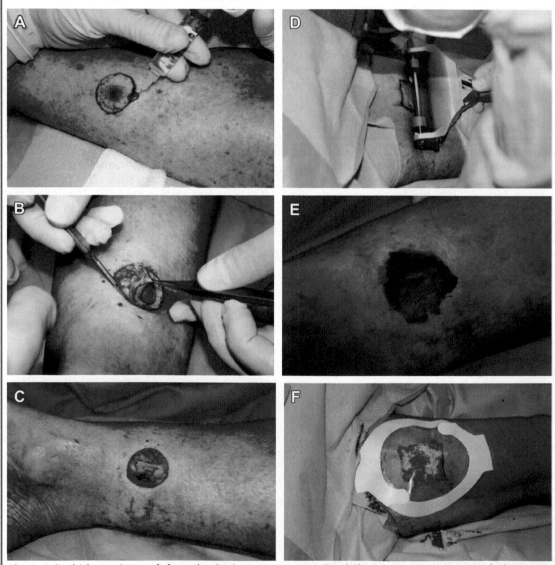

Fig. 1. Split-thickness skin graft from the thigh to reconstruct a distal tibial defect after excision of a basal cell carcinoma (1.5 × 1.5 cm) using local anesthetics. (*A*) Application of local anesthetic to the recipient site, (*B*) excision of the lesion with 5-mm margins, (*C*) donor defect measuring 3 × 3 cm, (*D*) harvesting of the skin graft from thigh with Zimmer dermatome, (*E*) reconstruction of the defect with graft, and (*F*) donor-site dressing using Tegaderm absorbent.

Case: Full-Thickness Skin Graft for Basal Cell Carcinoma on the Nose

The second case demonstrates excision of a BCC from the dorsum of the nose and reconstruction with an FTSG (**Fig. 2**). The procedure was done with LA with anesthesia staff on standby to give sedation, owing to the patient's anxiety. Similar to the previous case, 1% lidocaine with epinephrine was injected into the donor and recipient site. The lesion was excised with 2-mm margins down to the nasalis muscle. Intraoperative frozen sections were used to ensure clear margins. The FTSG measuring 2.5 × 3 cm was harvested and defatted. The donor site was closed primarily. The skin graft was then conformed to the defect on the right side of the nose and then sutured in place with nylon, and a tie-over dressing was applied.

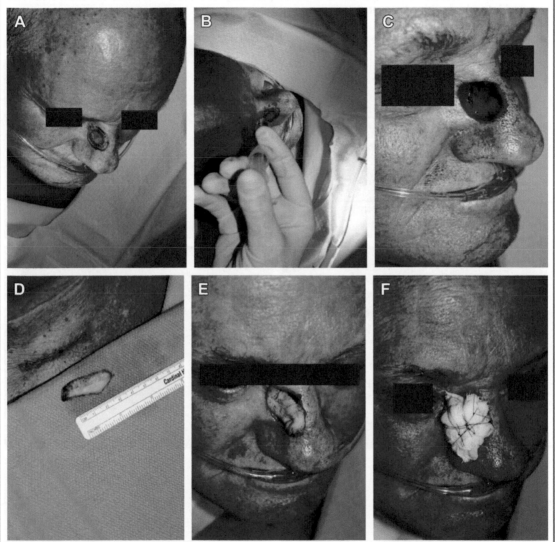

Fig. 2. Full-thickness skin graft (FTSG) from the neck to reconstruct the nose after excision of a basal cell carcinoma (1.0 × 1.5 cm) using local anesthetics. (*A*) The lesion and resection margins of 2 mm, (*B*) application of local anesthetic to the recipient site, (*C*) donor defect, (*D*) harvesting of the FTSG from the neck (2.5 × 3 cm), (*E*) reconstruction of the defect with FTSG, and (*F*) bolster dressing.

Case: Full-Thickness Skin Graft for Basal Cell Carcinoma in Temporal Region

The third case concerns an FTSG from the neck to reconstruct a defect after excision of a BCC in the left preauricular and temporal region (**Fig. 3**). The lesion extended into the root of the helix and portion of the tragus. With anesthesia staff on standby, the procedure was done in the MOR using LA and frozen section. From the technical point of view this could have been done in an MPR, but the need for frozen section, which was not available in the MPR, precluded this. Both the donor and recipient site were infiltrated with 1% lidocaine with epinephrine. To obtain clear margins, dissection was carried down to the level of the temporal muscle. The final defect size was 6 × 4 cm. An FTSG was harvested from the neck and defatted. The donor site was closed primarily. The FTSG was fitted for the defect and secured into place with a tie-over dressing.

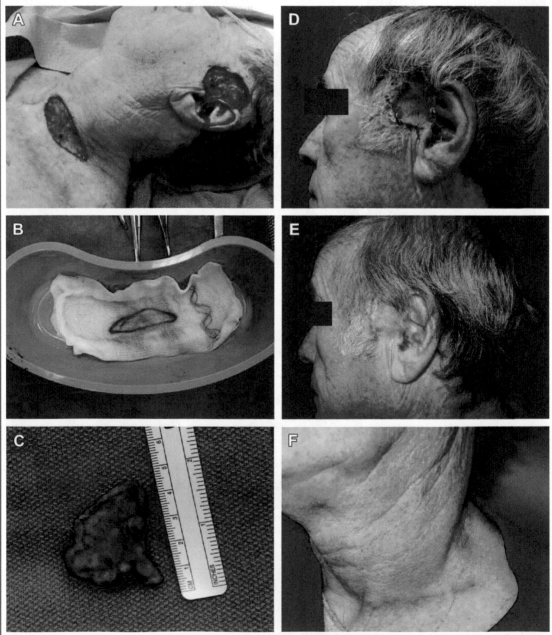

Fig. 3. FTSG from the left neck to reconstruct the preauricular and temporal region after excision of a basal cell carcinoma (6 × 4 cm). (*A*) Recipient and donor site, (*B*) FTSG, (*C*) resected tumor, and (*D*) postoperative status. (*E*) Two weeks postoperatively, (*F*) 6 weeks postoperatively.

Case: Flap for Excision of Squamous Cell Carcinoma of Temporal Region

This case involves an excision of an SCC from the left preauricular and temporal region (2.5 × 2 cm) and reconstruction with a Limberg flap (**Fig. 4**). The operation was done in the MPR with 1% lidocaine with epinephrine to infiltrate the tissue for resection and reconstruction. The lesion was excised with 5-mm margins and included the underlying fascia. A posteriorly based Limberg flap was rotated to fill the defect and secured into place with a nylon stitch, and covered with dressing. **Fig. 5** demonstrates a V-Y advancement flap to close the defect after excision of a BCC performed in the MPR under LA.

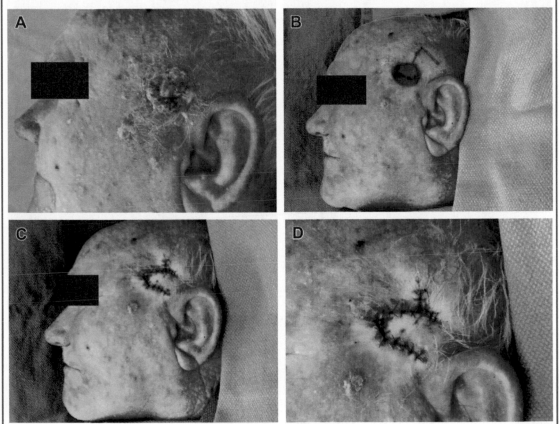

Fig. 4. Limberg flap to reconstruct a defect after excision of a squamous cell carcinoma (2.5 cm × 2 cm) using local anesthetics. (*A*) The lesion, (*B*) defect size and the Limberg flap, and (*C, D*) final closure.

(continued on next page)

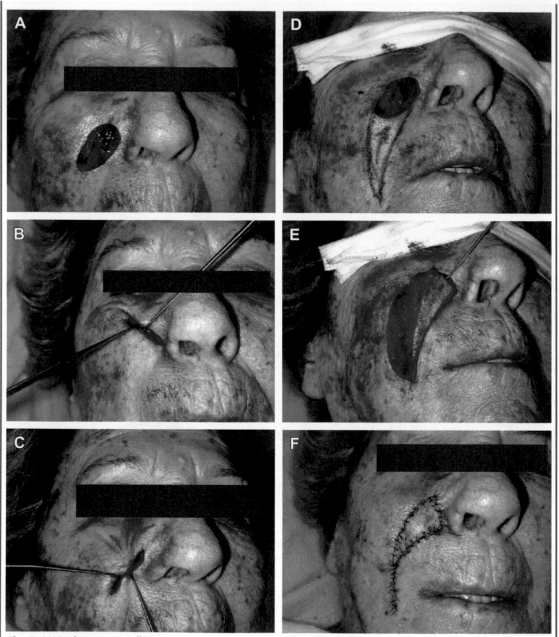

Fig. 5. V-Y advancement flap to reconstruction defect after excision of basal cell carcinoma from the right nasolabial area. (*A*) The defect, (*B, C*) inability to close defect primarily, (*D*) surgical markings for V-Y advancement flap, (*E*) mobility of the flap, and (*F*) final closure.

POTENTIAL COMPLICATIONS AND MANAGEMENT

The surgeon is expected to manage any postoperative complication specific to using LA, including management of allergic reaction or drug toxicity associated with lidocaine and/or epinephrine. In brief, if lidocaine toxicity is encountered, the first step in management is recognition of the toxicity and the basic principle of ABCs (Airway/Breathing/Circulation). If the patient is significantly affected, prompt consultation with a specialist unit may be required. Another important complication is the potential vasoconstrictor effect of epinephrine, especially in the digits. In the case of a procedure in the hand, there are studies showing that epinephrine can safely be injected into the fingers, and it has been documented that the ischemic effects attributed to epinephrine were actually derived from the acidic pH of the procaine.[18–20] However, if the surgeon considers the digits to be in jeopardy, phentolamine (1 mg in 1 mL of saline) should be injected into the area of concern.

The postoperative complications related to the specific surgical intervention are the same regardless of whether this is done with LA or general anesthetic. Typically complications with STSG include pain and minor bleeding at the skin donor site, which can be treated with oral analgesics and controlled with dressing care, respectively. With the use of local skin flaps there is risk of tissue necrosis, but generally the rotation flaps are designed in a manner that does not restrict blood flow.

POSTPROCEDURAL CARE

All postprocedure care is communicated to the patient in the form of oral and written instructions.

> ### Box 3
> ### Measures to reduce patient discomfort during injection of local anesthetic
>
> *Techniques*
>
> Distraction techniques (eg, scratching skin adjacent to the injection site)[23]
>
> Warming the solution to higher than room temperature[24]
>
> Buffering the local anesthetic[10]
>
> Slowing the injection rate[25]
>
> Injecting into subdermal plane[26]

The authors' typical postoperative care of skin grafts for the donor site includes an occlusive dressing such as Tegaderm absorbent for 3 weeks. If there any leaks from the dressing, one would need to simply reinforce the dressing. The bolster dressing applied to the recipient site is removed at 10 to 14 days. By this time the skin graft is adherent, and often the patient can return to daily functioning. However, if the bolster dressing is removed earlier there is a risk of lifting the skin graft from the bed. For local flaps, the postoperative care often depends on the specific flap design. Certain flaps such as the cross-finger flap may require an additional procedure that will be divided at 2 weeks. For more simple flaps, the authors remove the sutures after an appropriate postoperative course. All patients are given a prescription for an analgesic and stool softener.

REHABILITATION AND RECOVERY

The rehabilitation after this procedure is the same regardless of whether it is done with LA or with

Table 3
Safety of epinephrine in local anesthesia for grafts and flaps

Authors,[Ref.] Year	Findings
Wolfort et al,[27] 1990 *Animal study*	Lidocaine vs lidocaine with 1:100,000 epinephrine No difference in STSG survival Significantly greater FTSG loss in epinephrine group
Fazio and Zitelli,[28] 1995 *Human study*	Lidocaine vs lidocaine with 1:100,000 epinephrine Significantly greater partial graft failures in epinephrine group No difference in final cosmetic outcomes
Atabey et al,[29] 2004 *Animal study*	Lidocaine vs lidocaine with epinephrine Higher flap necrosis in groups injected with lidocaine with 1:100,000 and 1:200,000 epinephrine
Blome-Eberwein et al,[30] 2012 *Human study*	Saline vs epinephrine/saline/local anesthetic tumescent No difference in healing of STSG donor sites

Abbreviations: FTSG, full-thickness skin graft; STSG, split-thickness skin graft.

sedation and general anesthesia, because the actual surgical intervention is the same in either situation. The recovery, however, is different, as ambulatory patients do not require admission, and thus discharge home is expedited.

OUTCOMES

The surgical outcome is similar whether the procedure is done with LA or general anesthesia.

CLINICAL RESULTS IN THE LITERATURE

Clinical results published in the literature are summarized in **Box 3** and **Table 3**.

SUMMARY

The cost of health care is one of the major determining factors in the allocation of health care resources. As surgeons, we contribute to cost reduction by devising unique ways of achieving the same surgical goal. This article describes the use of LA for the application of skin grafts and local flaps. As ascertained in a recent Royal College of Physician and Surgeons conference in Ottawa, there is no more money available in health care, and the onus is on surgeons to find more ways to become efficient.[21] The use of LA, especially in the MPR, may become the standard of care in the face of long waiting times and high patient demands. It is our responsibility as surgeons to take an active role in allocating operative time effectively and efficiently.

ACKNOWLEDGMENTS

Special thanks to Manraj Kaur, MSc, for contributing time & resources towards the effort of writing this chapter.

REFERENCES

1. Ministry of Finance Public Accounts of Ontario 2011-2012: Annual report and consolidated financial statements. Available at: http://www.fin.gov.on.ca/en/budget/paccts/2012/12_ar.html. Accessed March 15, 2013.
2. The price of excess: identifying waste in healthcare spending. Available at: www.pwc.com/us/en/healthcare/publications/the-price-of-excess.jhtml. Accessed December 19, 2011.
3. Organization for Economic Cooperation and Development (OECD) health care systems: efficiency and policy settings. http://www.oecd.org/eco/healthcaresystemsefficiencyandpolicysettings.htm. Accessed on March 15, 2013.
4. The World Health Report—Health systems financing: the path to universal coverage. Available at: www.who.int/whr/2010/en/index.html. Accessed January 26, 2012.
5. Leblanc MR, Lalonde J, Lalonde DH. A detailed cost and efficiency analysis of performing carpal tunnel surgery in the main operating room versus the ambulatory setting in Canada. Hand (N Y) 2007;2: 173-8.
6. CanMEDS: better standards, better physicians, better care. Available at: http://www.royalcollege.ca/portal/page/portal/rc/canmeds. Accessed March 10, 2013.
7. Ahlstrom KK, Frodel JL. Local anesthetics for facial plastic procedures. Otolaryngol Clin North Am 2002;35:29-53, v-vi.
8. Marx JA, Hockberger RS, Walls RM, editors. Rosen's emergency medicine. Philadelphia: Mosby/Elsevier; 2010. p. 45-8.
9. Koay J, Orengo I. Application of local anesthetics in dermatologic surgery. Dermatol Surg 2002;28:143-8.
10. Cepeda MS, Tzortzopoulou A, Thackrey M, et al. Adjusting the pH of lidocaine for reducing pain on injection. Cochrane Database Syst Rev 2010;(12): CD006581.
11. Zaiac M, Aguilera SB, Zaulyanov-Scanlan L, et al. Virtually painless local anesthesia: diluted lidocaine proves to be superior to buffered lidocaine for subcutaneous infiltration. J Drugs Dermatol 2012;11: e39-42.
12. Quaba O, Huntley JS, Bahia H, et al. A users guide for reducing the pain of local anaesthetic administration. Emerg Med J 2005;22:188-9.
13. Harmatz A. Local anesthetics: uses and toxicities. Surg Clin North Am 2009;89:587-98.
14. Eidelman A, Weiss JM, Lau J, et al. Topical anesthetics for dermal instrumentation: a systematic review of randomized, controlled trials. Ann Emerg Med 2005;46:343-51.
15. Walsh A, Walsh S. Local anaesthesia and the dermatologist. Clin Exp Dermatol 2011;36:337-43.
16. Klein JA. Tumescent technique for regional anesthesia permits lidocaine doses of 35 mg/kg for liposuction. J Dermatol Surg Oncol 1990;16:248-63.
17. McKee DE, Lalonde DH, Thoma A, et al. Optimal time delay between epinephrine injection and incision to minimize bleeding. Plast Reconstr Surg 2013;131:811-4.
18. Lalonde DH. Reconstruction of the hand with wide awake surgery. Clin Plast Surg 2011;38:761-9.
19. Mustoe TA, Buck DW, Lalonde DH. The safe management of anesthesia, sedation, and pain in plastic surgery. Plast Reconstr Surg 2010;126:165e-76e.
20. Thomson CJ, Lalonde DH, Denkler KA, et al. A critical look at the evidence for and against elective epinephrine use in the finger. Plast Reconstr Surg 2007;119:260-6.
21. The 2012 Human Resources for Health (HRH) Dialogue and Specialty Medicine Summit, Royal

College, Ottawa, Ontario, Canada. December 4–5, 2012.

22. Brown RS, Rhodus NL. Epinephrine and local anesthesia revisited. Oral Surg Oral Med Oral Pathol Oral Radiol Endod 2005;100:401–8.

23. Ong EL, Lim NL, Koay CK. Towards a pain-free venepuncture. Anaesthesia 2000;55:260–2.

24. Hogan ME, vanderVaart S, Perampaladas K, et al. Systematic review and meta-analysis of the effect of warming local anesthetics on injection pain. Ann Emerg Med 2011;58:86–98.e1.

25. Serour F, Mandelberg A, Mori J. Slow injection of local anaesthetic will decrease pain during dorsal penile nerve block. Acta Anaesthesiol Scand 1998; 42:926–8.

26. Arndt KA, Burton C, Noe JM. Minimizing the pain of local anesthesia. Plast Reconstr Surg 1983;72:676–9.

27. Wolfort S, Rohrich RJ, Handren J, et al. The effect of epinephrine in local anesthesia on the survival of full- and split-thickness skin grafts: an experimental study. Plast Reconstr Surg 1990;86:535–40.

28. Fazio MJ, Zitelli JA. Full-thickness skin grafts. Clinical observations on the impact of using epinephrine in local anesthesia of the donor site. Arch Dermatol 1995;131:691–4.

29. Atabey A, Galdino G, El-Shahat A, et al. The effects of tumescent solutions containing lidocaine and epinephrine on skin flap survival in rats. Ann Plast Surg 2004;53:70–2.

30. Blome-Eberwein S, Abboud M, Lozano DD, et al. Effect of subcutaneous epinephrine/saline/local anesthetic vs only saline injection on split thickness skin graft donor site perfusion, healing, and pain. J Burn Care Res 2013;34:e80–6.

Peripheral Nerve Blocks for Distal Extremity Surgery

Chris Offierski, MD, FRCS

KEYWORDS

- Anesthesia • Local anesthesia • Regional anesthesia • Nerve blocks • Peripheral nerve blocks
- Foot surgery • Distal extremity

KEY POINTS

- Peripheral nerve block is well suited for distal extremity surgery.
- Blocking nerves in the distal extremity is safe with a low risk of toxicity as a result of smaller dosing of the anesthetic agents required for the smaller diameter and superficial nerves in the distal extremity.
- Blocking the nerves at the distal extremity is easily done, because the nerves are superficial and landmarks easily palpable for safe needle placement.

INTRODUCTION

Peripheral nerve block is well suited for distal extremity surgery of the hands and feet.[1-5] The technique is simple, safe, and effective for obtaining anesthesia in the outpatient clinic or office.

Blocking the nerves at the distal extremity is easily done, because the nerves are superficial and landmarks easily palpable for safe needle placement. It does not require the use of ultrasound or stimulators to identify the nerve.

Blocking nerves in the distal extremity is safe with low risk of toxicity as a result of smaller dosing of the anesthetic agents. Nerves in the distal extremity are smaller in diameter, more superficial, and require less volume to achieve a good block. The effect of the nerve block is limited to the distribution of the nerve only, sparing the other functions in the extremity.

The distal nerves in the lower extremity are sensory branches of the sciatic nerve. This provides a sensory block only and leaves the motor function intact. This has the advantage of allowing the patient

to actively contract tendons in the foot, which is useful when doing tenotomies to correct deformities in toes (ie, claw toes or hammer toes). This also allows the patient to ambulate more quickly after surgery and shortens postoperative recovery times.

PATIENT SELECTION

Patient selection is critical to the success of nerve block anesthesia. The use of a nerve block requires that the patient is agreeable to the procedure, understands the nature of nerve block anesthesia, and is cooperative. This technique is not suitable for patients with language barriers, because cooperation of the patient and verbal feedback are required for this method to be successful. Children and anxious patients are not good candidates for nerve block anesthesia. Mild anxiety can be treated with a mild preoperative sedative to make the patient relaxed. I have learned that patients who say they have difficulty with dental freezing are better suited to general or neuraxial anesthesia.

Orthopedic Surgery, Greater Niagara General Hospital, 6453 Morrison Street, Suite 300, Niagara Falls, Ontario L2E 7H1, Canada
E-mail address: dr.offierski@bellnet.ca

Clin Plastic Surg 40 (2013) 551–555
http://dx.doi.org/10.1016/j.cps.2013.07.005
0094-1298/13/$ – see front matter © 2013 Elsevier Inc. All rights reserved.

plasticsurgery.theclinics.com

INDICATIONS

Most patients undergoing surgery to the foot desire a limited regional anesthesia rather than a general or neuraxial anesthesia.

Infection is a predominant cause of surgery of the foot. Extensive cellulitis or ascending lymphangitis at the site of the nerve block would preclude utilizing a nerve block technique.

Peripheral vascular ischemia, a common reason for foot surgery, is suitable for nerve block anesthesia as long as no epinephrine is added to the blocking agent. Because the distal nerves are small in diameter and easily accessible, epinephrine is not required to augment the distal nerve block.

Distal extremity nerve block is best suited to operative procedures of 30 minutes or less. Although the nerve block will last for a few hours, the patient will become uncomfortable from positioning the leg for an extended time and not moving. The use of a tourniquet becomes more painful with time when only part of the foot is blocked. Procedures longer than 30 minutes duration are better done under general or neuraxial anesthesia.

TECHNIQUE

The peripheral sensory nerves are superficial and well localized by easily identifiable landmarks. This allows the Xylocaine to be infiltrated around the nerve for optimal blocking concentration. Not infrequently, Paraesthesia may be elicited if the nerve is touched. The risk of traumatizing the nerve is minimized by ensuring that the bevel of the needle is parallel to the alignment of the nerve being blocked. Smaller-gauge needles minimize damage to the nerve if accidentally touched. It is important to stop injection immediately and withdraw the needle slightly if the patient experiences paraesthesia and pain with infiltration.

To minimize the discomfort associated with injecting Xylocaine, the Xylocaine can be buffered with 2 mL sodium bicarbonate 8.4% in 20 mL of Xylocaine. This reduces the acidity of the Xylocaine and takes away the sting associated with the infiltration. This makes the infiltration of the anesthetic much more tolerable to the patient, who feels a sensation of pressure rather than stinging.

Surgery is done with tourniquet of the extremity (**Fig. 1**A). Using a tourniquet restricts the time

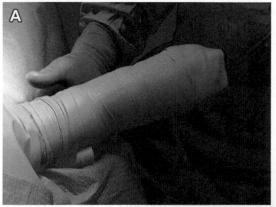
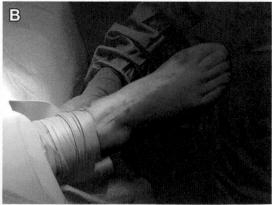
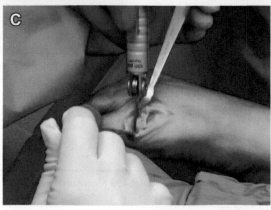

Fig. 1. (*A*) Tourniquet of the extremity. (*B*) Elastic bandage tight around the ankle as a tourniquet. (*C*) Surgical procedure on foot following nerve blocks.

of surgery to less than 30 minutes, after which the pressure of the tourniquet becomes painful to the patient. A blood pressure cuff can be used around the calf for a short period of time, but this can be uncomfortable because of compression of the calf muscles. An Esmark elastic bandage can be used to exsanguinate the foot and remain tight around the ankle as a tourniquet (see **Fig. 1**B). This is better tolerated by the patient, because the tourniquet pressure is applied to the distal tibia and ankle, minimizing soft tissue and muscle compression, which can be uncomfortable. **Fig. 1**C shows the beginning of surgery.

ANKLE BLOCK

The classic technique for local anesthesia in the foot is to utilize an ankle block. This technique involves blocking up to 5 nerves at the level of the ankle joint (**Fig. 2**). The multiple injection sites may be a little uncomfortable to the patient and require a larger volume of local anesthetic to achieve adequate anesthesia. If surgery is confined to only 1 part of the foot, fewer nerves can be blocked for the procedure. The blocks used in an ankle block include the posterior tibial nerve, sural nerve, saphenous nerve, superficial peroneal nerve, and the deep peroneal nerve.

POSTERIOR TIBIAL NERVE BLOCK

The posterior tibial nerve is easily located behind medial malleolus of the ankle (**Fig. 3**). The nerve is part of the neurovascular complex as it passes behind the medial malleolus. The anatomy of the complex at the level of the ankle can be described as the posterior tibial artery is anterior; the posterior tibial vein is immediately behind the artery, and the posterior tibial nerve is behind the vein. The nerve is located less than 1 fingerbreadth behind the palpable artery. Because of the close proximity of the blood vessels, it is important to aspirate the syringe before injecting the nerve block. About 5 cc of buffered Xylocaine are sufficient for a block. A successful block will give anesthesia to the sole of the foot, extending from the heel to all the toes. This block is very useful for reducing the pain associated with hydrocortisone injection for plantar fasciitis, as well for surgical release of the plantar fascia. This block alone is sufficient to allow surgery on the sole of the foot (ie, plantar fibromas, calluses, or flexor tenotomies).

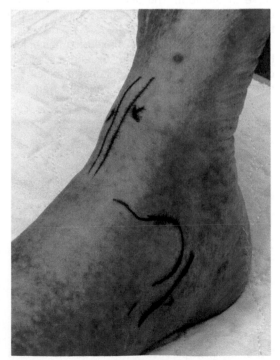

Fig. 2. Ankle block. Up to 5 nerves at the level of the ankle joint are blocked.

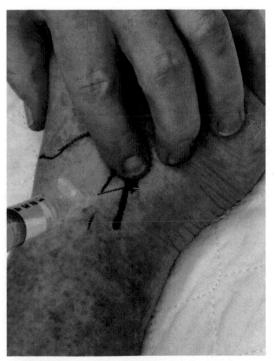

Fig. 3. Posterior nerve block. Part of the neurovascular complex as it passes behind the medial malleolus.

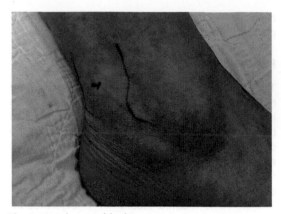

Fig. 4. Sural nerve block.

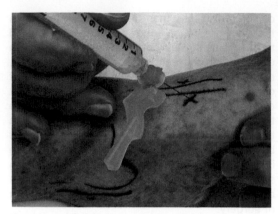

Fig. 5. Superficial peroneal nerve block.

SURAL NERVE BLOCK

The sural nerve is located behind the lateral malleolus. It is situated superficially under the skin midway between the lateral border of the Achilles tendon and the posterior edge of the distal fibulae (**Fig. 4**).

The area is infiltrated with 5 to 7 cc of buffered Xylocaine. A successful block will give good anesthesia along the lateral border of the foot extending out to the fifth toe. Surgery on the fifth metatarsal and toe will require augmentation with posterior tibial nerve block. This will give adequate anesthesia for excising bunionette, percutaneous pinning fifth metacarpal fractures, partial amputation, or tenotomies.

DEEP PERONEAL NERVE BLOCK

Sensation to the dorsum of the foot is through 2 branches of the peroneal nerve. It requires that both nerves be blocked simultaneously. The deep peroneal nerve is located between the extensor hallux longus and the extensor digitorum longus tendons, which are easily palpable at the front of the ankle. The nerve is located just lateral to the dorsalis pedis artery, deep to the extensor retinaculum. The needle is advanced through the extensor retinaculum to deposit 5 cc of buffered Xylocaine around the deep peroneal nerve. Because of the close proximity of the dorsalis pedis artery, it is important to aspirate the syringe before injecting. A successful block will give anesthesia in the first web space and is required for any surgery involving the first and second ray of the foot.

SUPERFICIAL PERONEAL NERVE BLOCK

The superficial branch of the peroneal nerve is located superficially overlying the extensor digitorum longus tendon (**Fig. 5**).

The area is infiltrated with 5 to 10 cc of buffered Xylocaine subcutaneously. A successful block provides anesthesia to the dorsum of the foot but must be combined with a deep peroneal block.

COMMON PERONEAL NERVE BLOCK

The common peroneal nerve can be blocked at the level of the neck of the fibulae for full anesthesia of the dorsum of the foot. This is my preferred block for all my foot surgery, because it eliminates the saphenous nerve block and the need to block both branches of the peroneal nerve in the foot. The sensory block is higher on the leg, reducing the discomfort of the tourniquet.

The nerve is located 1 to 2 fingerbreadths below the head of the fibulae (**Fig. 6**), and it is easily palpated in the thin leg. A successful block will give both an immediate motor block to anterior

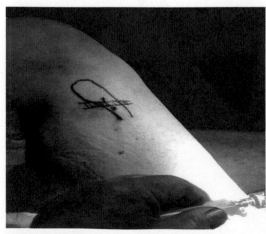

Fig. 6. Common peroneal nerve block. The nerve is located 1 to 2 fingerbreadths below the head of the fibulae.

tibial muscles (a drop foot) and sensory block over the front of the tibia and the dorsum of the foot. This reduces any discomfort arising from the tourniquet around the ankle. Bunion surgery can be done with only 2 blocks, to the common peroneal and the posterior tibial nerves.

REFERENCES

1. Davies RJ. Buffering the pain of local anaesthetics: a systemic review. Emerg Med (Fremantle) 2003; 15(1):81–8.

2. Klien EJ, Shugermann RP, Leigh-Taylor K, et al. Buffered lidocaine: analgesia for intervenous line placement in children. Pediatrics 1995;5:709–12.

3. Morgan GE, Mikhail M. Peripheral nerve blocks. In: Morgan GE, editor. Clinical anesthesiology. 4th edition. New York: Lange Medical Books; 2006.

4. Russon K, Findley H, Harclerode Z. Peripheral nerve blocks "getting started". In: Anaesthesia tutorial of the week. vol. 134. 2009.

5. Wedel DJ, Horlocker TT. Peripheral nerve blocks. In: Longnecker DE, et al, editors. Anesthesiology. New York: McGraw-Hill Medical; 2008.

Cubital Tunnel Release Using Local Anesthesia

Nasim S. Huq, MD, FRCSC, MSc, FACS, CAQHS, DABPS*,
Naweed Ahmed, BSc, MD, Mehdi Razeghi, MD

KEYWORDS

- Cubital tunnel syndrome • Cubital tunnel release • Local anesthesia • Ulnar nerve
- Decompression surgery • Nerve entrapment

KEY POINTS

- The procedure results in an anterior transposition of the ulnar nerve in the subcutaneous plane while still under local anesthesia.
- Patients benefit from walking in and out of a minor procedure suite without any exposure to the risks of general anesthesia.
- There is no difference in our patient outcomes between performing cubital tunnel release under local anesthesia in a minor operating setting compared with the results obtained under general anesthesia in a main operating room.

INTRODUCTION

Cubital tunnel syndrome is one of the most common nerve entrapment syndromes, second only to carpal tunnel syndrome.[1] It often results in such symptoms as complaints of numbness and tingling in the ulnar half of the hand, and can extend to more severe symptoms, such as wasting of intrinsic muscles. In many cases, treatment of cubital tunnel syndrome requires surgical intervention. Today, the most recognized surgical interventions are in situ decompression, medical epicondylectomy, subcutaneous anterior transposition, and submuscular transposition. Most of these procedures require general anesthesia and an operating room environment.[2]

CUBITAL TUNNEL RELEASE WITH LOCAL ANESTHESIA

Cubital tunnel syndrome can be treated in many ways including conservative measures, in situ decompression, medial epicondylectomy, direct release with subcutaneous anterior transposition, and submuscular anterior transposition.[2] Cubital tunnel release, with or without anterior transposition, can easily be performed under local anesthesia without the need for intravenous sedation.

Although carpal tunnel decompression is one of the most common operations performed in the world, the cubital tunnel release is much less common because of the belief held by many surgeons that general anesthesia is required. The surgery can be performed with a brachial plexus block or even an intravenous Bier block; however, it is difficult to obtain a complete release proximally, if two blood pressure cuffs are applied to the arm.

The ulnar nerve originates in the brachial plexus and passes through the cubital tunnel. The elbow joint is very dynamic, with a range of approximately 150 degrees.[3] The ligaments over the ulnar nerve stretch and move with elbow motion.[4] Vanderpool and colleagues[4] indicated that there is a significant stretch of the aponeurosis around the

The authors have nothing to disclose.
Niagara Plastic Surgery Centre, McMaster University, 5668 Main Street, Suite 1, Niagara Falls, Ontario L2G 5Z4, Canada
* Corresponding author.
E-mail address: Niagaraplasticsurgery@gmail.com

Clin Plastic Surg 40 (2013) 557–565
http://dx.doi.org/10.1016/j.cps.2013.08.003

elbow with flexion. In full flexion, the cubital tunnel has been shown to be compressed and narrowed by approximately 55%.[5] It is thought that this decreased volume predisposes the ulnar nerve to compression.[4,6,7]

Flexion at the elbow results in the ulnar nerve having to travel a greater distance as opposed to extension of the elbow (**Figs. 1** and **2**). With elbow flexion, intraneuronal pressure of the ulnar nerve increases significantly.[8–10] It has also been shown that excursion of the ulnar nerve around the elbow occurs with shoulder and elbow motion.[11,12] Repetitive motion or dynamic traction and excursion may cause some inflammation around the nerve, which has been validated with histology and imaging studies.[11,12] Blood flow and axoplasmic flow is affected by compression of the ulnar nerve at the elbow.[13] The ulnar nerve is located superficially at the elbow and mechanical compression may be common when there is very little soft tissue for padding over the nerve.[12] Of course, directly leaning on the elbow and the cubital tunnel can produce a direct mechanical compression on the ulnar nerve. Other sources include soft tissue masses, such as ganglions or lipomas, and direct bony abnormalities, such as cubitus valgus or fractures.[11,12] Rheumatoid disease, diabetes, and hypothyroidism have all been associated with peripheral neuropathies.[11]

ULNAR NERVE ANATOMY AND SITES OF COMPRESSION

The ulnar nerve originates in the brachial plexus from C8 and T1 nerve roots. The ulnar nerve containing sensory and motor nerve fibers exits the brachial plexus as a branch of the medial cord and travels from the axillary region to the medial arm.

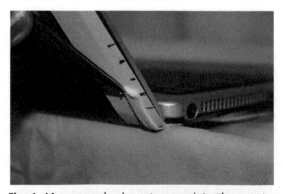

Fig. 1. Many people do not appreciate the greater distance the ulnar nerve must travel when the elbow is flexed as opposed to extended. Illustration by the computer represents the elbow and the string represents the ulnar nerve. Markings shown are 1 cm apart.

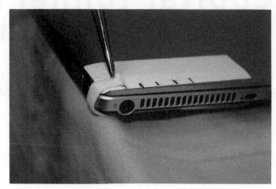

Fig. 2. Illustration by the computer represents flexion of the elbow resulting in the ulnar nerve traveling an extra 1 to 2 cm in length represented by the string. Markings shown are 1 cm apart.

The first site of compression of the ulnar nerve occurs as it passes posterior to the medial intermuscular septum of the arm. Continuing on its path, the ulnar nerve then passes through the arcade of Struthers, approximately 8 to 10 cm proximal to the medial epicondyle.[14] This arcade lies just anterior to the ulnar nerve and is almost 5 cm in length.[12]

The second site of potential entrapment of the ulnar nerve at the elbow is the medial intermuscular septum. This potential site of compression exists only if there is an anterior transposition of the ulnar nerve or if the ulnar naturally subluxes anterior to the medial epicondyle. As the ulnar nerve approaches the medial epicondyle, it may be entrapped under an anomalous anconeus epitrochlearis muscle, which has been identified as a cause of ulnar compression.[15,16]

The senior author has performed more than 200 cubital tunnel release procedures and has found that approximately 20% of these patients have had a prominent anconeus epitrochlearis. It is therefore suspected that patients who are symptomatic with ulnar compression at the elbow are more likely to have this anomalous muscle than the general population.

The ulnar nerve then continues toward the elbow and passes underneath the cubital tunnel retinaculum or Osborne ligament. The nerve travels beyond the deep fascia, which is also known as Osborne fascia. The third site of frequent ulnar compression lies deep to Osborne fascia, at the distal aspect of the cubital tunnel.[12,17]

The ulnar nerve then passes between the ulnar and radial heads of the flexor carpi ulnaris (FCU) muscle. Approximately 5 cm beyond the medial epicondyle, the ulnar nerve penetrates deep to the fascia to lie between the FCU and the flexor digitorum profundus (FDP) muscle bellies. The ulnar nerve provides motor branches to the FCU in this area. The fascial bands between the two heads of the FCU can contribute to the fourth site of compression.[17]

The anterior branch of the medial brachial cutaneous (MBC) nerve and the medial antebrachial cutaneous (MABC) nerve are very important structures in cubital tunnel release surgery. The MBC can sometimes be found just at the proximal edge of the incision, roughly 2 to 5 cm from the medial epicondyle.[18] There is considerable variability in the location of the MABC nerve because it has multiple branches that may pass proximal, over, or distal to the medial epicondyle. These cutaneous branches must be protected when performing cubital tunnel release to avoid iatrogenic injury.[19] The incidence of neuroma formation after cubital tunnel release has been reported to be as high as 30%.[18]

The surgical approaches to cubital tunnel include in situ decompression, which may be performed in an open or endoscopic fashion.[20] The nerve may require anterior transposition to a subcutaneous position or submuscular position. It is difficult to perform a submuscular anterior transposition of the ulnar nerve entirely under local anesthesia.

HISTORY AND PHYSICAL EXAMINATION AND INVESTIGATIONS

It is important to obtain an accurate history before performing surgery. In cubital tunnel surgery, in particular, it is important to distinguish proximal and distal entrapments, including double crush-type syndrome.[21] Furthermore, it is important to determine if the patient has any further entrapment at the wrist in or around Guyon canal. Document any penetrating trauma, traction-injuries, masses, or history of direct trauma.[11,12,22] Other important historical information includes metabolic diseases, such as diabetes, hypothyroidism, and rheumatoid disease. Grading symptom severity is important in terms of evaluating the degree to which the patient has been affected by the disorder.[11,12,22]

Importantly, the internal typography of the ulnar nerve explains the relative sparing of the flexi carpi ulnaris and the flexi digitorum profundus because these motor fibers often are found to lie deep within the nerve.[4] The motor branches to the intrinsic muscles are similarly affected in chronic and severe acute compression. The more superficially located sensory fibers are likely to be more susceptible to earlier forms of compression injuries.[4] **Tables 1** and **2** respectively describe a nonnumerical grading system of nerve compression at the elbow and a numerical grading system for ulnar nerve compression at the elbow.[22–26]

Table 1
McGowan grading system

Grade I	Mild symptoms, intermittent paresthsia/hypesthsia, no motor changes
Grade II	Persistent symptoms of paresthsia/hypesthsia, varying degrees of mild weakness/atrophy, ulnar innervated muscles
Grade III	Persistent sensory symptoms, marked atrophy, or weakness

Adapted from Refs.[23,25,26]

On physical examination, the ulnar nerve needs to be palpated in flexion and extension for enlargement or subluxation around the medial elbow. Tinel sign is tested over the cubital tunnel and direct manual pressure may be applied over the

Table 2
Staging of ulnar nerve compression at the elbow

Mild compression	
Sensory	Paresthesias come and go, vibratory perception increased
Motor	Subjective weakness, clumsiness, or loss of coordination
Tests	Elbow flexion or Tinel sign may be positive
Moderate compression	
Sensory	Paresthesias come and go, vibratory perception decreased of normal
Motor	Measurable weakness in pinch or grip strength
Tests	Elbow flexion test or Tinel sign are positive, finger crossing might be abnormal
Severe compression	
Sensory	Paresthesias are persistent, vibratory perception decreased, abnormal two-point discrimination (static $\geq$6 mm, moving $\geq$4 mm)
Motor	Measurable weakness in pinch and grip muscle atrophy
Tests	Positive elbow flexion test or positive Tinel sign may be present, finger crossing may be abnormal

Adapted from Refs.[22,24,26]

ulnar nerve for 1 minute to test the ulnar nerve for paresthesias or numbness within the hand. Full elbow flexion with hyperextended wrist may also test the traction on the ulnar nerve.[27–29]

Motor function, however, is tested through examination of the intrinsic muscles of the hand. There may also be a positive Froment paper sign (ie, flexion of the interphalangeal (IP) joint of the thumb is elicited with a side pinch). Furthermore, a positive Wartenberg sign may be present when there is abnormal abduction of the small finger caused by a weakened third palmar interossei muscle. A distinguishing factor for compression within Guyon canal may be weakness of the extrinsic flexors, such as the FDP.[21]

Contraindications for cubital tunnel release may include a brachial plexus compression caused by a Pancoast tumor or C8-T1 radiculopathy. In the senior author's experience, these conditions are very uncommon in patients presenting with cubital tunnel syndrome.

CONSERVATIVE TREATMENT

Conservative measures do not have the potential complications of surgery; however, they also do not necessarily have the same results. In very mild disease, conservative measures are often a very good choice. In most cases, acceptable improvement occurs with simple modifications, such as splinting or environmental adaptations. Eighty-six percent improvement in severity of symptoms was found in 73 patients who underwent splinting without surgery.[30] Simple modifications, such as changing sleeping positions or using elbow padding, may have a significant effect and may help avoid surgery. Optimizing medical management of diabetes, thyroid disease, or rheumatoid disease may ameliorate symptoms. Radiographic examination of the elbow may also aid in making the decision for surgery. It is important to rule out thoracic outlet syndrome, which may present in a similar way as cubital tunnel syndrome.[3,31]

Diagnostic imaging plays an important role in the diagnosis of cubital tunnel syndrome. Some centers have found ultrasonography useful in helping to diagnose cubital tunnel syndrome.[31] Magnetic resonance imaging has also been studied as a diagnostic test in cubital tunnel syndrome. However, although easily available, magnetic resonance imaging may not be the most cost-effective or the most convenient test because of its limitations of static testing and false-negative rates.

Night splinting has been the mainstay of conservative measures for cubital tunnel syndrome.[3,32] This improvement can even be confirmed with electrodiagnostic testing. Patients are also reminded not to rest their elbows on hard surfaces. There are a variety of splints available for conservative management.[3,32] Cortisone injections, in conjunction with splinting, have not been found to add any significant advantage in the treatment of the symptoms of cubital tunnel syndrome.[33–35] In our center, we recommend wrapping a light pillow, a light sleeping bag, or egg crate cushion foam around the elbow. The cushioning material may then be taped or tied in place with shoelaces. Patients find this method to be more comfortable than rigid splints; however, some patients do feel warm or uncomfortable, regardless of the type of splint used.

Conservative measures are a useful option in the management of cubital tunnel syndrome, especially in milder cases or presentations with reversible etiologies. Patient education also plays an important role in treating mild forms of cubital tunnel syndrome.

SURGICAL TREATMENT

In 1989, Dellon published a key review paper that analyzed 50 studies conducted from 1898 to 1988, with 1435 patients classified into a staging system (see **Table 2**).[22,24,26] After stratifying the patients based on minimal, moderate, and severe disease stages, the authors concluded that there was no difference in outcomes achieved between the various types of surgical procedures, if the patients had minimal disease.[26] For moderate compression, the anterior transposition worked about 80% of the time and for severe compression, no method was highly successful.[26]

There have been many debates regarding whether anterior transposition of the ulnar nerve is required or whether simple in situ ulnar nerve decompression is sufficient. If anterior transposition is required, should it be submuscular or will subcutaneous transposition be sufficient? In the senior author's opinion, the answer to this should be determined partly by the skill and the experience of the surgeon. The senior author has performed more than 200 ulnar nerve decompressions. More than half of them have been undertaken under general anesthesia in a main operating room using the method of subcutaneous anterior transposition of the ulnar nerve. More recently, we have been performing this procedure under local anesthesia in the minor operating procedure suite starting with in situ ulnar nerve decompression. Anterior transposition is undertaken only if the ulnar nerve subluxes naturally anteriorly to the medial epicondyle with full elbow flexion.

The senior author has found that most patients are able to tolerate the tourniquet time of about 20 to 25 minutes for ulnar nerve decompression at the elbow. If needed, a carpal tunnel release is also performed at the same time as the cubital tunnel procedure.

OPERATIVE PROCEDURE

Before embarking on the surgical procedure, the patient confirms the correct limb, and we review the procedure again, thus facilitating the answering of all questions. The patient's weight is recorded in kilograms. The ulnar nerve is examined and marked externally. The bony landmarks of the olecranon and medial epicondyle are also marked with the elbow at 90 degrees (**Fig. 3**). Initial nerve blocks are instituted with solution #1 (1% xylocaine with adrenaline diluted 50% with normal saline in a 1:1 ratio) infiltrated over the path of the ulnar nerve. A second syringe with solution #2 (9 mL and 1% xylocaine with adrenaline mixed with sodium bicarbonate) is prepared on the high stand. The normal path for an open cubital tunnel release is marked and infiltrated with the first solution in case the limited incision technique needs to be converted to an open incision.

Some surgeons use a more posterior approach in keeping with the open midposterior incision similar to that used for open reduction of an olecranon fracture. This incision does heal well, and requires a larger dissection, which is difficult to perform under local anesthesia. It is important to note the normal location of the MBC and the MABC nerves. Generally, for most elbows the senior author is able to place the incision just proximal and posterior to the medial epicondyle; he does not cross into the forearm. A 5-cm incision is usually sufficient for adequate visualization (**Fig. 4**). A tourniquet is applied as high onto the arm as possible, and the entire limb is prepared and draped in a sterile fashion.

Under tourniquet control, the 5-cm incision is made proximal and posterior to the medial epicondyle. Blunt dissection is directed down to the ulnar nerve and any branches of the MABC nerve are identified and preserved, if possible. The ulnar nerve is easily identifiable and traced proximally (**Fig. 5**). The fascial plane is just superficial to the ulnar nerve and is released at least 10-cm proximal to the medial epicondyle. As soon as the ulnar nerve is identified under local anesthesia, solution #2 is injected with a 25-gauge needle into the epineurium of the ulnar nerve. The senior author has found that a dilated solution of less than this concentration does not produce adequate anesthesia of the ulnar nerve. After solution #2 is injected, the area around the medial epicondyle and proximally in the area of the arcade of Struthers is also infiltrated with this solution.

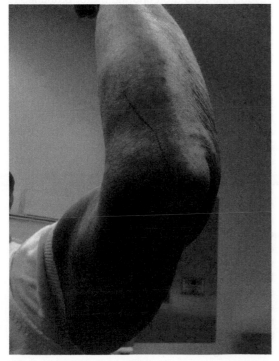

Fig. 3. Preoperative marking.

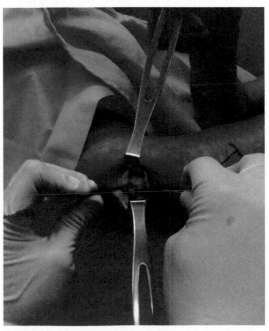

Fig. 4. Anconeus epitrochlearis is identified intraoperatively.

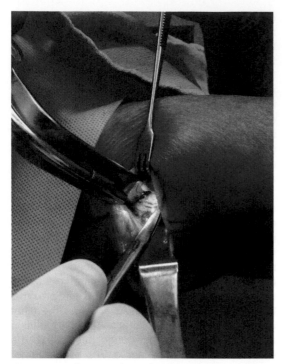

Fig. 5. Muscle is released and nerve is traced proximally.

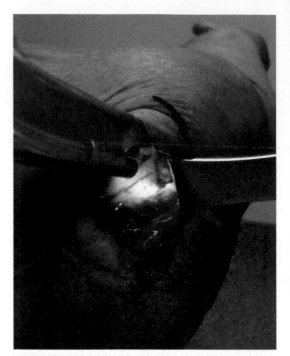

Fig. 6. Nerve is released distally.

While this local anesthetic is taking effect, the ulnar nerve is traced over the Osborne ligament on to the volar antebrachial fascia into the forearm. The sensory branches of the MABC are in the superficial fat and in the flap above the volar antebrachial fascia. This full-thickness flap is elevated to approximately 10-cm distal to the medial epicondyle. The sensory nerves are usually not encountered but an occasional perforating vein may be identified and cauterized under direct visualization. More of the local anesthetic is infiltrated over the path of the ulnar nerve into the forearm flap and into the muscle, as needed.

The ulnar nerve is then traced proximally. Under direct visualization with a lighted right angled retractor, the arcade of Struthers is released until there is no remaining ligament and a finger is able to pass well proximal to the preoperative markings. The surgeon can palpate the ulnar nerve completely unrestricted in this area.

The ulnar nerve is then traced distally and Osborne ligament and Osborne fascia are released under direct visualization at the elbow (**Fig. 6**). The senior author does not attempt any type of neurolysis at this point. If an accessory muscle of anconeus epitrochlearis is identified, this muscle is also infiltrated with local anesthetic. The nerve is then traced down into the forearm. The volar antebrachial fascia is released 10 cm distal to the medial epicondyle with a long pair of Metzenbaum scissors. The ulnar nerve is then traced below into the volar forearm muscle and the FCU arch is identified and released under direct visualization.

After the ulnar nerve is traced distally and beyond the FCU arch and the motor branches to the FCU are preserved, the muscle is split with a gentle sweeping position of the finger. The muscle itself can be infiltrated with additional local anesthetic just before this maneuver. Small vessels are cauterized during the procedure if seen within the operative field. The lighted retractor is used to trace the ulnar nerve as it runs under the FCU and the FDP. The lighted retractor ensures direct visualization of the ulnar nerve at all times because it is imperative not to cause any direct injury to the ulnar nerve.

The senior author does not dissect the ulnar nerve out the groove unless necessary. The elbow is flexed, and if the ulnar nerve remains naturally in its posterior position, the procedure is ready to be completed. If the ulnar nerve naturally subluxes out of the groove because of the significant tension on the ulnar nerve with elbow flexion, then the senior author proceeds with external neurolysis (**Fig. 7**). The ulnar nerve must be protected and immobilized; use just a small right angle retractor. More local anesthetic may be required because the nerve block must be fully effective at this stage of the procedure. The soft tissue is elevated over the medial epicondyle leaving the

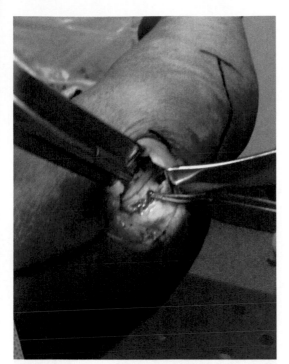

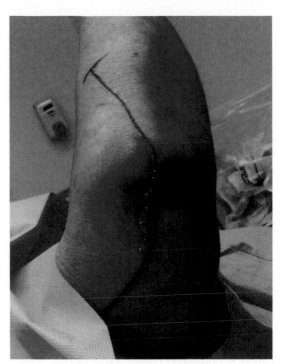

Fig. 7. The elbow is flexed and after decompression in situ the ulnar nerve does not sublux anteriorly. The accessory muscle is left transected.

Fig. 8. Immediate postoperative closure.

fascia intact, and a large rectangular fascial sling is elevated off the muscle. The external neurolysis has to be completed to ensure preservation of any motor branches to the FCU. Then the ulnar nerve can be transposed anterior to the medial epicondyle without difficulty. The elbow is subsequently flexed and extended to confirm no kinking of the ulnar nerve occurs.

The fascial sling is sutured to the dermis with the ulnar nerve transposed anteriorly. 4-0 Monocryl is used to suture the fascial sling to the dermis in a very large bed to allow the nerve to glide without any entrapment. The senior author prefers to deflate the tourniquet before closure, so that hemostasis can be rechecked. No drains are used. The skin is closed with buried Monocryl in a subcutaneous fashion followed by over-and-over Vicryl Rapide (Ethicon Inc., Somerville, NJ, USA) in the skin. Cutaneous staples may also be used (**Fig. 8**).

If the ulnar nerve is transposed, the intermuscular septum of the triceps muscle must be released. Cautious dissection is performed with either incision or excision of a few centimeters of this band. A very significant venous collection is located just at the base of this band and careful attention is required to preserve these vessels because they can be difficult to control.

COMPLICATIONS

Painful or symptomatic neuromas of the MABC or the MBC are important to avoid. In the senior author's experience, neuromas are very uncommon if the dissection is limited to the 5 cm described and the sensory nerves are protected in the superficial flaps. If the incision does require further dissection, then sensory nerves should be identified and preserved. The senior author has encountered one patient who had several sensory-type neuromas in usual places around the forearm. However, she had an untreated congenital, bilateral, radial ulnar synostosis. As an adult, she required multiple peripheral nerve releases. As a result, her sensory nerves in and around the elbow were not in predictable positions. On revision surgery, the senior author opened the entire area. The sensory nerves were identified and two small neuromas were buried leading to symptom improvement.

The senior author has found that in patients who have had repeat decompression after previous anterior transposition of the ulnar nerve by other surgeons, on exploration, the release needs to be extended more proximally and distally. This maneuver may decrease the kinking in the area or any entrapment from a fascial band.

Even with this new technique, the senior author encountered one patient who required a repeat release because of scarring down in the subcutaneous plane, even though there had been an adequate bed and a large fascial flap. For this reason, the senior author encourages early active range of motion of the elbow with ulnar decompression alone and with anterior transposition of the ulnar nerve.

Direct nerve injury may occur or a cutaneous neuroma may develop. Other complications include slow resolution of symptoms because it often takes several months to a year or more for the ulnar nerve to regenerate all the way down to the hand. There is a possibility of infection, hematoma, or delayed wound healing. Fortunately, in the senior author's experience, this is collectively less than 5% of all voiced complications.

Recurrent or worsening symptoms may occur if there is incomplete release of the ulnar nerve or if further scarring prevents adequate excursion of the nerve. The nerve may become unnaturally immobilized again.

Failed surgery may be caused by preoperative problems, such as an incorrect diagnosis. Another cause is unrealistic patient expectations. Intraoperative complications may occur, as previously discussed. Other postoperative complications may include perineural scarring, elbow stiffness, or contracture.

OUTCOMES

Most patients experience improved sensation to the hand with decreased pain and improved fine motor manual dexterity. Depending on severity of the preoperative symptoms, range of motion also improves. For patients with significant intrinsic atrophy, the remaining fibers are at least preserved and further atrophy is halted with surgical intervention.

Patients who have mild to moderate severity of symptoms of cubital tunnel syndrome and those who fail conservative measures may be candidates for cubital tunnel release under local anesthesia. The procedure can be converted to an anterior transposition in the subcutaneous plane while the patient is still under local anesthesia. This procedure is well tolerated under local anesthesia with a tourniquet time of less than 30 minutes. If necessary, the tourniquet may be deflated and the rest of the procedure may be completed with the tourniquet down. Otherwise, the senior author has found no difference in patient outcomes between performing cubital tunnel release under local anesthesia in a minor operating setting compared with outcomes when the procedure is performed in the main operating room **(Fig. 9)**.

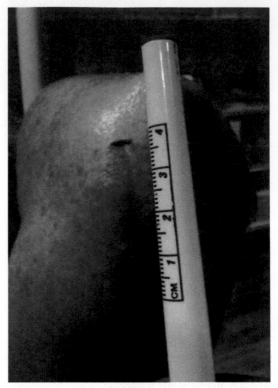

Fig. 9. Incision site after 2 years.

REFERENCES

1. Bozentka DJ. Cubital tunnel syndrome pathophysiology. Clin Orthop Relat Res 1998;351:90–4.
2. Bartels R, Verhagen W, van der Wilt G, et al. Perspective randomized control study comparing simple decompression versus anterior subcutaneous transposition for idiopathic neuropathy of the ulnar nerve at the elbow: part 1. Neurosurgery 2005; 56(3):522–30.
3. Szabo R, Kwak C. Natural history and conservative management of cubital tunnel syndrome. Hand Clin 2007;23:311–8.
4. Vanderpool DW, Chalmers J, Lamb DW, et al. Peripheral compression lesions of the ulnar nerve. J Bone Joint Surg Br 1968;50(4):792–803.
5. Apfelberg DB, Larson SJ. Dynamic anatomy of the ulnar nerve at the elbow. Plast Reconstr Surg 1973;51(1):79–81.
6. Feindel W, Stratford K. Cubital tunnel compression in tardy ulnar palsy. Can J Surg 1958;1(4):287–300.
7. Pechan J, Julius I. The pressure measurement in the ulnar nerve: a contribution to the pathophysiology of the cubital tunnel syndrome. J Biomech 1975;8(1): 75–9.
8. Gelberman RH, Yamaguchi K, Hollstein SB, et al. Changes in interstitial pressure and cross-sectional area of the cubital tunnel and of the ulnar nerve

with flexion of the elbow: an experimental study in human cadaver. J Bone Joint Surg Am 1998;80(4): 492–501.

9. Patel VV, Heidenreich FP Jr, Bindra RR, et al. Morphologic changes in the ulnar nerve at the elbow with wrist flexion and extension: a magnetic resonance imaging study with 3-dimensional reconstruction. J Shoulder Elbow Surg 1998;7(4): 368–74.

10. Schuind FA, Goldschidt D, Bastin C, et al. A biomechanical study of the ulnar nerve at the elbow. J Sports Med 1977;5:182–5.

11. Posner MA. Compressive ulnar neurophathies at the elbow. I. Etiology and diagnosis. J Am Acad Orthop Surg 1998;6(5):282–8.

12. Polatsch D, Melone C, Beldner S, et al. Ulnar nerve anatomy. Hand Clin 2008;23:283–9.

13. Catalano L, Barron O. Anterior subcutaneous transposition of the ulnar nerve. Hand Clin 2008; 23:339–44.

14. Pfaeffle H, Waitayawinyu T, Trumble T. Ulnar nerve laceration and repair. Hand Clin 2007;23:291–9.

15. Tiong W, Kelly J. Ulnar nerve entrapment by anconeus epitrochlearis ligament. Hand Surg 2012; 17(1):83–4.

16. Miller T, Reinus W. Nerve entrapment syndromes of the elbow, forearm, and wrist. Am J Roentgenol 2010;195:585–94.

17. Amadio PC, Beckenbaugh RD. Entrapment of the ulnar nerve by the deep flexor-pronator aponeurosis. J Hand Surg Am 1986;11(1):83–7.

18. Sarris I, Gobel F, Gainer M, et al. Medial brachial and antebrachial cutaneous nerve injuries: effect on outcome in revision cubital tunnel surgery. J Reconstr Microsurg 2002;18(8):665–70.

19. Williams E, Dellon A. Anterior submuscular transposition. Hand Clin 2007;23:345–58.

20. Tsai T, Chen I, Majid ME, et al. Cubital tunnel release with endoscopic assistance: results of a new technique. J Hand Surg 1999;24:21–9.

21. Cutts S. Cubital tunnel syndrome. Postgrad Med J 2007;83(975):28–31.

22. Waugh R, Zlotolow D. In situ decompression of the ulnar nerve at the cubital tunnel. Hand Clin 2007; 23:319–27.

23. Mackinnon SE. Surgery of the peripheral nerve. New York: Thieme Medical Publishers; 1998.

24. Dellon AL. Clinical grading of peripheral nerve problems. Neurosurg Clin N Am 2001;12(2):229–40.

25. McGowen A. The results of transposition of the ulnar nerve for traumatic ulnar neuritis. J Bone Joint Surg Br 1950;32(3):293–301.

26. Dellon AL. Review of treatment results of ulnar nerve entrapment at the elbow. J Hand Surg 1989;14(4): 688–700.

27. Rayan GM, Jensen C, Duke J. Elbow flexion test in the normal population. J Hand Surg Am 1992; 17(1):86–9.

28. Buehler MJ, Thayer DT. The elbow flexion test. A clinical test for the cubital tunnel syndrome. Clin Orthop Relat Res 1998;233:213–6.

29. Novak CB, Lee GW, Mackinnon SE, et al. Provocative testing for cubital tunnel syndrome. J Hand Surg Am 1994;19(5):817–20.

30. Dimond M, Lister G. Cubital tunnel syndrome treated by long-term splintage. Proceedings of the 1985 American Society for Surgery of the Hand Annual Meeting. J Hand Surg Am 1985;10:430.

31. Wiesler ER, Chloros GD, Cartwright MS, et al. Ultrasound in the diagnosis of ulnar neuropathy at the cubital tunnel. J Hand Surg Am 2006;31(7):1088–93.

32. Seror P. Treatment of ulnar nerve palsy at the elbow with a night splint. J Bone Joint Surg Br 1993;75(2): 322–7.

33. Hong CZ, Long HA, Kanakamedal RV, et al. Splinting and local steroid injection for the treatment of ulnar neuropathy at the elbow: clinical and electrophysiological evaluation. Arch Phys Med Rehabil 1996;77(6):573–7.

34. McPherson SA, Meals RA. Cubital tunnel syndrome. Orthop Clin North Am 1992;23(1):111–23.

35. Lund AT, Amadio PC. Treatment of cubital tunnel syndrome: perspectives for the therapist. J Hand Ther 2006;19(2):170–8.

Hand Surgery Using Local Anesthesia

King H. Wong, MB BCh, FRCS[a],
Nasim S. Huq, MD, FRCSC, MSc, FACS, CAQHS, DABPS[b],*,
Aqib Nakhooda, MD[b]

KEYWORDS

- Dupuytren disease • Fractures • Dislocations • Flexor and extensor tendons • Arthrodesis
- Ganglions • Carpal tunnel release • Hand trauma

KEY POINTS

- Local anesthesia as a field block or regional nerve block is a simple and useful tool and an adjuvant in the management of hand surgery problems.
- Many patients can tolerate local anesthesia procedures in the hand with a tourniquet time of up to 30 minutes.
- A wide variety of hand surgery problems, both elective and traumatic, can be treated with local anesthesia without the need for any sedation and general anesthesia.

INTRODUCTION

Hand surgery is unique because it is a field whereby the OHIO principle can be easily applied: only handle it once. This is a simple principle that is applicable to many aspects of life, including hand surgery. A once-in-and-once-out approach is a simple way to treat most hand traumas in a weekly fracture clinic. It is easier for patients to be assessed and treated in one visit without undergoing the inconvenience of preoperative fasting, taking time from work, or rescheduling family commitments.

What proportion of our day is spent in bringing patients into procedure rooms, asking them when they last ate, whether they have allergies, and in moving to different rooms for terminal cleaning and changeover? Trainees and staff can help leverage our time. Perhaps we focus on how we can explain postoperative care, prescriptions, and follow-up visits during the course of operating under local anesthesia. The authors use 3 procedure rooms and a consultation room concurrently in a fully accredited private facility. This practice allows a surgeon to perform a high number of new consultations annually and operate on most of these individuals, often on the same day, which permits direct and internal marketing for a minimal external marketing budget. Most of the authors' overhead expenses are spent on staff salaries to help ensure high-quality patient-centered care. A comprehensive electronic medical record system helps in scheduling, tracking outcomes, managing specimens, dictating consultation and operative reports, submitting billings, and communicating to other health care providers.

The World is Flat: A Brief History of the 21st Century by Thomas Friedman (2007) explains how and why the world has changed in the last 2 decades. The Internet permits almost anyone to

The authors have nothing to disclose.
[a] Toronto, Ontario, Canada; [b] Niagara Plastic Surgery Centre, McMaster University, 5668 Main Street, Suite 1, Niagara Falls, Ontario L2G 5Z4, Canada
* Corresponding author.
E-mail address: Niagaraplasticsurgery@gmail.com

Clin Plastic Surg 40 (2013) 567–581
http://dx.doi.org/10.1016/j.cps.2013.08.004

research their diagnosis, treatment, and even their surgeon. Patients as consumers or customers are now more informed than ever before.

In a time of fiscal restraint in the health care profession, it behooves us all to provide timely and effective care in a cost-effective manner. Surgery of the hand under local anesthetics can not only avoid the adverse effects of general anesthesia and the hospital cost of both preoperative and postoperative care as well as the administration and paperwork but there is also great convenience for both the surgeon and patients. Many common hand surgical procedures can be performed under local anesthesia in a minor operative suite with minimal intervention and monitoring.

Simple, elective surgery is not likely to threaten a person's life, but it is the general anesthetic that poses the greater overall health risk. Readers are directed to the article by Chung and Harris elsewhere in this issue. The avoidance of general anesthesia when reasonably possible may be, at times, uncomfortable for patients; however, the relative trade for a lower health risk is worthwhile if the patients' health demands it. Present patients with all options.

LOCAL ANESTHETIC IN HAND SURGERY

The use of a local anesthetic in hand surgery has recently increased, as indicated by increasing published reports in the literature.[1–4] The advantages are its increased safety profile, ease of use, and effectiveness in providing painless anesthesia. Wide-awake surgery also allows surgeons to check their work, as in gapping in flexor tendon repairs.[1] In addition, a recent study shows that patients preferred local anesthetic to intravenous regional anesthesia in a randomized controlled trial for carpal tunnel release because of better intraoperative and postoperative pain control.[2]

An important consideration when using local anesthetic is hemostasis control. Although tourniquets can still be applied and used, local anesthetic with epinephrine has repeatedly been shown to be efficacious and safe.[5,6] A prospective multicenter study following 3110 patients showed no complications of epinephrine (1:100,000 concentration or less) when used in finger and hand surgery. If a tourniquet is preferred, a randomized controlled study of forearm versus upper arm tourniquet showed that the former is better tolerated even with a mean time of 25 minutes.[7] In addition, the use of topical or injectable anesthetic under the tourniquet can be used to reduce tourniquet-associated pain.[8]

DIGITAL BLOCKS

Numerous techniques have been described for digital block. These techniques include transthecal versus 2 dorsal or web space injections.

Chiu[9] originally described the transthecal technique in 1990. He injected 2 mL of lidocaine into the potential space of the flexor tendon sheath at the level of the palmar crease. Of the 420 patients, only 4 required supplemental local anesthetic infiltration; there were no observable complications. In 1991, Harbison[10] described a variation of this technique whereby lidocaine was injected into the subcutaneous tissues of the proximal flexion crease of the target finger. A randomized control study comparing these two techniques showed that injection into the subcutaneous tissues was easier to administer and better tolerated by patients.[11]

The 2-injection dorsal or web space injection was advocated to be less painful than the volar injections.[12] The local anesthetic is injected into the web space on either side of the finger to be anesthetized (**Fig. 1**). The question of whether it is less painful was recently contraindicated by a study showing that 27 volunteer patients preferred the single volar subcutaneous injection versus the 2-injection dorsal method.[13,14]

WRIST BLOCK

There are variations of how the median, ulna, and radial nerves contribute to sensory innervation of the hand. A comprehensive wrist block must

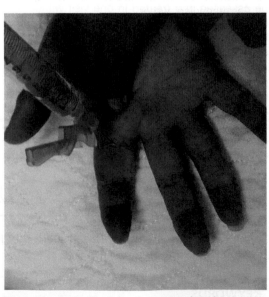

Fig. 1. The nerve block is administered to this patient.

anesthetize all 3, including their cutaneous branches.

A study of 825 patients by Klezl and colleagues[15] (2001) showed that partial wrist blocks led to more failures than complete wrist blocks, 18% in the former versus 2% in the latter. Knowing the anatomic landmarks of where these nerves are located is essential to providing a good block. In addition, a good technique includes aspirating before injecting, stopping if you feel resistance or patients complain of radiating pain, injecting the anesthetic slowly, and infiltrating the skin around the injection site (**Fig. 2**).

Blockade of the median nerve is done by the injection of local anesthetic between the palmaris longus (PL) and the flexor carpi radialis (FCR) or ulnar to the FCR if the PL is absent. The nerve is deep to the fascia. For the palmar cutaneous branch, this branches from the radial side of the median nerve at an average of 4.9 cm from the wrist flexion crease range, with a range of 4.1 to 7.8 cm.[16] In the same study, 3 variations of the palmar cutaneous branch of the ulna nerve were described in frequency: the classic palmar branch arising approximately 4.6 cm proximal to the pisiform (4 of 25 specimens), the nerve of Henle (14 of 25 specimens), and a transverse branch that originates distal to the proximal wrist flexion crease. A local anesthetic injection to block the ulnar nerve can be done by injecting deep and ulnar to the flexor carpi ulnaris (FCU) tendon. An additional injection to the subcutaneous tissue radial to the FCU should also be done to block the ulnar cutaneous branch to the palm. In a cadaveric study of 32 specimens, the dorsal branch of the ulnar nerve originated approximately 5.1 cm proximal to the ulnar styloid, crossing the subcutaneous border about 0.2 cm proximal to ulnar process.[17] Therefore, infiltration of the subcutaneous tissues just proximal to the ulnar styloid process should provide anesthesia to the dorsal ulna aspect of the hand. A field block is usually recommended for the superficial branch of the radial nerve because of its variation in anatomy and multiple divisions into smaller cutaneous branches.[18]

FIELD BLOCK

Infiltrative field block can be done using tumescent or a large amount of local anesthetic.[1] This technique helps to spread the local anesthetic to as much tissues as possible and should be done by using diluted local anesthetic. Lalonde[1] (2009) advises starting from proximal to distal, infiltrating the subcutaneous tissues and recommends waiting at least 15 minutes so the epinephrine can have its maximum effect.

The senior author routinely performs approximately 1000 local anesthetic blocks per year, with a combination of 9 mL of 1% lidocaine with epinephrine followed by 0.25% bupivacaine with epinephrine about 2 minutes later. Surgery is started within minutes after the second block, and it is very rare to have any difficulty with this method because the second injection is testing the field treated by the first block.

FRACTURES
Overview

The total annual incidence of hand fractures has been estimated to be about 36 per 10,000 per year.[3] In the same study, metacarpals were the most affected, and there was an 8% incidence of multiple fractures in the hand. Operative management for unstable patterns may be necessary to obtain and maintain an acceptable reduction. A variety of anesthetic options are available, including local anesthesia. Most closed hand fractures can be very successfully treated without the need for open reduction.[4] In the authors' institute, they open less than 1% of all closed hand fractures.

Operative Technique

Local anesthesia can be sufficient to perform operative management of most metacarpal or phalangeal fractures. Adequate anesthesia is crucial to obtain the reduction because relaxation of deforming muscle forces is necessary. For middle and distal phalanx fractures, a digital block with epinephrine or digital tourniquet can be

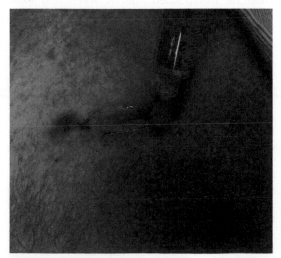

Fig. 2. There is greater ease for the surgeon sometimes to bend the injection needle.

performed. For proximal phalanx and metacarpal fractures, a wrist or elbow block can be performed. Supplemental infiltrative local anesthetic and/or sedation can also be used to ensure adequate anesthesia.

Obtaining anatomic reduction can be obtained by several methods. Closed reduction maneuvers can be performed to reduce shaft or neck fractures. Other adjuncts to obtaining reduction include the manipulation of the fragments using reduction clamps, or Kirschner (K) wires as joysticks.

Metacarpal Fractures

Certain indications for fixation of metacarpal fractures include intraarticular incongruity of more than 1 mm, shortening of more than 3 mm because this can create an extensor lag, scissoring as shown on clinical examination indicating malrotation, any subluxation at the carpal metacarpal (CMC) joint, and an unacceptable angulation of the fracture. For metacarpal neck and shaft fractures, the intrinsic muscles cause an apex dorsal angulation. The Jahss reduction maneuver was first described in 1938[19] and involves flexion of the metacarpophalangeal joint (MCPJ) and proximal interphalangeal joint (PIPJ) while a dorsally directed force is applied to reduce the metacarpal neck fracture.[20] Traction with a dorsal-to-volar directed force can also be used to correct CMC dislocations and shaft fractures. Often, the manipulation of intraarticular fractures can be successfully done with a K-wire joystick to help anatomically reduce the fragment under fluoroscopic guidance. Metacarpal head fractures can be fixed with K-wire or screw fixation. A variety of options exists for neck and shaft fractures. Closed reduction with the Jahss maneuver allows the reduction and correction of rotational deformity while percutaneous pinning can be accomplished. K-wire fixation to the adjacent metacarpals requires at least one, preferably 2, pins in each of the fragments. Cross K-wire fixation can also be done, ensuring that the pins do not cross at the fracture site in order to avoid rotational instability. Intramedullary (IM) nailing with IM rods or multiple K wires can be accomplished with minimal soft tissue damage. However, intramedullary K-wire fixation has described complications, including pin tract infections, extensor tendon ruptures, shortening, and malrotation.[21] CMC dislocations or subluxations may require transarticular pinning to maintain the reduction. Open reduction internal fixation (ORIF) can be done with plate and screws or with 2 screws alone in oblique fractures whereby the length is twice the diameter of the metacarpal shaft. Fixation with plates and screws offers the most rigid construct.[22] A recent study favored bicortical screw fixation showing that they were significantly stronger than unicortical screws in a cyclical loading biomechanical study.[23]

Fractures at the thumb metacarpal and small metacarpal base have distinct patterns. Bennett fractures are simple intraarticular fractures whereby the volar ulnar corner fragment is held in the joint via the anterior oblique ligament while the rest of the metacarpal fragment is pulled proximally and dorsal via the abductor pollicis longus and adducts because of the adductor pollicis muscle. A closed reduction maneuver involves traction, abduction, and pronation with a simultaneous volar-directed force on the fragment. The fragments are then held with K-wire fixation inserted in a percutaneous manner. The K wires can be transfixed into the second metacarpal and/or in a transarticular manner into the trapezium. Alternatively, ORIF can also be performed. Reverse Bennett fractures are also prone to subluxation because of the deforming force of the extensor carpi ulnaris. Closed reduction is, thus, achieved by traction, ulnar deviation, and radially directed pressure on the subluxed metacarpal fragment.

Proximal and Middle Phalanx

Proximal and middle phalangeal fractures can be classified according to their anatomic location: condylar (unilateral or bilateral), neck, shaft, or base fractures. Displaced condylar fractures can often be manipulated with K wires and fixed with the K wires or with percutaneous screws. Should the condylar fracture be very comminuted, one can contemplate arthrodesis of the joint. Shaft and neck fractures can be described according to the fracture pattern: transverse, oblique, spiral, or comminuted. Similar to the metacarpal fractures, indications to operate include marked angulation or displacement at the fractures site, any clinical malrotation, articular incongruity, and marked comminution leading to shortening. A variety of treatment options are available and include closed reduction and percutaneous pinning (CRPP), intramedullary nailing devices, ORIF with screw or plates, and external fixator devices.

Fractures of the base can be volar, dorsal, or involve the entire articular surface (pilon fractures). Dorsal base fractures of the middle phalanx compromise the integrity of the central slip and can lead to instability. Operative fixation can be accomplished through screws, hook plate devices, K wires, and intraosseous (IO) suture fixation.[20] Supplemental transarticular pinning is also usually performed to help maintain joint reduction. Because of the more distal flexor digitorum superficialis (FDS) insertion on the middle phalanx, volar base fractures can lead to dislocation because of the loss of the bony buttress and dissociation of the dorsal fragment from the volar plate/collateral complex. Operative fixation options include dorsal blocking pin, transarticular pinning, volar plate arthroplasty, hemihamatearthroplasty, articulated external fixator devices, CRPP, or ORIF.

Intraarticular PIPJ fractures can be a very challenging aspect of hand surgery. Although many of the aforementioned techniques have been used, closed reduction and dynamic traction have recently been described with comparable outcomes (**Fig. 3**).[1,2,9,24] Final active and passive range of motion was similar to other studies, and there is no need for an operating room or even a K-wire insertion and subsequent removal (**Fig. 4**).

Distal Phalanx Fractures

Distal phalanx fractures can be classified according to their anatomic location, such as tuft, shaft,

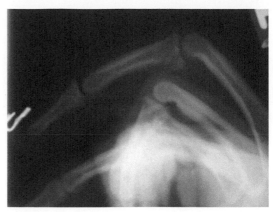

Fig. 4. The same patient after 1 week of elastic traction.

or intraarticular, and whether they are simple or comminuted.

Tuft fractures may or may not result in nail bed injuries. Treatment of nail bed injuries usually involves removing the nail and suturing any nail bed laceration with fine absorbable sutures under loupe magnification and administration of antibiotics and tetanus immunization, if necessary. One can also drill a hole into the nail plate to decompress the hematoma. One study of open distal phalanx fractures managed operatively with and without antibiotics showed an infection rate of 3% and 30%, respectively.[25] These injuries can be splinted up to, but not including, the PIPJ to avoid stiffness at that joint for 2 to 3 weeks. The authors have very rarely ever taken these injuries to a main operating room, and their infection rate is well less than 2% without the use of antibiotics in most cases.

Shaft fractures can be classified according to the fracture pattern: longitudinal, transverse, or comminuted. If the fracture pattern is stable and undisplaced, a mallet type of splint can be used. For unstable fractures, antegrade cross K-wire pinning, retrograde transarticular pinning through the distal interphalangeal joint (DIPJ), or screw fixation can all be considered (**Figs. 5–8**).

Intraarticular avulsions are caused by the extensor terminal tendon or the flexor digitorum profundus. Acutely, these can be fixed with either internal fixation or pullout wires. Usually, the authors use transarticular pinning for additional protection. Small avulsions on the extensor side can be treated nonoperatively with a mallet splint. Arthrodesis of severely comminuted fractures or those diagnosed very late can be considered as an alternate treatment.

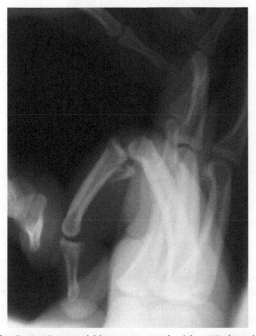

Fig. 3. A 16-year-old boy presented with a 17-day-old fracture/dislocation of the long finger PIPJ. It was not reducible with closed techniques, and the finger was placed into traction for 1 week.

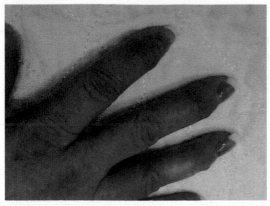

Fig. 5. This patient requests fusion of the right index finger DIPJ.

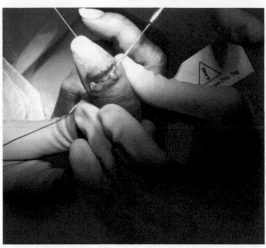

Fig. 6. The intraosseous wire is inserted with a threading technique of an 18-gauge needle and a K-wire driver.

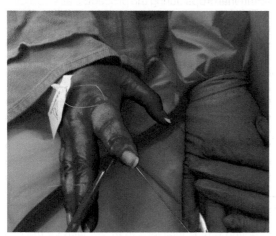

Fig. 7. The intraosseous (IO) wire is tightened with the distal K wire ready for retrograde insertion.

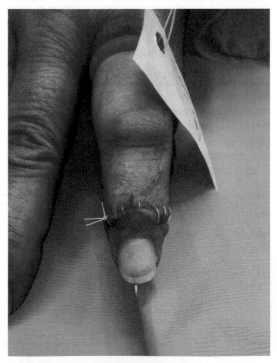

Fig. 8. The same patient postoperatively.

Complications

There are many possible unique complications in the treatment of fractures in the hand. In addition to the usual complications of delayed unions, non-unions, malunions, infections, and nerve damage, one must also be vigilant that the hand is particularly prone to stiffness secondary to tendon adhesions. Because of the close proximity to tendons, hardware irritation and tendon ruptures may occur. Adequate fixation should be achieved to allow early range of motion to help prevent tendon adhesions. The use of lower profile plate and screws, allows a greater respect for soft tissues can also help to minimize complications and achieve the best outcome (**Fig. 9**).

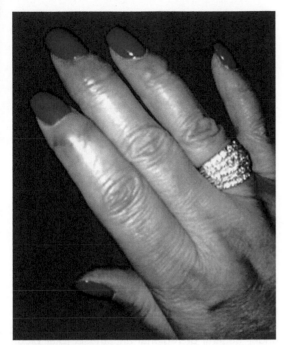

Fig. 9. The patient returned to the clinic after infusion 24 weeks after surgery.

DUPUYTREN CONTRACTURE
Synopsis

Local anesthetic can be used for both percutaneous fasciotomy and open partial fasciectomy. Numerous studies demonstrate the safety of these techniques as well as the lower complication rate.[26–31]

Operative Technique

For percutaneous needle fasciotomies, multiple anesthesia techniques have been described. Eaton[29] (2011) described "pinpoint" surface anesthesia by injecting into each portal at the depth of the subcutaneous tissues. Foucher and colleagues[27] (2003) used local or regional anesthetic with a forearm tourniquet.

In his review article, Eaton[29] (2011) states that his indications for needle aponeurectomy are cooperative patients with a palpable cord and adequate skin. Technical recommendations for needle placements to minimize skin tears and damage to flexor tendons include placement directly over diseased cords over unblanched skin, portal placements at least 5 mm apart, and going on the convex side of flexion creases.[29]

Adjuncts to improve the safety of the procedure include needle placement with the use of Doppler to avoid the digital vessel especially when transecting spiral cords; repeated fingertip sensory examination (with pinpoint anesthesia); and active flexion/extension of the finger to check the placement of the needle and to keep the finger extended, thereby making the cords more prominent.[27,29] The sectioning is done in a distal-to-proximal direction because going the opposite direction may reduce the prominence of the digital cords (**Fig. 10**).[27,29] The recommended sizes of needle gauge vary from 19 to 25 mm.[27,29] The following technique, is described by Eaton[29] (2011), includes

1. Clearing: The needle is inserted first with the bevel parallel to the cord to make a plane between the dermis and cord.
2. Perforating: The needle is turned so the bevel is perpendicular to the cord. The width of the cord is estimated by a perforating motion.
3. Sweeping: Once the edges of the cord have been estimated, the cord is then cut with the needle in a sweeping fashion. This action translates into a crunching feeling.

Foucher and colleagues[27] (2003) recommended a pie-crusting technique for finger cords, whereas a complete sectioning was done for palmar cords. They averaged 2 levels each of sectioning for both the finger and the palm. After needle aponeurectomy, passive extension of the fingers with the wrist flexed is performed to straighten the fingers,[29] which may require additional intraarticular anesthetic or a wrist block.

Limited or partial fasciectomies have also been performed under local anesthetic with or without a tourniquet.[30,31] In Denkler's[30] (2005) series of 40 patients undergoing a fasciectomy with local anesthetic, a mixture of 3 mL of 1% lidocaine with 1:100,000 epinephrine, 3 mL of 1% lidocaine plain, and another 3 mL of bupivacaine

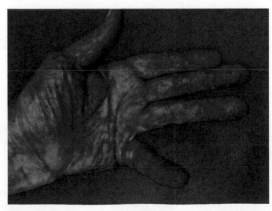

Fig. 10. Patient in for preoperative of Dupuytren contracture.

hydrochloride (Marcaine) 0.5% was used.[30] When the amounts were recorded, an average of 8.7 mL was used per finger and palm to perform both a finger block and local infiltration directly under a Bruner type of incision. Another published technique is wrist blocks to the median and/or ulna nerves with a mixture of 1% lidocaine and 0.5% bupivacaine, dependent on the affected digits with an upper arm tourniquet.[31] Additional local anesthetic was injected to the incision sites, and the total amount used in the study was routinely approximately 10 mL.[31] A tourniquet in the upper arm was also used, with an average time of 25 minutes (range 10–40 minutes). They also preferred a longitudinal incision with Z-plasties performed at the creases and full-thickness grafting from the wrist as necessary (**Fig. 11**). Another series used infiltrative local anesthetic of 1% lidocaine and 1:100,000 epinephrine with no tourniquet or sedation.[32]

The senior author has performed more than 1000 open fasciectomies, serially, entirely under local anesthesia (**Fig. 12**). There has been a reported ulnar digital nerve injury. The overall complication rate, including flap necrosis, wound infection, and hematoma, is less than 3%.

Outcomes

In Foucher and colleagues'[27] (2003) series of patients who underwent percutaneous fasciotomies, extension improved on average 38° for the MCPJ and 24° for the PIPJ at the short-term follow-up. One complete nerve injury, 3 cases of hemi digital paresthesia, one preoperative failure, and 19 skin incisions were among the list of complications.

For Denkler's[30] (2005) series of 60 digits undergoing open fasciectomies under local anesthetic,

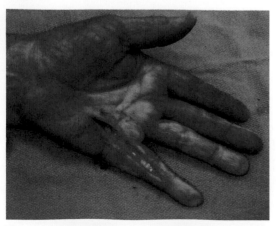

Fig. 11. Same patient after release of Dupuytren contracture.

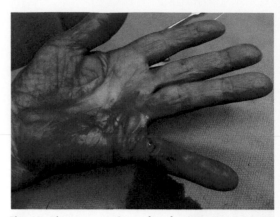

Fig. 12. The same patient after fasciectomy.

the average time for follow-up was 9.3 months. The MCPJ and PIPJ extension improved on average 29.8° and 25.3°, respectively. These results are comparable with the 42 digits operated on under general or regional anesthesia (Bier block or axillary), whereby the MCPJ and PIPJ extension improved at an average of 30.2° and 22.5°, respectively. Complications were similar with 2 nerve injuries in the local anesthetic group versus one in the other group. Both groups had one artery damage and an infection rate of 8.5% (local anesthetic group) or 11.5% (general/regional/Bier block group).

In a prospective trial, Tate and colleagues[32] (2011) reported their mean improvement in total passive extension deficit was 70° at 2 months in 230 patients. Complications included nerve injury (4%), delayed wound healing (2%), and one patient had partial necrosis of their skin graft. Satisfaction rates averaged 7 on a scale of 1 to 10. Complaints included local anesthetic injection (9%), 2 complaints of tourniquet discomfort, and 3 patients (2%) indicated they would prefer a general anesthetic for future surgeries.

Another case control series of local anesthetic versus general anesthetic showed no significant difference in extension improvement for any digit or joint or total active movement.[9] Complications and the length of postoperative therapy were also similar between the two groups.

Using local anesthetic as the choice of anesthetic in the treatment of Dupuytren disease is both efficacious and safe.[1,2,5–9] Two case control series have shown similar improvement in finger posture and complication rates. They also highlight some of the advantages, including cost benefits and eliminating the use and risks of tourniquets and general anesthetic.

EXTENSOR TENDON INJURIES
Overview

The extensor mechanism of the hand receives contributions from both intrinsic and extrinsic systems. Proper examination is essential to identify extensor tendon injuries. Extension of the individual joints of each digit should be documented, in addition to strength testing. Clinical examinations, like the Elson test for acute central slip injuries and isolating the MCPJ extension via interphalangeal joint (IPJ) flexion, help to focus the clinician to the nature of the injury. Additional vigilance is often required because of the high rate of associated injuries that have been reported with extensor tendon injuries; one study reported it to be as high as 46.7%.[33] Extensor tendon disruptions can also commonly occur in closed injuries (**Fig. 13**).

Surgical Technique

Infiltration of local anesthetic into the zone of injury, with or without digital blocks and/or wrist blocks, to the dorsal ulna branch and superficial radial nerve can give adequate anesthesia. The advantages of epinephrine to the site of injury will help hemostasis, making the identification of key structures and their treatment easier.

As previously mentioned, associated injuries are common; one should be prepared to do additional procedures, such as irrigation and debridement, bony stabilization, and repair of other soft tissue, such as sagittal bands.

For injuries in zones 1 through 3, a digital block can easily be used. Epinephrine is preferred to a digital tourniquet, which may limit the excursion of any tendon requiring repair. Open injuries can also be treated with a splint; however, if a repair is done, tenodermodesis is preferred in zone 1 and 2 because of the thin nature of the tendon at these locations (**Fig. 14**).[34] Supplemental K-wire fixation across the DIPJ may also be required (**Fig. 15**).

Zone 3 injuries can lead to acute boutonniere deformities. If there is enough tendon length distally, a suture repair can be done. This repair can be done with a 2-stitch core suture, with or without an epitendinous repair. When there is no distal stump remaining, reconstruction rather than repair may be necessary such as using the lateral bands as described by Aiche et al (1970) technique of using the lateral bands,[35] Snow's

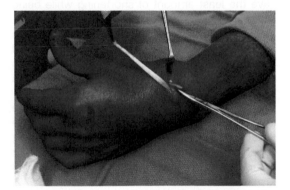
Fig. 14. The tendons are aligned with tension.

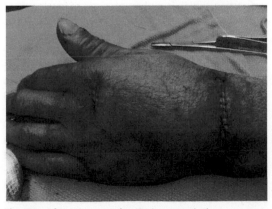
Fig. 15. After closure, the IPJ is extended.

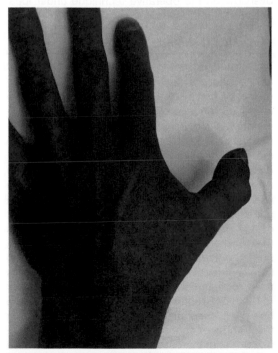
Fig. 13. This patient had an extensor pollicis longus rupture.

technique of using a tendon turndown,[36] or the use of a suture anchor or bony tunnels. Treatment options for bony avulsions include splinting if minimally displaced, excision of a fracture fragment if it is too small to fix, and reattachment of the tendon with suture anchors or fixation of the fracture fragment if it is large enough. Again, K-wire fixation across the joint can also be performed to protect the repair, after which it can be removed after approximately 6 weeks.

Injuries to zone 4 through 7 can be anesthetized via a wrist block and infiltrative local anesthetic to the site of the injury. Zone 4 injuries can usually accommodate a core suture repair technique, such as the modified Bunnell or Kessler stitch with a 4-0 nonabsorbable suture. The aforementioned techniques have been shown biomechanically to be the strongest while producing minimal shortening of the tendon.[37] Shortening the tendon can lead to reduced flexion at the PIPJ and MCPJ in zones 4 through 7.[37–39]

As the tendon girth increases, one can consider using 3-0 nonabsorbable sutures in zones 5 through 7. Again, Newport and Williams'[38] (1992) study showed the modified Bunnell technique to have the least amount of shortening while being in the strongest in terms of gap prevention.

Special considerations should include the exclusion of an intraarticular penetration caused by a bite in zone 5, sagittal band ruptures in zone 5, and ensuring smooth excursion of a repaired tendon under the extensor retinaculum in zone 7.

Repairs at zone 8 and 9 are difficult because they are through muscle tissue. It may be possible distally because the overlying fascia may be strong enough. Otherwise, consideration should be given to tendon transfers that may give better functional results if there is substantial muscle belly loss.

The key difference for thumb extensor injuries is that the extensor pollicis longus (EPL) is a more substantive tendon throughout its course and may accommodate a core suture repair distally (**Fig. 16**). K-wire fixation across the joint is usually not required.

Postoperative Course and Outcomes

Multiple postoperative regimens exist after extensor tendon repair, including static splinting, dynamic splinting, and early active motion protocols. A recent literature review by Hammond and colleagues[39] examined these differing protocols and their complication rates. A limitation highlighted by their study was the variability of outcome measures used by the various studies. A long-term study of extensor tendon results showed that poor prognostic factors were associated injuries

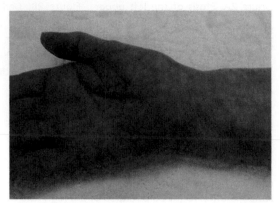

Fig. 16. This patient requested right carpal tunnel release with abductorplasty.

and an injury to more distal zones (1–4 as compared with 5–8).[40] They also showed that flexion loss was greater than extension loss.

FLEXOR TENDON REPAIR
Overview

The treatment of flexor tendon injuries has greatly improved over the last several decades. The idea that primary repair cannot be done in zone 2 led to the term *no man's land*. This thought has now been abandoned through an improved understanding of flexor tendon physiology and improved surgical techniques. This section includes a brief overview on the operative technique under local anesthetic and postoperative care.

Operative Technique

The stated advantages of awake tendon repair are to observe any gapping of the repair, triggering of the tendon within the pulleys, and an improved understanding of the repair to formulate an individualized postoperative therapy regimen.[1,41] The reported flexor tendon rupture rate was 3%, with all of them occurring in noncompliant patients. However, the low follow-up rate was a limitation in the study.[41] Lalonde (2009) describes his preferred method for local anesthetic delivery whereby a tumescent amount of 1% lidocaine with 1:100,000 epinephrine is used if the amount required is less than 50 mL. For quantities of 100 to 200 mL, a solution of 0.25% lidocaine and 1:400,000 epinephrine is used for injection.

The type of suture and the suture technique have been well researched. Biomechanically, increasing the number of core sutures helps to resist gap formation and increase the ultimate force of the repair.[42] Suture caliber of at least 4-0 has also been recommended by several studies.[43,44] Newer suture material, such as FibreWire (Arthrex, Naples, Florida USA), a braided polyblend polyethylene suture, has been shown in experimental studies to have a higher ultimate force and stiffness.[43,45]

After allowing a minimum of 10 to 15 minutes after the local anesthetic injection, a Bruner type of incision is made in the fingers while the use of palmar creases helps to guide the incision in zone 3 injuries (**Fig. 17**). The tendon ends are retrieved and freshened up and approximated by the use of 25-gauge needles (**Figs. 18** and **19**). The core sutures are then placed, approximating the tendon ends. The knots are buried within the tendon ends, a practice that has been shown in a canine model to have equal tensile strength to knot placement outside the tendon at 6 weeks.[46] Finally, the epitendinous stitch is placed as the final step of the repair. Wade and colleagues[47] showed the epitendinous repair helped to resist gap formation while increasing the strength of the repair. The most common epitendinous technique is a simple running stitch, which can be further strengthened by deeper placement of the suture,[48] increasing the number of passes,[49] or implantation of a locking technique.[50]

Postoperatively, all fingers and wrist are placed in a dorsal extension-blocking splint with the fingers and wrist flexed. Several investigators have advocated for an early motion protocol,[51] but there are insufficient data to show superiority

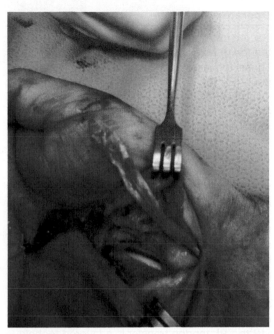

Fig. 18. The palmar fascia is isolated. Note the severe deformity of the medial nerve.

of one postoperative rehabilitation protocol to another.[52–54]

TENDON TRANSFER
Overview

Tendon transfers allow the restoration of useful function in otherwise nonfunctioning or paralyzed parts of the limb. Important consideration must be given not only to technical details but also to patient factors. One of the most important intraoperative technical factors is optimal tensioning of the transferred tendon.

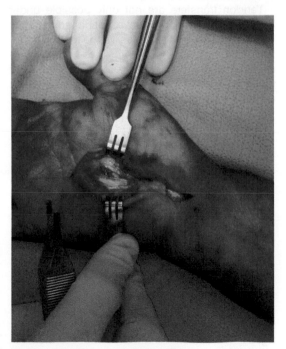

Fig. 17. The palmaris fascia is isolated.

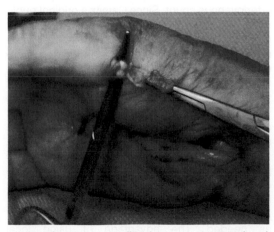

Fig. 19. The abductor pollicis brevis tendon is isolated.

Operative Technique

Recent case series have described techniques for tendon transfer surgery under local anesthetic.[55,56] These techniques included extensor indicis proprius (EIP) to EPL transfers and opponensplasty using FDS of the ring finger. The stated technical advantage was observation of the tendon transfer in action, helping to define the location of the optimal anchor point and tension. The wide-awake approach also demonstrates how quickly patients are able to use the transfer. No tourniquet was necessary in either study, further aiding in judging the tendon excursion.

EPL ruptures can occur after blunt and open trauma, distal radius fractures, and synovitis; but spontaneous cases have been reported in the literature, with mechanical and vascular theories proposed as the pathophysiology.[24,57,58] A recent study showed an EPL rupture incidence rate of 5% after nondisplaced distal radius fractures, occurring an average of 6.6 weeks after the injury. EIP to EPL tendon transfer is a favored technique with a good success rate and minimal complications.[59] In their case series of EIP to EPL transfers, Bezuhly and colleagues[55] (2007) described a field block with 1% lidocaine and 1:200,000 epinephrine. This area encompassed all potential incisions, and they advised to wait at least 30 minutes in order for the epinephrine to work.

The first described tendon transfer for severe thenar atrophy associated with long-standing carpal tunnel was in 1929 by Camitz.[60] In the authors' literature search, one of the first studies to use local anesthetic in tendon transfers was published by Terrono and colleagues[61] in 1993. This cases series included 29 patient with 33 hands who underwent the Camitz palmaris longus abductorplasty, of which a significant but unspecified number of patients had it done under local anesthetic because of the presence of an ipsilateral arteriovenous shunt. Since Camitz's original publication, many types of opponensplasties and/or modifications to Camitz's original described technique have been published.[62-68] In their case series of 9 opponensplasties under local anesthetic, Okutsu and colleagues[56] (2011) used a mixture of 1.0% to 1.5% lidocaine and 1:100,000 epinephrine with infiltration to the thumb and proximal phalanx of the ring finger in combination with a median nerve block.

In both of the aforementioned case series, the patients actively ranged the tendon transfer intraoperatively in order to help judge what the tension should be set at. The surgeons were also able to judge the alignment of the insertion and adjust it as needed. The advantage of using local anesthetic with epinephrine was that there were no tourniquets used; therefore, tendon excursion was not affected.[56,61]

The senior author of this article has done a series of patients who had Camitz abductorplasty (see **Fig. 16**) or EIP to EPL transfers done under local anesthetic. For the abductorplasty, infiltration of local anesthetic is done at the median nerve and its palmar cutaneous branch and the dorsal and radial aspect of the thumb and wrist and around the PL near its insertion into the palmar fascia. If done concomitantly, an open carpal tunnel is performed, extending the incision into the distal forearm (see **Figs. 17** and **18**). The PL is freed up with a strip of palmar fascia of approximately 5 to 6 cm in length. A second incision on the radial side of the MCPJ of the thumb is made, and the PL is passed through a subcutaneous tunnel. The PL is then temporarily fixed to the abductor pollicis brevis (APB) tendon (see **Fig. 19**), and the patient is asked to palmar abduct the thumb. After optimizing the tension of the transfer, the PL is then weaved into the APB tendon in a Pulvertaft fashion and reinforced into the dorsoradial capsule (**Fig. 20**).

Postoperative Care and Outcomes

The hand is usually splinted for approximately 4 weeks postoperatively, after which patients are allowed to start range-of-motion exercises. Formal therapy, in addition, may not be necessary[61] because the function is quickly learned.[55,56]

Tendon transfers are not only possible under local anesthetic but also have distinct advantages because it allows one to observe the tendon transfer function. Whether this translates into any clinical advantage is difficult to ascertain because of the limited amount of patients and studies, but it remains a promising technique.

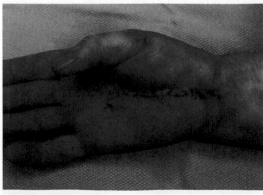

Fig. 20. The tendon is transferred with the thumb in good position, and the skin is closed.

REFERENCES

1. Lalonde DH. Wide-awake flexor tendon repair. Plast Reconstr Surg 2009;123(2):623–5.
2. Sorensen AM, Dalsgaard J, Hansen TB. Local anesthesia versus intravenous regional anesthesia in endoscopic carpal tunnel release: a randomized controlled trial. J Hand Surg Eur Vol 2013;38(5): 481–4.
3. Freeland AE. Closed reduction of hand fractures. Clin Plast Surg 2005;32(4):549–61.
4. Feehan LM, Sheps SB. Incidence and demographics of hand fractures in British Columbia, Canada: a population-based study. J Hand Surg Am 2006;31(7):1068–74.
5. Lalonde D, Bell M, Sparkes G, et al. A multicenter prospective study of 3,110 consecutive cases of elective epinephrine use in the fingers and hand: the Dalhousie Project clinical phase. J Hand Surg Am 2005;30A:1061–7.
6. Thomson CJ, Lalonde DH, Denkler KA, et al. A critical look at the evidence for and against elective epinephrine use in the finger. Plast Reconstr Surg 2007;119:260–6.
7. Maury AC, Roy WS. A prospective randomized controlled trial of forearm versus upper arm tourniquet tolerance. J Hand Surg Br 2002;27B(4): 359–60.
8. Inal S, Er M, Ozsoy M, et al. Comparison of two different anesthesia techniques for tourniquet pain with the use of forearm tourniquet. Iowa Orthop J 2009;29:55–9.
9. Chiu D. Transthecal digital block: flexor tendon sheath used for anesthetic infusion. J Hand Surg Am 1990;15A:471–3.
10. Harbison S. Transthecal digital block: flexor tendon sheath used for anesthetic infusion [letter]. J Hand Surg Am 1991;16:957.
11. Low CK, Vartany A, Engstrom JW, et al. Comparison of transthecal and subcutaneous single-injection digital block techniques. J Hand Surg Am 1997;22:901.
12. Braun H, Harris ML. Operations on the extremities. In: Braun H, Harris ML, editors. Local anesthesia: its scientific basis and practical use. 2nd edition. New York: Lea &Febiger; 1924. p. 366–7.
13. William JG, Lalonde DH. Randomized comparison of the single-injection volar subcutaneous block and the two-injection dorsal block for digital anesthesia. Plast Reconstr Surg 2006;118: 1195–200.
14. McCahon RA, Bedforth NM. Peripheral block at the elbow and wrist. Cont Educ Anaesth Crit Care Pain 2007;7(2):42–4.
15. Klezl Z, Krejca M, Simcik J. Role of sensory innervation variations for wrist block anaesthesia. Arch Med Res 2001;32:155–8.
16. Martin CH, Seiler JG 3rd, Lesesne JS. The cutaneous innervation of the palm: an anatomic study of the ulnar and median nerves. J Hand Surg Am 1996;21(4):634–8.
17. Puna R, Poon P. The anatomy of the dorsal cutaneous branch of the ulnar nerve. J Hand Surg Eur Vol 2010;35(7):583–5. http://dx.doi.org/10.1177/1753193410373186.
18. Goldstein B. Musculoskeletal upper limb pain. In: Loeser JD, editor. Bonica's management of pain. 3rd edition. Philadelphia: Lippincott-Raven; 2001. p. 1032.
19. Jahss S. Fractures of the metacarpals: a new method of reduction and immobilization. J Bone Joint Surg Am 1938;20A:178–86.
20. Siddiqui F, Huq N, Hossain S. Nail hooks and elastic bands external dynamic traction for fractures of the proximal interphalangeal joint. Tech Hand Up Extrem Surg 2012;16(3):148–52. http://dx.doi.org/10.1097/BTH.0b013e31825bd4da.
21. Manueddu CA, Della Santa D. Fasciculated intramedullary pinning of metacarpal fractures. J Hand Surg Br 1996;21B:230–6.
22. Massengill JB, Alexander H, Langrana N, et al. A phalangeal fracture model— quantitative analysis of rigidity and failure. J Hand Surg Am 1982;7: 264–70.
23. Afshar R, Fong TS, Latifi MH, et al. A biochemical study comparing plate fixation using uni-cortical and bi-cortical screws in transverse metacarpal fracture models subjected to cyclic loading. J Hand Surg Eur Vol 2012; 37(5):396–401. http://dx.doi.org/10.1177/1753193411424557.
24. Bjorkman A, Jorgsholm P. Rupture of the extensor pollicis longus tendon: a study of aetiological factors. Scand J Plast Reconstr Surg Hand Surg 2004;38:32–5.
25. Sloan JP, Dove AF, Maheson M, et al. Antibiotics in open fractures of the distal phalanx. J Hand Surg Br 1987;12(1):123–4.
26. Cheng HS, Hung LK, Tse WL, et al. Needle aponeurotomy for Dupuytren's contracture. J Orthop Surg 2008;16:88–90.
27. Foucher G, Medina J, Navarro R. Percutaneous needle aponeurotomy: complications and results. J Hand Surg Br 2003;28B:427–31.
28. Van Rijssen AL, Werker PM. Percutaneous needle fasciotomy in Dupuytren's disease. J Hand Surg Br 2006;31B:498–501.
29. Eaton C. Percutaneous fasciotomy for Dupuytren's contracture. J Hand Surg Am 2011;36(5): 910–5.
30. Denkler K. Dupuytren's fasciectomies in 60 consecutive digits using lidocaine with epinephrine and no tourniquet. Plast Reconstr Surg 2005; 115(3):802–10.

31. Tate R, Mackay D, Broome G. A prospective study of limited palmar and digital fasciectomy under local anaesthetic wrist block and upper arm tourniquet. J Hand Surg Am 2011;36(9):811–2.

32. Nelson R, Higgins A, Conrad J, et al. The wide awake approach to Dupuytren's disease: fasciectomy under local anesthetic with epinephrine. J Hand Surg Am 2010;5(2):117–24.

33. Patillo D, Rayan GM. Open extensor tendon injuries: an epidemiologic study. J Hand Surg Am 2012;17(1):37–42.

34. McFarlane RM, Hampole MK. Treatment of extensor tendon injuries of the hand. Can J Surg 1973;16:366–75.

35. Aiche A, Barsky AJ, Weiner DL. Prevention of boutonnière deformity. Plast Reconstr Surg 1970; 46:164–7.

36. Snow JW. Use of a retrograde tendon flap in repairing a severed extensor at the PIP joint area. Plast Reconstr Surg 1973;51:555–8.

37. Newport ML, Pollack GR. Biomechanical characteristics of suture techniques in extensor zone IV. J Hand Surg Am 1995;20:650–6.

38. Newport ML, Williams CD. Biomechanical characteristics of extensor tendon suture techniques. J Hand Surg Am 1992;17:1117–23.

39. Hammond K, Starr H, Katz D, et al. Effect of aftercare regimen with extensor tendon repair: a systematic review of the literature. J Orthop Surg 2012;21(4):246–52.

40. Newport ML, Blair WF, Steyers CM Jr. Long-term results of extensor tendon repair. J Hand Surg Am 1990;15(6):961–6.

41. Higgins A, Lalonde D, Bell M, et al. Avoiding flexor tendon repair rupture with intraoperative total active movement examination. Plast Reconstr Surg 2010;126(3):941–5.

42. Viinikainen A, göransson H, Huovinen K, et al. A comparative analysis of the biomechanical behavior of five flexor tendon core sutures. J Hand Surg Br 2004;29B:536–43.

43. Lawrence TM, Davis TR. A biomechanical analysis of suture materials and their influence on a four-strand flexor tendon repair. J Hand Surg Am 2005;30A:836–41.

44. Taras JS, Raphael JS, Marczyk SC, et al. Evaluation of suture caliber in flexor tendon repair. J Hand Surg Am 2001;26A:1100–4.

45. Miller B, Dodds SD, deMars A, et al. Flexor tendon repairs: the impact of fiberwire on grasping and locking core sutures. J Hand Surg Am 2007;32A: 591–6.

46. Pruitt DL, Aoki M, Manske PR. Effect of suture knot location on tensile strength after flexor tendon repair. J Hand Surg Am 1996;21A:969–73.

47. Wade PJ, Wetherell RG, Amis AA. Flexor tendon repair. Significant gain in strength from the Halsted peripheral suture technique. J Hand Surg Br 1989; 14B:232–5.

48. Diao E, Hariharan JS, Soejima O, et al. Effect of peripheral suture depth on strength of tendon repairs. J Hand Surg Am 1996;21A:234–9.

49. Kubota H, Aoki M, Pruitt DL, et al. Mechanical properties of various circumferential tendon suture techniques. J Hand Surg Br 1996;21B: 474–80.

50. Lin GT, An KN, Amadio PC, et al. Biomechanical studies of running suture for flexor tendon repair in dogs. J Hand Surg Am 1988;13A:553–8.

51. Thien TB, Becker JH, Theis JC. Rehabilitation after surgery for flexor tendon injuries in the hand. Cochrane Database Syst Rev 2004;(4):CD003979.

52. Strickland JW, Cannon NM. Flexor tendon repair – Indiana method. Indiana Hand Center Newsletter 1993;1–19.

53. Silfverskiöld KL, May EJ. Flexor tendon repair in zone II with a new suture technique and an early mobilization program combining passive and active flexion. J Hand Surg Am 1993;19: 53–60.

54. Osada D, Fujita S, Tamai K, et al. Flexor tendon in zone II with 6 strand technique and early active mobilization. J Hand Surg Am 2006; 31(6):987–92.

55. Bezuhly M, Sparkes GL, Higgins AH, et al. Immediate thumb extension following extensor indicis proprius-to-extensor pollicis longus tendon transfer using the wide-awake approach. Plast Reconstr Surg 2007;119:1507–12.

56. Okutsu I, Hamanaka I, Yoshida A. Opponoplasty without postoperative immobilization. Hand Surg 2011;16(3):295–300.

57. Choi JC, Kim WS, Na HY, et al. Spontaneous rupture of the extensor pollicis longus tendon in a tailor. Clin Orthop Surg 2011;3:167–9.

58. Roth KM, Blazar PE, Earp BE, et al. Incidence of extensor pollicis longus tendon rupture after nondisplaced distal radius fracture. J Hand Surg Am 2012;37(5):942–7.

59. Gelb RI. Tendon transfer for rupture of the extensor pollicis longus. Hand Clin 1995;11(3): 411–22.

60. Camitz H. Uber die Behandlung der Oppositionslahmung. Acta Chir Scand 1929;65:77–81.

61. Terrono AL, Rose JH, Mulroy J, et al. Camitz palmaris longus abductorplasty for severe thenar atrophy secondary to carpal tunnel syndrome. J Hand Surg Am 1993;18A:204–6.

62. Bunnell S. Opposition of the thumb. J Bone Joint Surg Am 1938;20:269–84.

63. Curtis RM. Opposition of the thumb. Orthop Clin North Am 1974;5(2):305–21.

64. Riordan DC. Tendon transfers in hand surgery. J Hand Surg Am 1983;8(5 Pt 2):748–53.

65. Thompson TC. A modified operation for opponens paralysis. J Bone Joint Surg 1942;24:632–40.
66. Littler JW, Li CS. Primary restoration of thumb opposition with median nerve decompression. Plast Reconstr Surg 1967;39:74–5.
67. Royle ND. An operation for paralysis of the intrinsic muscles of the thumb. JAMA 1938;111:612–3.
68. Naeem R, Lahiri A. Modified Camitz opponensplasty for severe thenar wasting secondary to carpal tunnel syndrome: case series. J Hand Surg Am 2013;38(4):795–8.

Breast Surgery Under Local Anesthesia
Second-stage Implant Exchange, Nipple Flap Reconstruction, and Breast Augmentation

Dimitri J. Koumanis, MD, FACS[a],*, Alex Colque, MD[b],
Michael L. Eisemann, MD[c], Jenna Smith[d]

KEYWORDS

- Breast reconstruction • Local anesthesia • Nipple • Areola • Nipple-areola complex (NAC)
- Star flap • Implant exchange • Silicon breast implant

KEY POINTS

- Local anesthetic as an alternative to general or monitored anesthesia care (MAC) has been used for the past 30 years.
- Several health risks associated with general anesthesia/MACs are not present with local sedation, providing a safer option for the patient as well as the surgeon.
- When attempting to perform surgery under local anesthesia, consider the patient's desires and tolerance to being awake for the procedure. If anxiety is associated with the procedure or the needle, intravenous sedation is added to the anesthetic plan. A neurologic assessment of the breast mound area is performed, evaluating for light touch and pressure as well as pain.
- The star flap and the tattoo method for nipple-areola complex reconstruction, in conjunction with the Keller Funnel sizer to tissue expander exchange to silicon implant performed under local anesthesia, allow a single-site wound and minimal stress, time, and financial burden to the patient, but provide optimal aesthetic results and psychological benefits.

INTRODUCTION

As of 2011, more than 93,000 patients were undergoing breast reconstruction. Of those 93,000 patients, two-thirds of the procedures were implant based.[1] More than 60,000 of these patients were postmastectomy breast reconstructions.[2]

Implant-based reconstruction is more frequently performed in 2 stages, with the first tissue expander stage performed immediately after the mastectomies. Results for implant reconstruction have become reliable and have even improved in the setting of radiation therapy in certain instances.[3] Although performing the first stage of reconstruction usually requires general anesthesia, the

second stage seems more amenable to performing the procedure under local anesthetic, which can be performed with small incisions with the techniques to be described in this article. Breast augmentation, which is more involved compared with second-stage breast implant reconstruction, has been shown to be performed successfully under local anesthetic.[4]

Reconstruction of the nipple-areola complex (NAC) is most frequently associated with breast cancer and, consequently, mastectomies, and it is also indicated in burn or trauma deformities, complications of reduction mammaplasties, and congenital or developmental disorders.[5] Increase in case

[a] Capital Area Plastic Surgery of New York, 377 Church Street, Saratoga Springs, NY 12866, USA; [b] Private Practice, 21675 E. Moreland Boulevard, Waukesha, WI 53186, USA; [c] Private Practice, 6550 Fannin Street, Suite 2119, Houston, TX 77030, USA; [d] Private Practice, Glens Falls Hospital, 100 Park Street, Glens Falls, NY 12801, USA
* Corresponding author.
E-mail address: jkoumanis@yahoo.com

Clin Plastic Surg 40 (2013) 583–591
http://dx.doi.org/10.1016/j.cps.2013.08.001
0094-1298/13/$ – see front matter © 2013 Elsevier Inc. All rights reserved.

numbers over the years has led to many techniques being developed and revised to accommodate the aesthetic objectives of a nipple-areolar reconstruction. The unique texture and color of the NAC makes developing an alternative challenging. Since first being documented by Adams[6] in 1949, the reconstruction of the areola has historically been accomplished via the nonoperative side sharing techniques, grafting from other sites, NAC saving or banking, dermabrasion, and tattooing. Some of these have been used in conjunction with ultraviolet light to facilitate better pigmentation. Reconstruction of the nipple has been achieved through grafting, centrally based flaps, subdermal pedicle flaps, internal nipple prostheses, or autogenous implants.[5] Although skin grafting in conjunction with areolar tattooing can provide an aesthetically pleasing result, it requires a skin graft to be harvested, which in turn produces an additional donor site wound. As an alternative, star flaps in combination with tattooing can provide an equally aesthetically pleasing result without the need for an added site wound.

Local anesthetic as an alternative to general or monitored anesthesia care (MAC) has been used for the past 30 years[4] and provides many benefits to the patient. Several of the health risks associated with general anesthesia/MACs are not present with local anesthetic, providing a safer option for the patient as well as the surgeon. In addition, as an outpatient procedure with no sedation, patients can go home immediately following the procedure, as opposed to general anesthesia/MACs with which the patients must recover from the anesthetic gasses in the postanesthesia care unit (PACU). Furthermore, patients are not required to abstain from the consumption of food or beverages after midnight on the night before their procedure, which alleviates the need for an additional change in the patient's routine. Patients benefit financially from the procedure being performed under local anesthesia as well. The costs to the patient are significantly less because an anesthesiologist is not necessary for the procedure; recovery in the PACU after stage 1, 2, or both is not necessary; and the only anesthetic is a local medication.

In breast reconstruction, it is therefore feasible to perform tissue expander exchange to permanent breast implant and third stage nipple flap reconstruction under local anesthesia with successful and reliable results. In our practice this is the usual method.

TREATMENT GOALS AND PLANNED OUTCOMES

Treatment goals for restoring the NAC and exchanging sizers for silicon implants are commonly the same regardless of the surgeon's technique. Position, size, shape, texture, pigmentation, permanent projection, scar position, and symmetry are essential components for aesthetically pleasing results. The end result must be created in a way that allows patients to readily incorporate the change into their healthy body images. This concentration on the optimization of psychological benefits has been shown to have a positive influence on the overall recovery course of women undergoing postmastectomy breast reconstruction.[7]

TISSUE EXPANDER EXCHANGE TO PERMANENT BREAST IMPLANT
Preoperative Planning

The patient is marked in the preoperative holding area with a surgical marker. We use an existing scar to make the incision and generally excise the scar with 1-mm margins in order to provide clean tissue for the subsequent closure. Patients are given 1 dose of prophylactic antibiotics covering gram positives, unless the patient has had a previous infection, in which case we refer to previous cultures to guide our choice of antibiotics. A recent analysis study that searched the literature for antibiotic regimens using 1 dose preoperatively, at 24 hours, and greater than 24 hours showed no significant difference between 24 hours and greater than 24 hours of antibiotic use after surgery. One dose was associated with higher infection rates.[1] However, the literature lacks any randomized trials to answer this question and most plastic surgeons continue to justify their antibiotic protocols based on their training and experience.

Patient Positioning and Procedure

Patients are placed on the operating room table in the supine position with their arms extended out on arm extensions and wrapped with gauze wraps to facilitate sitting the patient up during the procedure to look for symmetry. A chlorhexidine skin preparation is used and, if the procedure requires only a small incision and a simple exchange from a tissue expander to a permanent implants, a small amount of 1% lidocaine with 1:100,000 epinephrine mixture is injected into the incision line and deeper as the surgeon dissects down toward the muscle and capsule/acellular dermal junction. If concomitant revisions of the breast flaps are needed, intravenous sedation and intercostal blocks can be injected, as described by in a recent study.[4] The blocks are injected into the intercostal spaces 3 to 7 with a 1% lidocaine and 0.25% bupivacaine with 1:100,000 equal parts mixture. This mixture is injected at the midaxillary line and the lateral border of the sternum if needed. Because of the added toxicity of both mixtures, we calculate the dose at 4 mg/kg, erring on the lower end for safe dosing.

The breast pocket is entered at this junction, which can typically be identified preoperatively by palpation with the patient flexing the pectoralis muscle. The tissue expander is deflated with a #15 blade over suction tubing and removed from the pocket. A minimal incision is used in order for the silicone gel implant to be inserted into the breast pocket. The size of the silicone gel implant is ascertained with silicone gel sizers. In our practice, we have been using the Keller Funnel to introduce the implant into the breast pocket. This funnel allows us to use a smaller incision per implant size. The funnel has standardized markings that represent a specific diameter opening of the funnel (**Fig. 1**). The funnel end is cut according to the implant size that the surgeon is planning to insert into the breast pocket. Along with changing gloves when handling the implant, and triple antibiotic wash of pocket, implants, and the funnel, a reduction in bacteria load and capsular contracture rates has been reported.[8,9] The incision is closed using a multilayer closure, and Steri-Strips and sterile gauze dressings are then applied.

NIPPLE-AREOLA RECONSTRUCTION
Preoperative Planning and Preparation

Several techniques have been described in nipple reconstruction, including nipple sharing techniques, local flaps, and grafts.[10–13]

In our practice, we almost always use the modified star flap as described by several investigators.[14,15] It has offered consistent results and satisfactory outcomes without the need for skin or other tissue grafts and the morbidity that can be associated with those methods. The star flap is also a flap that is easily executed under local

anesthetic conditions, circumventing the need for general anesthesia and its associated higher costs and potential morbidity (nausea, vomiting and so forth).

When attempting to perform any operation under local anesthetic, we consider the patient's desires and tolerance to being awake for the procedure. If there is some anxiety associated with the procedure or the needle, intravenous sedation is added to the anesthetic plan. In addition, a neurologic assessment of the breast mound area is performed, evaluating for light touch and pressure as well as pain. Many patients have decreased or little sensation in this area because of the previous mastectomy and reconstructive procedures.

We begin our planning of the modified star flap reconstruction with several key measurements based on specific anatomic points. The suprasternal notch, the midclavicular line, and the inframammary fold are all marked or taken into consideration when placing our nipple. Most of our nipple measurements are within the meridian of the breast and form close to an equilateral triangle in relation to the sternal notch, the nipples on each side, and the lines connecting both nipples on the horizontal. The patient is involved in the final decision of the nipple position by asking her to look into a mirror with us and comment on the placement of the circles we have drawn. If it is a unilateral, the native nipple is used as a reference point. We typically do our mastopexy or reduction symmetry operations in the second stage of an implant breast reconstruction when performing the exchange from tissue expander to permanent implant. The native nipple has therefore settled to a more stable position.

The 3 limbs of the flap are drawn, with the lateral and medial limbs having 2-cm lengths and a 1-cm to 1.5-cm width at their bases. The inferior limb is drawn shorter, to about 1.5 cm, with a width of 2 cm at the base as well (**Fig. 2**). The inferior limb can sometimes be referred to a superior limb depending on the direction of the blood supply to the flap. As described by Gurunluoglu and colleagues,[16] the horizontal or vertical scar is incorporated into the flap design so that the limb making up the cap of the nipple flap is the one that may cross a preexisting scar. A vertical scar incorporation means that the star flap is designed medially or laterally, and an inferior-based or superior-based flap in relation to a horizontal mastectomy scar.

Patient Positioning and Procedure

Once on the operating room table, the patient is placed in the supine position and chlorhexidine

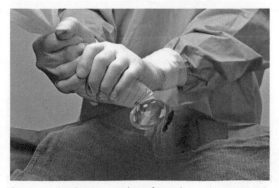

Fig. 1. Keller breast implant funnel.

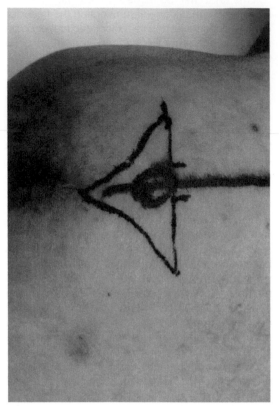

Fig. 2. Modified star flap design with a superior-based pedicle.

skin preparation is applied and our sterile field is secured. A single preoperative prophylactic dose of intravenous antibiotic is given if the reconstruction is associated with an implant.

Local anesthetic is prepared with a 1% lidocaine with 1:100,000 epinephrine mixture. If the patient has sensation to the skin involved, we add 1 mL of bicarbonate for every 9 mL of lidocaine drawn into our 10-mL syringe. Because nipple flap surgery encompasses a small surface area and little local anesthetic is used, we add 0.25% bupivacaine at the end of the procedure for longer-acting analgesia. However, if we are doing a larger area because of breast flap revisions, we do not use bupivacaine because of its lower lethal dose calculations compared with lidocaine (maximum dose 2–3 mg/kg bupivacaine with epinephrine vs 5–7 mg 1% lidocaine with epinephrine). Animal studies have also shown that mixing the two local anesthetics has an additive toxicity, making calculations of toxic levels more difficult.[17] In addition, cardiotoxicity related to bupivacaine is generally unresponsive to resuscitation efforts according to some animal studies.[18,19] Therefore, we tend to use lidocaine instead of bupivacaine in procedures requiring large volumes of local anesthetic. If our calculations bring us anywhere near toxic

doses of local anesthesia use, we opt for general anesthesia.

The skin incisions are performed with a #15 scalpel blade and are raised with sufficient subcutaneous thickness and kept thickest when dissecting near the base of the pedicle. The medial and lateral flap limbs are set with an interdigitating pattern to form the cylindrical base of the flap, whereas the inferior limb makes up the superior cap of the flap. We use 5-0 chromic sutures to sew the limbs together. The donor site is undermined full thickness just above the pectoralis muscle fascia and the defect is closed in 2 layers with 3-0 Monocryl for the deep dermal stitches and running or interrupted 4-0 nylon stitches to close the skin defect. The base of the flap is secured to the skin and closed off with 5-0 chromic interrupted sutures as well (**Fig. 3**). We then dress the flap and its donor areas with Xeroform strips 1 layer thick and a nipple protective cup as a dressing (**Fig. 4**). We keep the dressings light without any increase in complications, including infection.

Approximately 3 to 6 months after the nipple reconstruction is complete, the patient is ready for nipple and areola tattooing. We use a professional medical tattoo artist to perform the tattoos. The artist is capable of recreating the small three-dimensional nuances of the female areola, including the areolar glands and the transitional nature of areolar tissue to regular skin. In addition, a good tattoo artist can use shading to accentuate the nipple from the areola and improve the appearance of projection. A satisfactory outcome can be obtained with these techniques, removing the need for areola skin grafts (**Figs. 5** and **6**).

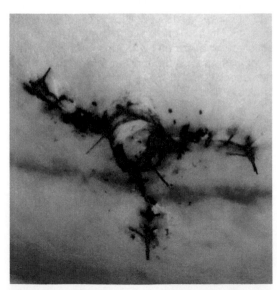

Fig. 3. Close-up of immediate postoperative result of nipple star flap.

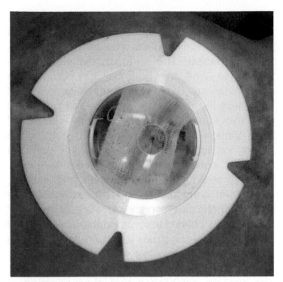

Fig. 4. Nipple flap dressed with Xeroform and nipple protecting cup.

BREAST AUGMENTATION
Preparation and Operative Method

Breast augmentation methods under local anesthesia were described by Colque and Eisemann.[4] The study was of 171 patients who underwent breast augmentation, all subpectoral, some with mastopexy. The procedures were all performed in an outpatient operating room in an office setting accredited by the American Association of Accreditation of Ambulatory Surgery Facilities. Patients were placed in the supine position and intravenous

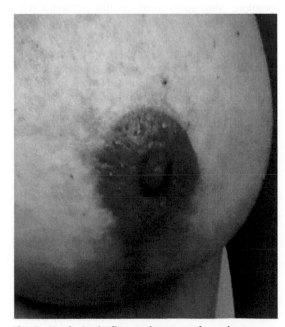

Fig. 5. Final nipple flap and tattoo of areola.

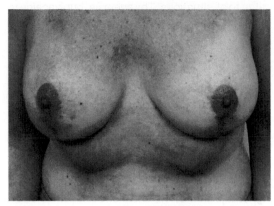

Fig. 6. Postoperative result of bilateral implant breast reconstruction with modified star nipple flap and areola/nipple tattoos.

sedation, directed by the surgeon, was started with 1 mg of midazolam, 50 μg of fentanyl, and 10 mg of ketamine. Appropriate additional doses were titrated to comfort by the circulating nurse, as directed by the surgeon. Patients' vitals and oxygen saturation were monitored throughout the case.

The local anesthetic consisted of a 1:1 solution of 0.25% bupivacaine and 1% lidocaine with 1:100,000 epinephrine. Lateral ribs 3 to 7 were marked at the midaxillary line and the intercostal spaces corresponding with those ribs were each injected with 2 mL of the anesthetic solution (Figs. 7 and 8). The lateral margin of the sternum was also injected with anesthetic solution, providing a lateral and medial block to the breast (Fig. 9).

The incisional approach was either inframammary or periareolar, depending on the patient's preference. Varying amounts of local anesthetic solution were also injected into the operative field if patients experienced intraoperative pain. The

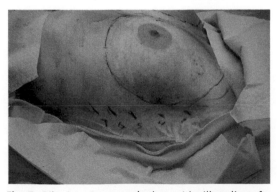

Fig. 7. Ribs 3 to 7 are marked at midaxillary lines for the lateral intercostal blocks. (Reprinted from Colque A, Eisemann ML. Breast augmentation and augmentation-mastopexy with local anesthesia and intravenous sedation. Aesthet Surg J 2012;32:304; with permission.)

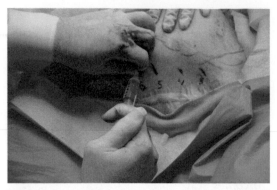

Fig. 8. Injection of 1:1 anesthetic solution of 0.25% bupivacaine and 1% lidocaine with 1:100,000 epinephrine solution, 2 mL in each intercostal space. (*Reprinted from* Colque A, Eisemann ML. Breast augmentation and augmentation-mastopexy with local anesthesia and intravenous sedation. Aesthet Surg J 2012;32:305; with permission.)

results of 2 patients undergoing a breast augmentation and a breast augmentation-mastopexy under local anesthesia are shown in **Figs. 10** and **11**.

Outcomes, Potential Complications, and Management

Surgical complications for breast reconstruction include infection, hematoma, flap necrosis, and capsular contracture. Unlike clean, elective surgery, breast reconstruction infection rates can exceed 20%. These rates are mainly attributed to the presence of prosthetic devices and drains. Preventative measures taken to avoid infection include diligent aseptic technique, the use of antibiotics,[1] and the Keller Funnel. The Keller Funnel is a medical device consisting of rip-stop nylon and a

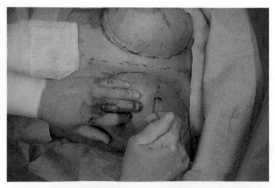

Fig. 9. Injection of 0.25% bupivacaine and 1% lidocaine with 1:100,000 epinephrine to the lateral sternal border. (*Reprinted from* Colque A, Eisemann ML. Breast augmentation and augmentation-mastopexy with local anesthesia and intravenous sedation. Aesthet Surg J 2012;32:304; with permission.)

hydrophilic inner coating. The function of the device is to reduce the amount of handling and skin contact between the implant, the surgeon, and the patient. The no-touch technique is intended to limit the potential for parenchyma contamination. Bacterial contamination was 2 times less likely with the Keller Funnel compared with the standard digital insertion technique.[8] Even though the cause of capsular contracture is not implicit, there is a correlation between capsular contracture and bacterial infection. Capsular contracture has long been, and remains, one of the commonly reported complications in both aesthetic and reconstructive breast surgery.[9] Adams and colleagues[20] conducted a study of optimal broad-spectrum antibacterial coverage for the organisms that are most frequently responsible for implant contracture and infection. The analysis established that a combination of povidone-iodine, gentamicin, and cefazolin provided optimal coverage.[20] To date, the use of triple-antibiotic irrigation has been clinically associated with low incidence of capsular contracture compared with other published reports.[9]

Anesthetic complications are also of significance. General anesthesia affects the entire body and presents the potential for aspiration, allergic reactions, increased blood pressure, increased heart rate, damage to teeth and lips, swelling of the larynx, nausea and vomiting, delirium, infection, heart attack, stroke, malignant hyperthermia, systemic toxicity, or (on extremely rare occasions) death, but locally infiltrated anesthetics are distributed only to the operative location, alleviating most of the potential risks associated with general or MAC anesthesia. Although risks associated with locally infiltrated anesthesia are minimal, local anesthetic's ability to cross the blood-brain barrier presents an absorption risk that can, in rare cases, lead to systemic reactions. In the presence of extremely high levels, coma, respiratory arrest, cardiac arrhythmia, hypotension, and cardiovascular collapse are possible. Prevention measures can be achieved through heart rate, blood pressure, and electrocardiogram monitoring, as well as an awareness of suggested dosing, frequent syringe aspiration for blood, and an initial test of a small sample dose. If systemic toxicity develops, local anesthetic injection should be stopped and oxygenation and ventilation should be maintained to resist hypoxemia, hypercarbia, and acidosis, because the presence of these increases systemic toxicity.[21–24]

Regarding the safety and efficacy of breast augmentation (with or without mastopexy) Colque and Eisemann[4] were able to show that the

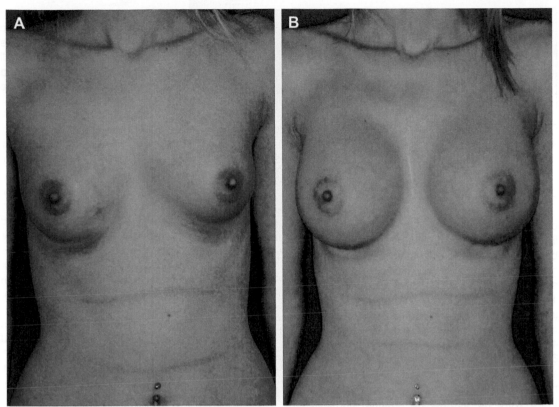

Fig. 10. An 18-year-old woman is shown (*A*) before and (*B*) 10 months after primary breast augmentation with 360-mL saline implants (Allergan, Inc; Irvine, CA). (*Reprinted from* Colque A, Eisemann ML. Breast augmentation and augmentation-mastopexy with local anesthesia and intravenous sedation. Aesthet Surg J 2012;32:303–7; with permission.)

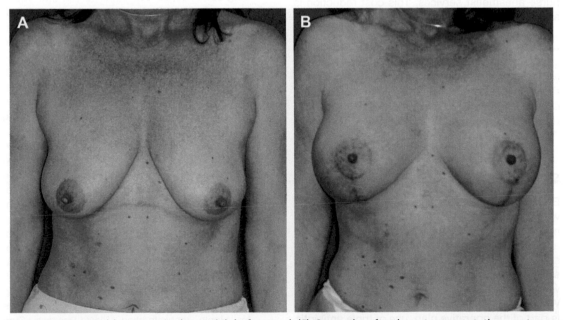

Fig. 11. A 40-year-old woman is shown (*A*) before and (*B*) 6 months after breast augmentation-mastopexy with 339-mL silicone gel implants (Allergan, Inc; Irvine, CA). (*Reprinted from* Colque A, Eisemann ML. Breast augmentation and augmentation-mastopexy with local anesthesia and intravenous sedation. Aesthet Surg J 2012;32:306; with permission.)

Table 1
Cost analyses of local versus general anesthesia for a 2-hour nipple-areola reconstruction (the table shows the amounts that were billed to insurance companies)

	Local (US$)	General (US$)
Operating room	2668.00	2817.00
Patient care unit	0.00	873.00
Medical supplies	489.00	710.00
Anesthesia	0.00	900.00
Total	3157.00	5300.00

operation can be performed successfully with a lidocaine/bupivacaine solution using intercostal blocks and surgeon-directed sedation. In the breast augmentation–only group (n = 132), the average 1% lidocaine/0.25% bupivacaine with 1:100,000 epinephrine mixture used was 79.6 mL (range, 25–120 mL) and, in the breast augmentation/mastopexy group, it was 90.9 mL (range, 45–144 mL). Average operating room time was 63.8 minutes and 134.7 minutes respectively for each group. There was some slight nausea (between 10% and 12.5%) across both groups and there were no deaths, no hospital admissions, and no serious complications in either group, underscoring the safety and efficacy of this approach. The investigators avoided propofol as a sedative and the need for anesthesiologist or nurse anesthetist services. This cost reduction is significant for the patient.

A cost analysis of our nipple-areola reconstruction under general versus local anesthetic, taking into account operating room, recovery room (PACU), medical supplies, pharmacy, and anesthesia fees, showed a local anesthetic procedural cost of US$3157 and a general anesthetic procedural cost of US$5300; a difference of US$2143 (**Table 1**).

SUMMARY

Breast reconstruction can be performed safely with local anesthesia, providing the patient with minimal discomfort, minimal complications, and a financially beneficial option. Utilization of the star flap method in conjunction with tattooing successfully provides optimal aesthetic results without the need for an additional donor site. When tissue expander to silicon implant exchange is part of the operative plan, use of triple antibiotic irrigation as well as the Keller Funnel is recommended to decrease both infection and capsular contracture. Breast augmentation and breast augmentation-mastopexy can also be performed safely and with good results under local anesthetic in a private operating room setting, with some sedation directed by the operative surgeon. All other operative conditions, including sterility and sound operative surgical techniques, should be the mainstay of any practice.

REFERENCES

1. Phillips BT, Bishawi M, Dagum AB, et al. A systematic review of antibiotic use and infection in breast reconstruction: what is the evidence? Plast Reconstr Surg 2013;131(1):1–13.
2. Bogue DP, Mungara AK, Thompson M, et al. Modified technique for nipple-areolar reconstruction: a case series. Plast Reconstr Surg 2003;112(5):1274–8.
3. Spear SL, Seruya M, Rao SS, et al. Two-stage prosthetic breast reconstruction using AlloDerm including outcomes of different timings of radiotherapy. Plast Reconstr Surg 2012;130:1.
4. Colque A, Eisemann ML. Breast augmentation and augmentation-mastopexy with local anesthesia and intravenous sedation. Aesthet Surg J 2012;32:303–7.
5. Farhadi J, Maksvytyte GK, Schaefer DJ, et al. Reconstruction of the nipple-areola complex: an update. J Plast Reconstr Aesthet Surg 2006;59:40–53.
6. Adams WM. Labial transplant for correction of loss of the nipple. Plast Reconstr Surg 1949;4:295.
7. Mohamed SA, Parodi PC. A modified technique for nipple-areola complex reconstruction. Indian J Plast Surg 2011;44(1):76–80.
8. Moyer HR, Ghazi B, Saunders N, et al. Contamination in smooth gel breast implant placement: testing a funnel versus digital insertion technique in a cadaver model. Aesthet Surg J 2012;32:194–200.
9. Adams WP, Rios JL, Smith SJ. Enhancing patient outcomes in aesthetic and reconstructive breast surgery using triple antibiotic breast irrigation: six-year prospective clinical study. Plast Reconstr Surg 2006;117:30–6.
10. Bhatty MA, Berry RB. Nipple-areola reconstruction by tattooing and nipple sharing. Br J Plast Surg 1997;50:331.
11. Losken A, Mackay GJ, Bostwick J. Nipple reconstruction using the C-V flap technique: a long-term evaluation. Plast Reconstr Surg 2001;108:361.
12. Kroll SS, Reece GP, Miller MJ, et al. Comparison of nipple projection with the modified double-opposing tab and star flaps. Plast Reconstr Surg 1997;99:1602.
13. Lesavoy M, Liu TS. The diamond double-opposing V-Y flap: a reliable, simple, and versatile technique for nipple reconstruction. Plast Reconstr Surg 2010;125:1643.
14. Anton MA. Nipple reconstruction with local flaps: star and wrap flaps. Perspect Plast Surg 1991;5:67.

15. Shestak KC, Gabriel A, Landecker A, et al. Assessment of long-term nipple projection: a comparison of three techniques. Plast Reconstr Surg 2002;110: 780–6.

16. Gurunluoglu R, Shafighi M, Williams SA, et al. Incorporation of a preexisting scar in the star-flap technique for nipple reconstruction. Ann Plast Surg 2012;68:17–21.

17. Mets B, Janicki PK, James MF, et al. Lidocaine and bupivacaine cardiorespiratory toxicity is additive: a study on rats. Anesth Analg 1992;75(4):611–4.

18. Albright GA. Cardiac arrest following regional anesthesia with etidocaine or bupivacaine. Anesthesiology 1979;51:285–7.

19. Marx GF. Cardiotoxicity of local anesthetics: the plot thickens. Anesthesiology 1984;60:3–5.

20. Adams WP, Conner W, Barton FE, et al. Optimizing breast pocket irrigation: an in vitro study and clinical implications. Plast Reconstr Surg 2000;105:334.

21. Barash PG, Cullen BF, Stoelting RK, editors. Clinical anesthesia. 4th edition. Philadelphia: Lippincott Williams and Wilkins; 2001. p. 459–62.

22. Laeken NV, Genoway K. Nipple reconstruction using a two-step purse-string suture technique. Can J Plast Surg 2001;19(2):56–9.

23. Mulroy MF. Systemic toxicity and cardiotoxicity from local anesthetics: incidence and preventative measures. Reg Anesth Pain Med 2002;27(6):556–61.

24. Boccola MA, Savage J, Rozen WM, et al. Surgical correction and reconstruction of the nipple-areola complex: current review of techniques. J Reconstr Microsurg 2010;26:589–600.

Tumescent Liposuction

Ala Lozinski, MD, FRCPC, DABD[a,*],
Nasim S. Huq, MD, FRCSC, MSc, FACS, CAQHS, DABPS[a,b,c]

KEYWORDS

- Local tumescent anesthesia • True or Pure tumescent liposuction • Megaliposuction
- Serial liposuction • Microcannulae • Hypodermoclysis • Hydrodissection • Absorption kinetics
- Lidocaine • Reservoir effect • Cytochrome P450 3A4 • Pharmacokinetics • Pharmacovigilance
- Adverse event reporting • Confounding factor

KEY POINTS

- It is no longer true tumescent liposuction if general anesthetic, sedatives/dissociative agents (propofol, ketamine, etomidate, midazolam), or analgesics that result in moderate or deep sedation (fentanyl, morphine, ketamine) are used.
- Pharmacovigilance is mandatory given that concurrent cytochrome P450 metabolic substrates can affect lidocaine metabolism.
- Infection rates associated with true tumescent liposuction have been rare, estimated at less than 1 per 2000 cases, and have been attributed to the antibacterial activity of lidocaine.
- There is significantly less potential for morbidity and mortality when general anesthetic and moderate or deep sedation during liposuction are avoided (consistent with criteria for true tumescent liposuction).
- For liposuction, it is not necessary to use local anesthetics, which are longer acting and potentially more cardiotoxic than lidocaine.
- Given that there is no anesthetist present in true tumescent liposuction, advanced cardiac life support certification for surgeon and assisting nursing staff is mandatory.

 Video of technique for tumescent liposuction of the neck accompanies this article at www.plasticsurgery.theclinics.com

EVOLUTION OF LIPOSUCTION

The history of liposuction is multidisciplinary, with multiple specialties responsible for its evolution. Lipectomy was introduced to the modern world by a French surgeon, Dujarier. It was an inauspicious beginning. In 1921, he used a uterine curette to extract fat from a ballerina's knees and calves. This procedure resulted in gangrene and leg amputation and extinguished interest in body contouring for several decades.[1]

In the early 1960s, Schrudde, a German plastic surgeon, proposed lipo-exeresis, wherein fat was suctioned via a specialized curette through small incisions. High blood loss and infection rates compelled further modifications.

Cannula liposuction was first described in the mid-1970s by Fischer, an Italian, whose early specialty training was in gynecology and otolaryngology. Soon after, Fournier, a French general surgeon, and Ilouz, who practiced obstetrics and gynecology in Paris, introduced blunt-tipped cannulae. Fournier developed the cross-tunneling technique as well as syringe liposuction. Ilouz was the first to inject hypotonic saline with

---

[a] Division of Dermatology, Department of Medicine, McMaster University, 1280 Main Street W, Hamilton, ON L8S 4L8, Canada; [b] McMaster University, Niagara Falls, Ontario, Canada; [c] Private Practice, Plastic, Reconstructive, Hand and Microsurgery, 5668 Main Street Niagara Falls, Ontario L2G 5Z4, Canada
* Corresponding author. Aestheticare, 15 Mountain Avenue South, Suite 312, Stoney Creek, Ontario L8G 2V6, Canada.
E-mail address: drlozinski@aestheticare.ca

Clin Plastic Surg 40 (2013) 593–613
http://dx.doi.org/10.1016/j.cps.2013.07.006
0094-1298/13/$ – see front matter © 2013 Elsevier Inc. All rights reserved.

epinephrine into the fat before liposuction (wet technique), thereby reducing blood loss to some extent. However, it did not entirely obviate post-operative blood transfusions in some cases. This situation, and significant procedural discomfort (necessitating general anesthesia), spurred further refinement.[2]

By the early 1980s, various American specialists had learned liposuction from the Europeans and introduced it to the United States. The first, in 1981, was performed in Los Angeles by Martin, an otolaryngologist. Shortly thereafter, Lytton was the first plastic surgeon to perform liposuction in Washington DC. Lawrence Field, a US dermatologist, was taught liposuction in Paris in 1977. He and Chrisman had introduced the technique to many dermatologists by the early 1980s.[3–5]

Anesthesia for Liposuction

1884 had marked the clinical introduction of pharmacologic local anesthesia, in the form of cocaine. Epinephrine was advanced as a chemical tourniquet in 1901. Procaine was created in 1904 and lidocaine in 1948.[6,7]

In 1987, a California dermatologist, Jeffrey Klein, described tumescent liposuction using exclusively local anesthesia. In 1988, an entire issue of *Journal of Dermatologic Surgery and Oncology* was devoted to liposuction. In 1995, Hanke and colleagues reported data on 15,336 patients who underwent true tumescent liposuction. There were no serious complications such as death, embolism (pulmonary or fat), thrombophlebitis, perforation of peritoneum or thorax, or hypovolemic shock. Blood transfusions were not required in any of these patients, and there were no admissions to the hospital for treatment of complications.[8,9]

DEFINITION OF TUMESCENT LIPOSUCTION

True tumescent liposuction, as defined by Klein, is not modified by the use of general anesthesia (intravenous [IV] or inhalational).[10] Only minimal sedation (anxiolysis, ie, 1–2 mg. lorazepam) is permitted. The addition of monitored anesthesia care (MAC) constitutes semitumescent rather than true tumescent technique. It is no longer true tumescent liposuction if sedatives/dissociative agents (propofol, ketamine, etomidate, midazolam) or analgesics that result in moderate or deep sedation (fentanyl, morphine, ketamine) are used. The addition of any other local anesthetic is strictly contraindicated. Some investigators

have referred to this technique as pure tumescent liposuction.[11]

In true tumescent liposuction, cannula size must be limited in order to be tolerated and the area treated limited by safe local anesthetic dose limits. True tumescent liposuction is not conducive to megaliposuction. Although there is no consensus among surgeons regarding the definition of megaliposuction, the maximum fat aspirate recommended by the American Academy of Dermatology (AAD) is 4.5 L.[8] The American Society of Dermatologic Surgery (ASDS) suggests an upper limit of 4 L per liposuction session.[9]

IV fluid replacement is considered unnecessary and undesirable by the AAD and ASDS.

In a liposuction variant, the super wet technique, wetting solution is infiltrated at a 1:1 ratio per mL of expected fat aspirate. The super wet technique involves the use of general anesthesia or MAC, thus carrying with it a more significant risk of respiratory depression. It also uses infiltrative fluid volumes of dilute epinephrine, with or without lidocaine, which may achieve less than tumescent effect (sufficient expansion and hydrostatic pressure for hemostatic effect) in the subcutaneous tissue. When associated with fat aspiration in the megaliposuction range, there is potential for significant fluid shifts. The super wet technique is not recommended in AAD and ASDS guidelines.

Clinical Pharmacology

Potential lidocaine toxicity is the most important consideration with true tumescent anesthesia. Its acceptance as a viable form of anesthesia has been impeded by a reluctance to accept that the absorption pharmacokinetics of dilute lidocaine infiltrated into the fat layer are at variance with that of dermally injected 1% or 2% preparations that are commercially available.

Lidocaine toxicity

Symptoms of lidocaine toxicity may occur at 6 μg/mL, but are more likely to manifest at concentrations exceeding 10 μg/mL. Drowsiness and lightheadedness can occur far below toxic concentration.[12] These symptoms would be difficult to evaluate with concurrent moderate or heavy sedation and impossible under general anesthesia. Localized muscle fasciculations are not uncommon at safe therapeutic levels.[13]

Central nervous system (CNS) toxicity occurs at lower levels than myocardial toxicity (**Table 1**).

Table 1
Effects of lidocaine on the CNS and cardiovascular system (CVS)

Concentration (µg/mL)	CNS Effect[a]	CVS Effect[a]
<5	Anticonvulsant activity Mild sedation Analgesia Circumoral paresthesiae	Antiarrhythmic activity Mild increases in mean blood pressure with similar increases in cardiac output or peripheral vascular resistance
5–10	Lightheadedness, slurred speech, drowsiness, restlessness, euphoria	Cardiovascular instability
10–15	Disorientation Uncontrollable tremors Respiratory depression Tonic-clonic seizures	
15–20	Coma Respiratory arrest	
>20		Profound myocardial depression, vasodilatation Cardiovascular collapse

[a] CNS and CVS effects are listed in approximate order of occurrence with increasing blood concentration.
Adapted from Yagiela JA. Local anesthetics. Anesth Prog 1991;38:128–41; and Butterwick KJ, Goldman MP, Sriprachya-Anunt S. Lidocaine levels during the first 2 hours of infiltration of dilute anesthetic solution for tumescent liposuction: rapid versus slow delivery. Dermatol Surg 1999;25(9):681–5.

Lidocaine safe dosing

Traditionally, 7 mg/kg of lidocaine (if given with epinephrine) was accepted as the maximum dose for dermal infusion, with only minimal data regarding how this level was ascertained.[14] Without epinephrine, 4 to 5 mg/kg has been quoted as the upper limit.[12]

It required a paradigm shift to accept that dilute lidocaine, when combined with dilute epinephrine, results in safe serum levels despite a higher dose of lidocaine. Klein showed that when the concentration of lidocaine was reduced to 0.1% or less in physiologic saline and in combination with 1:1,000,000 epinephrine, serum peak concentrations are decreased and delayed and resulted in a longer duration of action. The first credible estimate of maximum safe tumescent lidocaine dose, 35 mg/kg, was published by Klein in 1990.[15] Sequential measurement of plasma lidocaine over more than 24 hours showed peak levels 12 to 14 hours after infiltration. The maximum plasma range was 0.8 to 2.7 µg/mL, well below the toxic levels. Clinical local anesthesia was evident for up to 18 hours. These paradoxic findings can be accounted for by several factors. Lidocaine is highly lipid soluble as well as strongly lipophilic. Sequestration in fat is further prolonged by epinephrine-induced vasoconstriction, augmented by tumescent hydrostatic pressure, and the fact that the subcutaneous fat compartment is relatively avascular.[10,16–20]

These factors contribute to the reservoir effect for lidocaine in adipose tissue.

Ostad and colleagues[22] have shown in 60 patients that liposuction with a lidocaine dose of 55 mg/kg is safe, with no evidence of lidocaine toxicity over a 24-hour period. The peak plasma lidocaine concentrations obtained from these patients was less than 5 µg/mL; less than the threshold for when recognizable signs of lidocaine toxicity develop. Butterwick and colleagues[21] noted a nonlinear relationship between lidocaine dosing up to 58.2 mg/kg and peak lidocaine serum concentrations. A patient who was given 58.2 mg/kg had a peak lidocaine measurement of 0.9 µg/mL. Another, who had been given 57.7 mg/kg, had a peak serum level of 1.6 µg/mL. Yet another who was given 36.7 mg/kg yielded a peak lidocaine level of 1.9 µg/mL. The same nonlinear relationship was seen in the Ostad study. These studies refer to tumescent liposuction without MAC or general anesthesia and in the absence of drugs that interfere with lidocaine metabolism.[22]

Cytochrome P450 3A4 and lidocaine metabolism

The main elimination route of the local anesthetic in tumescent liposuction is resorption, hepatic metabolism, and excretion. Drainage through open insertion sites also lessens the systemic absorption, but by a minimal amount.

Given that lidocaine is cleared by de-ethylation in the liver by cytochrome P450 3A4 (CYP450), concurrent medications that are similarly metabolized must be noted, otherwise lidocaine toxicity might result. Hepatic CYP450 1A2 plays a role as well but the notable P450 1A2 inhibitors are already red-flagged as concurrent 3A4 inhibitors.

Commonly used medications known to inhibit CYP450 3A4 are listed in **Box 1**.

Specific potent inhibitors of CYP450 3A4 that have been associated with clinically relevant interactions include several benzodiazepines (particularly diazepam) and antidepressants, itraconazole, ketoconazole (azole antifungals), erythromycin, clarithromycin (macrolides), cimetidine, cyclosporin, amprenavir, indinavir, nelfinavir, ritonavir (human immunodeficiency virus [HIV] protease inhibitors), diltiazem, and mibefradil (calcium channel blockers).

Box 1
Drugs that inhibit CYP450 3A4

Antibiotics
  erythromycin, clarithromycin, tetracycline
  ciprofloxacin, isoniazid, metronidazole, miconazole
  ketoconazole, itraconazole, fluconazole

Analgesics
  alfentanil
  methadone
  fentanyl

Antiarrhythmic
  amiodarone

Anticonvulsants
  carbamazepine
  valproic acid

Antihistamines
  terfenadine (Seldane)[23]

Antihypertensives
  dihydralazine
  losartan
  propranolol
  calcium channel blockers
  amlodipine
  nifedipine
  diltiazem
  verapamil

Antidepressants
  sertraline (Zoloft)
  fluoxetine (Prozac)
  amitryptiline
  nefazodone

Benzodiazepines
  alprazolam
  diazepam
  flurazepam
  triazolam
  midazolam (Versed)[24]

Histamine 2 Receptor Antihistamine
  cimetidine

Hypnotic
  propofol

Immunosuppressants
  cyclosporine

Phosphodiesterase inhibitors
  sildenafil (Viagra)

Proton Pump Inhibitors
  omeprazole

Statins
  atorvastatin
  lovastatin
  pravastatin
  simvastatin

Adapted from Klein JA. Tumescent technique: tumescent anesthesia & microcannular liposuction. St Louis (MO): Mosby; 2000.

Some CYP450 3A4 metabolic substrates such as thyroxine may not significantly affect lidocaine metabolism on their own, but in combination with other drugs in this class may have an additive effect.

Naringenin (grapefruit juice) is a potent inhibitor of primarily enteric rather than hepatic CYP3A4, and therefore not a significant factor in the metabolism of lidocaine in tumescent liposuction.[10]

There are herbal constituents (eg, bergamottin and glabridin) that have been identified as CYP450 inhibitors.[25] Given the paucity of studies in this field; it is recommended that all herbal medications be avoided before tumescent liposuction.

β-Blockers may decrease blood flow to the liver. They are therefore best avoided before purely tumescent liposuction as well.

Overall, it is prudent to discontinue medications that may interfere with lidocaine metabolism 2 weeks before tumescent liposuction. If this is not possible, then the maximum lidocaine dose should be limited to 35 mg/kg. If there is potential for exceeding the maximum dose, the planned liposuction should be divided into separate procedures.

Volume infusion

Traditional liposuction assumes significant tissue trauma such that intravascular fluids are lost interstitially (third-space phenomenon), requiring volume replacement. Third spacing is not seen when using the true tumescent technique, given that the interstitial tissue is already filled with isotonic solution and tissue trauma is greatly minimized with strict adherence to the use of microcannulae. The profound hemostasis associated with true tumescent liposuction (see epinephrine section) further reduces the need for volume replacement. This degree of hemostasis is made possible by dilute epinephrine as well as hydrostatic pressure achieved by adequate tumescence.

The correct volume of tumescent solution for any given volume of targeted fat is the minimal volume that achieves complete local anesthesia and tumescence, usually twice the volume of estimated fat aspirate, but the ratio may safely approach or reach 3:1 in smaller (fat aspirate) volume cases.

Fluid loss is replaced by hypodermoclysis. Further IV fluid infusion is not necessary and potentially dangerous, given the potential for hypervolemia and pulmonary congestion.[10]

Rate of infusion

In Ostad and colleagues[22] study showing safe lidocaine dosing at 55 mg/kg, total infiltration times were 90 to 120 minutes, corresponding roughly to 25 to 35 mg/min. Nontoxic serum lidocaine levels were measured at 4, 8, 12, and 24 hours. Levels peaked earlier (4–8 hours) than in previous studies.[15,21]

Because a tumescent liposuction patient is minimally sedated at most, very rapid infiltration (which would be painful) is not possible. Extremely rapid infusion is also undesirable, because it tends to be less uniform. Unevenly distributed anesthetic solution results in suboptimal hemostasis and anesthesia. Postoperative analgesia is compromised as well. Uneven expansion of the fat compartment when suctioning predisposes to uneven liposuction results.[10]

Tumescent temperature

Tumescent infiltrate is ideally warmed to 37°C to 40°C to decrease the potential for hypothermia.

Kaplan and Moy[20] also reported that warmed tumescent solutions were judged by patients to be significantly more comfortable than when at room temperature.

Antibacterial properties of local anesthetic

Infection rates associated with true tumescent liposuction have been rare, estimated at less than 1 per 2000 cases.[26] This situation has been attributed to the antibacterial activity of lidocaine.[27] Bactericidal activity has been clearly shown at undiluted concentrations of lidocaine.[28,29] Another supporting study made note that greater microbial growth inhibition was seen at higher temperatures.[28]

Craig and colleagues[30] studied the antibacterial effect of the dilute lidocaine concentrations used in tumescent fluid and reported no bacterial inhibition. However, this study used inoculi of 1×10^8 colony forming units (CFU)/mL, whereas the recommended inoculum density for evaluating bactericidal effects of antimicrobial agents is 5×10^5 CFU/mL.[31]

In **Table 2**, Gajraj and colleagues[32] clearly show the bacteriostatic properties of dilute lidocaine. Most of the CFU/mL (which were found in Diprivan) are also considerably higher than ideal for studying bactericidal efficacy.

Table 2
Colony counts of gram-positive and gram-negative bacteria after 24 hours of incubation in Diprivan and in mixtures of lidocaine (L) and Diprivan.
The mood median test ($P<.05$) was used to compare colony counts. Lidocaine-Diprivan mixtures with colony counts that were not significantly lower (ns) than the corresponding colony counts in Diprivan alone are indicated

Organism	Colony Count in			
	Diprivan	0.05% L	0.1% L	0.2% L
Bacillus subtilis	9,700,000	6000	947	0
Staphylococcus aureus	199,333	59,667	17,333	913
Staphylococcus epidermidis	206,667	95,667	36,567	993
Escherichia coli	15,766,667	5,266,667	3,840,000	2,100,000
Moraxella osloensis	1,733,333	1,633,333 (ns)	593,333	103,000
Serratia marcescens	30,000,000	20,000,000	8,100,000	5,866,667
Burkholderia cepacia	36,333,333	37,000,000 (ns)	43,333,333 (ns)	12,200,000

From Gajraj RJ, Hodson MJ, Gillespie JA, et al. Antibacterial activity of lidocaine in mixtures with Diprivan. Br J Anaesth 1988;81:444–8; with permission.

Local anesthetic resistance

Experienced clinicians are aware that a small percentage of patients are a challenge to anesthetize with local anesthetic. It is often their dentist who has first brought this situation to their attention, and it is prudent to question them regarding this. In an uncontrolled single-blinded study, Trescot found that at least 3.8% of 1198 patients presenting to a Florida pain clinic over 1 month were hypoesthetic to lidocaine.[33] A poor response to lidocaine did not always correlate with resistance to mepivicaine or bupivacaine. Kavlock and Ting[34] hypothesized that local anesthetic receptor mutations or genetic variations in the sodium channel may account for this resistance.

Epinephrine

The addition of epinephrine to tumescent fluid is key for hemostasis, lower peak lidocaine levels, and prolonged anesthesia.

Previously, the end point of liposuction was primarily dictated by blood loss. The dry technique of liposuction was associated with blood loss of 20% to 45% of the aspirate and the wet technique, 4% to 30%.[35] With both, patients were prudently prepared with blood banking, and autologous transfusions were frequently required.

In contradistinction, the blood-tinged infranatant of the true tumescent liposuction aspirate has a hematocrit of less than 1%. Less than 12 mL of whole blood is lost per liter of fat extracted.

Epinephrine constricts arterioles, decreasing intravascular hydrostatic pressure, which in turn decreases local hemorrhage and distal transcapillary leakage of plasma; the tumescent hydrostatic pressure compresses the vasculature and further decreases hemorrhage. These factors minimize absorption of dilute tumescent anesthetic, resulting in prolonged anesthesia with lower peak serum levels of lidocaine. Altogether, these factors allow for the removal of larger volumes of fat than previous liposuction methods.[14] The epinephrine may also increase the cardiac output, which, in turn, hastens the hepatic metabolism of the lidocaine.

Klein has shown that epinephrine (0.65 mg/L = 1:1,500,000) provides consistently excellent vasoconstriction for many hours, with a low incidence of tachycardia. In areas that tend to be associated with increased intraoperative bleeding, such as upper abdomen, back and flank, and especially fibrous areas of fat, it is reasonable to use 1 mg of epinephrine/L (= 1:1,000,000) tumescent anesthetic solution.[10,14] AAD liposuction guidelines stipulate a maximum epinephrine dose of 50 µg/kg.

Sodium bicarbonate

In true tumescent liposuction, sodium bicarbonate is absolutely necessary to neutralize the acidic pH of commercially available lidocaine preparations. By eliminating the stinging and burning otherwise associated with this entity, the need for narcotic analgesia and moderate or deep sedation is eliminated.

A low pH in the extracellular space impairs the ability of local anesthetics to cross the nerve sheath and membrane, because it reduces the proportion of anesthetic in the lipophilic, free base form. A decrease in pH from 7.4 to 6.4, for instance, reduces the proportion of the base form of lidocaine in the extracellular fluid from 28% to 4%, a 7-fold reduction.[6]

Ten milliequivalents of sodium bicarbonate is added per liter of most tumescent formulations (see section on surgical technique). For more potent mixtures, 6 mEq sodium bicarbonate is added per 250 mL.[10]

Ancillary Pharmacy

Patients may receive 1 to 2 mg lorazepam sublingually and 0.1 mg clonidine orally before tumescent infiltration, but this decision is left to the discretion of the practitioner.[10]

The routine use of clonidine (0.1 mg) given preoperatively to patients without bradycardia or hypotension has greatly reduced the incidence of intraoperative and postoperative tachycardia with tumescent local anesthesia. A central α-agonist is often used as an antihypertensive agent. Clonidine acts primarily as a presynaptic CNS α_2-agonist, stimulating receptors in the nucleus tractus solitarii of the medulla oblongata. This situation inhibits sympathetic outflow, which results primarily in a reduction of sympathetically mediated vasoconstriction, cardiac inotropy, chronotropy, and mild drowsiness.[10]

Prophylactic antibiotics have been recommended for all larger volume liposuction.[26] The chosen antibiotic must not inhibit CYP3A4. Of the macrolide antibiotics, azithromycin is unique in that it does not inhibit CYP3A4. A 5-day course (500 mg. 1 day preoperatively followed by 250 mg once daily for days 2–5) of Zithromax is user friendly. β-Lactam antibiotics, including cephalosporins or cloxacillin, are among other options.[10,36]

Although the addition of hyaluronidase may hasten the diffusion of anesthetic, this addition may allow for increased absorption, different peak levels, and duration of anesthetic effect and is therefore not recommended. The addition of corticosteroid is also avoided, because it has not been found to decrease postoperative soreness and because it may increase the risk of infection.[10]

Because the postoperative analgesia of tumescent anesthetic has an 18-hour duration, bupivacaine is not needed, and it creates an added risk of cardiotoxicity.[10]

PATHOPHYSIOLOGY AND COMPLICATIONS

Worldwide, of all the advanced cosmetic surgeries, liposuction is the most commonly performed. It is worth focusing on how to maximize the safety of this procedure.[26]

When the guidelines for true or pure tumescent liposuction are strictly followed, morbidity and mortality are greatly reduced (**Box 2**, **Table 3**). Nevertheless, many surgeons and anesthesiologists who are not well versed in true or pure tumescent liposuction still believe that general anesthetic offers the safest option.[14]

Box 2
Factors associated with increased morbidity after liposuction

1. Large-volume liposuction (>5000 mL)
2. Multiple procedures (in addition to liposuction)
3. Cumulative surgical trauma
4. Increased levels of IV saline
5. General anesthesia without appreciation of early signs of lidocaine toxicity

From Kucera IJ, Lambert TJ, Klein JA, et al. Liposuction: contemporary issues for the anesthesiologist. J Clin Anesth 2006;18(5):379–87; with permission.

Safety Studies

Interdisciplinary safety studies are summarized in **Table 4**.

The safety of pure or true tumescent liposuction (TTL) is well documented.[18,26,37,38] In 1988, Bernstein and Hanke surveyed 55 dermatologists, who had performed 9478 cases.[39] The systemic complication rate was 0.7%. Hanke's later 1996 survey of the ASDS evaluated 15,336 TTL cases and found no serious complications.[42] A national survey in 2002 of more than 66,570 TTL procedures carried out by 261 dermatologic surgeons cited no deaths and a serious adverse event rate of 0.68 per 1000 TTL surgeries.[46]

Table 3
Lidocaine guidelines for a 70-kg patient with a 55-mg/kg limit in tumescent liposuction

Tumescent Solution (%)	mg	mL of 1% Lidocaine Used/L	Maximum Volume Recommended (L)	Total mL of 2% Lidocaine Recommended
0.1	3850	100	3.85	192
0.08	3850	80	4.81	192

Table 4
Liposuction safety studies

Reference	Number of Cases	Citation Source	Fatality Rate
Bernstein & Hanke,[39] 1988	9478	Journal of Dermatologic Surgery and Oncology	0
Teimourian & Rogers,[40] 1989	112,756	Plastic and Reconstructive Surgery	12.7/100,000
Dillerud,[41] 1991	3511	Plastic and Reconstructive Surgery	0
Hanke et al,[42] 1995	15,336	Dermatologic Surgery	0
American Society of Plastic and Reconstructive Surgeons Task Force on Liposuction,[43] 1997	24,295	American Society of Plastic and Reconstructive Surgeons	20.6/100,000
Grazer & de Jong,[44] 2000	496,245	Plastic and Reconstructive Surgery	19.1/100,000
Hughes,[45] 2001	94,159	Aesthetic Surgery Journal	Liposuction only 1/47,415 Liposuction + other procedures 1/17,314 Liposuction + abdominoplasty 1/3281
Housman et al,[46] 2002	66,570	Dermatologic Surgery	0
Hanke et al,[47] 2004	668	Dermatologic Surgery	0
Habbema,[48] 2009	3240	Dermatologic Surgery	0

In 1999, Coleman and colleagues[49] reviewed the National Database of the Physicians Insurance Association of America regarding malpractice data between 1995 and 1997. Their objective was to determine the influence of (1) location of the liposuction surgery and (2) specialty of the physician on the incidence of malpractice claims. Hospital-based liposuction had 3 times the rate of malpractice settlements when compared with office-based liposuction surgery. This finding contradicts the common belief that hospital-based liposuction is safer. Their study showed that fewer than 1% of the defendants were dermatologic surgeons, even although dermatologic surgeons performed about 33% of liposuctions in the United States.

Coldiron, in a review of Florida adverse event data, found that there were no TTL deaths. There were 2 deaths related to liposuction under general anesthesia.[50,51]

Table 5 summarizes Grazer and de Jong's 2000 survey results.

Deep venous thrombosis, associated with pulmonary embolism and death, is the most frequent serious complication of liposuction. In its evidence-based clinical practice guidelines, the American College of Chest Physicians has stated that the risk of venous thromboembolism may be reduced by more rapid postoperative mobilization and greater use of regional anesthesia.[52] True tumescent liposuction with minimal sedation affords the best opportunity for early and frequent postoperative ambulation.

Table 5
Liposuction fatal outcomes

Cause of Death	% (of 95 Total Fatalities)
Thromboembolism	23.1
Abdominal viscus perforation	14.6
Anesthesia/sedation/ medication	10.0
Fat embolism	8.5
Cardiorespiratory failure	5.4
Massive infection	5.4
Hemorrhage	4.6
Unknown	28.5

Data from Grazer FM, deJong RH. Fatal outcomes from liposuction: census survey of cosmetic surgeons. Plast Reconstr Surg 2000;105:436–46.

Table 6
Evidence rating scale for studies reviewed

Level of Evidence	Qualifying Studies
I	High-quality, multicentered or single-centered, randomized controlled trial with adequate power; or systematic review of these studies
II	Lesser quality, randomized controlled trial; prospective cohort study; or systematic review of these studies
III	Retrospective comparative study; case-control study; or systematic review of these studies
IV	Case series
V	Expert opinion; case report or clinical example; or evidence based on physiology, bench research, or first principles

Adapted from Haeck PC, Swanson JA, Gutowski KA, et al. Evidence-based patient safety advisory: liposuction. Plast Reconstr Surg 2009;124(4 Suppl):29S; with permission.

In the context of evidence-based medicine, the level of evidence of these large safety surveys is level IV (**Table 6**). However, within Haeck and colleagues[53] scale for grading recommendations (**Table 7**), they may be graded A or B recommendations.

CONFOUNDING FACTORS

A confounding factor is a variable that lies in the causal pathway of association between the exposure variable and outcome variable such that the presumed/reported association is invalid.[54]

This phenomenon has often clouded the perception of tumescent liposuction in medical literature.

For example, Rao's 1999 *New England Journal of Medicine* article has frequently been cited as evidence of death caused by tumescent anesthesia. However, closer examination shows that this conclusion is incorrect (**Table 8**).[55,56] Additional IV fluids were given to patient 1 (3 L), patient 2 (1.7 L), and patient 3 (7.3 L). Patient 1 had general anesthetic. Patient 2 was given midazolam, fentanyl, methohexital, and droperidol. Patient 3 had augmentation mammoplasty along with liposuction, with estimated blood loss of 700 mL and a postoperative hemoglobin of 5.8 g/dL. The fourth

Table 7
Scale for grading recommendations

Grade	Descriptor	Qualifying Evidence	Implications for Practice
A	Strong recommendation	Level I evidence or consistent findings from multiple studies of levels II, III, or IV	Clinicians should follow a strong recommendation unless a clear and compelling rationale for an alternative approach is present
B	Recommendation	Levels II, III, or IV evidence and findings are generally consistent	Generally, clinicians should follow a recommendation but should remain alert to new information and sensitive to patient preferences
C	Option	Levels II, III, or IV evidence, but findings are inconsistent	Clinicians should be flexible in their decision making regarding appropriate practice, although they may set bounds on alternatives; patient preference should have a substantial influencing role
D	Option	Level V: little or no systematic empirical evidence	Clinicians should consider all options in their decision making and be alert to new published evidence that clarifies the balance of benefit vs harm; patient preference should have a substantial influencing role

Adapted from Haeck PC, Swanson JA, Gutowski KA, et al. Evidence-based patient safety advisory: liposuction. Plast Reconstr Surg 2009;124(4 Suppl):29S; with permission.

Table 8
Confounding factors: deaths incorrectly attributed to tumescent liposuction

Patient Number Sex/Age (y)	Anesthesia (Primary)	Anatomic Site Surgery	Lidocaine Dose (mg/kg)	Aspirate (L)	Cause Death
1. Male/33	General	Flanks, abdomen	10	4.0	Bradycardia hypotension asystole
2. Female/40	IV sedation	Flanks, back	14.2	2.4	Bradycardia asystole
3. Female/33	IV sedation	Thorax, arms, back, abdomen, thighs, buttocks, knees	31.4	6.7	Pulmonary edema
4. Female/54	IV sedation	Back, flanks, abdomen, thighs	40	5.6	Pulmonary embolism

Data from Rao RB, Ely SF, Hoffman RS. Deaths related to liposuction. N Engl J Med 1999;340:1472; and Hanke CW, Sterling JB, Melton JL, et al. Review of liposuction safety studies. In: Hanke CW, Sattler G, editors. Procedures in cosmetic dermatology series–liposuction. London: Elsevier Saunders; 2005. p. 145.

had megaliposuction (back, flanks, abdomen, and thighs). For clarity, cases like these should be described as semitumescent liposuction.

Another example of a confounding factor is found in a 2008 case report ("Reporting a fatality during tumescent liposuction").[57,58] In this instance, toxicologic analyses revealed that the patient had lidocaine as well as mepivacaine *heart blood* concentrations of 4.9 and 16.2 μg/mL, respectively. In true tumescent liposuction, lidocaine alone is the preferred type of local anesthetic according to current AAD and ASDS guidelines of care for liposuction.[8,9] Adding other local anesthetics is not recommended. For liposuction, it is not necessary to use local anesthetics, which are longer acting and potentially more cardiotoxic than lidocaine.

EDUCATION/TRAINING/FACILITY

AAD guidelines of care for liposuction stipulate that the surgeon be board certified (or completed residency) in a recognized specialty that provides education in liposuction. For example, tumescent liposuction is a clearly designated part of the dermatology residency curriculum in Canada and the United States.[8]

Given that there is no anesthetist present in true tumescent liposuction, advanced cardiac life support certification for surgeon and assisting nursing staff is mandatory.

After an exhaustive review of these studies in 2002, the California Medical Board concluded that surgical centers are as safe as, and possibly safer than, hospital settings for liposuction.[59]

Although maintaining high standards in out-of-hospital premises is a laudable goal, restricting access to true or pure tumescent liposuction may, paradoxically, increase the morbidity and mortality associated with liposuction.

Surgical Technique

Indications
Preoperative patient evaluation includes a thorough history and physical examination. Patients should be in either American Society of Anesthesiologists Physical Status (ASA PS) class I or class 2 (**Table 9**).

Table 9
ASA PS classification system

ASA PS Category	Preoperative Health Status	Comments, Examples
ASA PS 1	Normal healthy patient	No organic, physiologic, or psychiatric disturbance; excludes the very young and very old; healthy with good exercise tolerance
ASA PS 2	Patients with mild systemic disease	No functional limitations; has a well-controlled disease of 1 body system (ie, controlled hypertension or diabetes without systemic effects, cigarette smoking without chronic obstructive pulmonary disease, mild obesity)

Laboratory studies

Complete blood count with quantitative platelet assessment, prothrombin time, partial thromboplastin time, and β-human chorionic gonadotropin in women of childbearing age are routinely obtained. History and systemic review may justify a chemistry profile, including liver function tests as well.

Local standards of care may vary and some surgeons may wish to obtain additional studies, including screening for HIV, hepatitis A, B, and C, and a urine pregnancy test on the day of the procedure.

Intraoperative and postoperative monitoring

The AAD recommends continuous monitoring of blood pressure, cardiac monitoring with pulse oximetry, and the availability of supplemental oxygen.[8]

Indications and formulations for tumescent anesthesia

The indications for tumescent anesthesia are ever expanding (**Table 10**).

It has proved useful for lipoma removal, Madelung disease, axillary hyperhidrosis, axillary bromhidrosis, laser removal of large tattoos, evacuation of hematomata, pseudogynecomastia, ambulatory phlebectomy, and endovenous laser treatment as well as to achieve hemostasis for more extensive surgeries such as mastectomies.

More recent novel uses include herniorrhaphy, treatment of pilonidal sinus, and revascularization of a coronary subclavian steal syndrome.[60–63]

Yet another reported application is for release of postburn contractures.[64]

Table 10
Recommended concentrations for effective tumescent anesthesia for liposuction

Areas	Lidocaine (mg/L)	Epinephrine (mg/L)	Sodium Bicarbonate (mEq/L)
Hips; lateral, medial, and anterior thighs; knees	700–750 (0.07%–0.075%)	0.65	10
Back; male flanks; arms	1000	0.65–1.0	10
Female abdomen (medial)	1000–1250	1.0	10
Male abdomen (medial) and male breasts	1250	1.0	10
Abdomen (lateral)	750	0.65	10
Female breasts; neck, cheek, and jowls	1500	1.5	10
Tumescent Anesthesia Other Indications			
Facial resurfacing (ablative CO_2 laser [ie, rhinophyma, deep acne scarring]) Dermabrasion Facial rhytidectomy Hair transplantation Platysmaplasty (with neck liposuction)	600–1000 mg/250 mL (0.24%–0.4%)	1 mg/250 mL	5 mEq/250 mL
Nonmelanoma skin cancer and thin malignant melanoma excision	600–1000 mg/250 mL	1 mg/250 mL	5 mEq/250 mL
Ambulatory phlebectomy Endovenous laser treatment[59]	1000–2000 (0.1%–0.2%)	1	10

Concentrations of lidocaine recommended range from 0.05% to 0.1% depending on the sensitivity of the area to be tumesced. On occasions, lidocaine 0.15% has been recommended in small quantities for very sensitive areas such as the female breast. Higher concentration lidocaine for more sensitive and fibrous areas. The most commonly used concentrations of lidocaine are 0.1%, 0.075%, and 0.05%.
Data from Klein JA. Tumescent technique: tumescent anesthesia & microcannular liposuction. St Louis (MO): Mosby; 2000.

Liposuction and full abdominoplasty under local anesthesia with mild sedation

Although abdominoplasty has traditionally been performed under general anesthesia or spinal anesthesia, there are some investigators who have routinely performed full abdominoplasty with IV sedation for many years. Kryger and colleagues[65] compared the outcomes of the abdominoplasties performed under these techniques over a 6-year experience and found that this type of procedure is well tolerated, has a high patient satisfaction rate and a low complication rate, and the patients were able to avoid general anesthesia. **Fig. 1** is of a patient who had liposuction alone. **Figs. 2** and **3** are patients who had full abdominoplasty.

The technique is performed in similar fashion to traditional abdominoplasty, except that the patient is awake throughout. Preoperative markings and calculations for allowable doses are essential. The area for excision is already preplanned and measured.

- Tumescent local anesthetic is infiltrated through the intended abdominal lipectomy site as well as the abdominal wall flap. It is essential to ensure that there are no abdominal hernias during this infiltration.[66]
- Liposuction can be performed at the beginning, during, or at the end of the abdominal lipectomy. The skin flaps are elevated up to the umbilicus, which is cored out, and the anterior abdominal wall flap is elevated up to the xiphisternum.
- During the flap elevation, the essential nerve blocks are performed and any perforating

sensory nerves may require some extra local anesthetic infiltration.

- The anterior abdominal wall is plicated in the usual fashion to improve the abdominal wall contour and to decrease the protuberance of the abdomen.
- The bed is still flexed at the hips and the knees and the new position of the umbilicus is measured and inset.

We prefer high lateral tension for our technique in abdominoplasty and the subscarpal fat is resected off the flap. Drains are no longer routinely used. The abdomen is closed in the standard fashion.[67] See **Fig. 1** is of a patient who had liposuction alone. **Figs. 2** and **3** are patients who had full abdominoplasty.

We have found that it is difficult to achieve a good anesthetic block on the anterior rectus sheath if the abdominal wall flap is large or thick. The local anesthetic works well for the thinner abdomen, where the appropriate wall structures can be easily identified.

Cutaneous surgery

Topologic transformation of tissues with mechanical elevation of skin from subjacent neurovascular structures can be achieved with tumescent anesthesia.

Tumescent anesthesia is an excellent alternative for outpatient skin cancer surgery of nonmelanoma skin cancers (NMSC) and thin melanomata as well as skin flap debulking and to harvest grafts.[68]

When tumescing outside adipose tissue, the benefits of lidocaine lipid solubility, lipophilicity, and prolonged sequestration no longer apply.

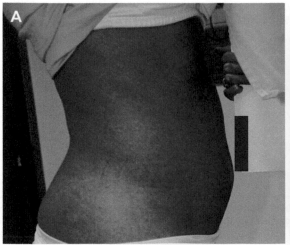
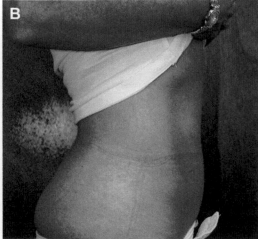

Fig. 1. (*A*) A 46-year-old woman who complained of abdominal prominence. (*B*) Three-month postoperative view after 2 L of liposuction fluid was removed.

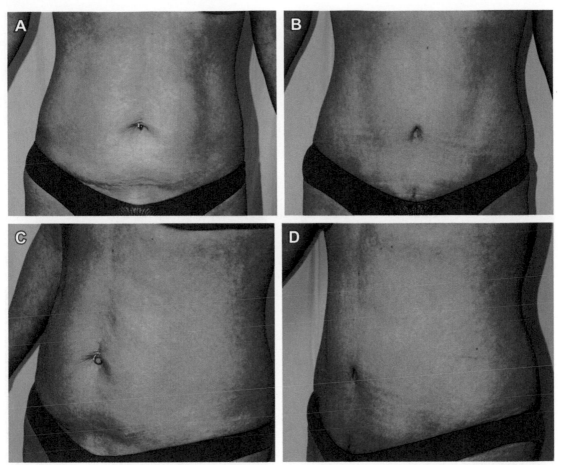

Fig. 2. (*A*) Preoperative view of a 42-year-old, gravida 3 patient who complained of excess skin and laxity in the anterior abdominal wall. She specifically requested local anesthesia only and would not accept general anesthesia for an abdominoplasty procedure. (*B*) Postoperative view. Lipoabdominoplasty with local anesthesia, no heavy sedation or inhalational or spinal anesthesia. (*C*) Preoperative oblique view. (*D*) Postoperative oblique view.

Assuming the traditionally accepted maximum safe dose of lidocaine (with epinephrine) of 7 mg/kg for primarily cutaneous injection, tumescent anesthesia is still of great benefit for NMSC and thin melanoma excisions. For a 70-kg patient in this cutaneous surgery scenario, using a standard commercial preparation of 2% lidocaine with 1:100,000 epinephrine, one would be limited to (7 × 70 = 490) 490 mg of lidocaine or 24.5 mL of this preparation. The concurrent epinephrine dose would be 0.245 mg.

If one were to infuse 490 mg of lidocaine using a 0.3% dilute lidocaine solution (750 mg lidocaine/250 mL with 1 mg epinephrine/250 mL), a maximum of 163 mL of tumescent fluid could be infused, allowing for significantly more extensive surgery in an alert patient than when using a commercially prepared 2% lidocaine solution.

The epinephrine dose (163 mL of 1 mg/250 mL) would be 0.652 mg.

STANDARDIZED TUMESCENT SOLUTION PREPARATION

It is essential that tumescent anesthetic fluid be mixed by trained personnel in accordance with the order of a physician, preferably on the day of surgery. The maximum dosage is calculated by multiplying the patient's weight in kilograms by the planned maximum lidocaine dose (35–55 mg/kg) to give the total lidocaine dosage. To calculate the safe number of liter bags containing the tumescent mixture, mg/L of lidocaine is divided into the maximum lidocaine dosage (mg) For example, a 70-kg patient has a maximum lidocaine dose by tumescent local anesthesia of

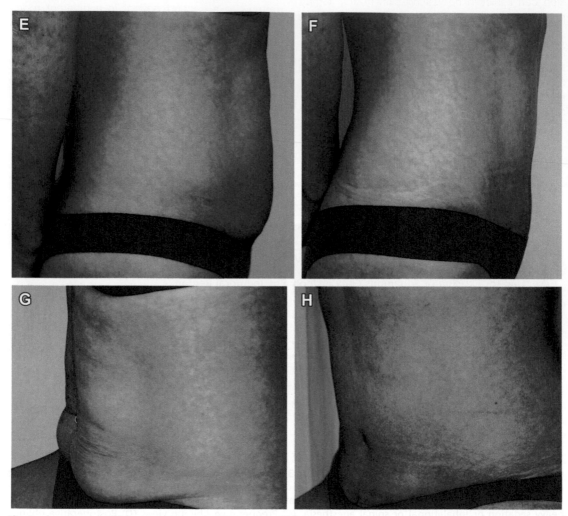

Fig. 2. (*continued*). (*E*) Preoperative right lateral view. (*F*) Postoperative right lateral view. (*G*) Preoperative seated view. (*H*) Postoperative seated view.

70 × 55 = 3850. If the concentration of the lidocaine solution in the tumescent bag is 0.05%, then there is 500 mg in each bag; therefore, 3850 is divided by 500 to give a total of 7.7 bags allowable in that patient. It is important that the physician standardizes the practice of mixing the solution in such a way that errors in lidocaine dosing do not occur. It is highly recommended that only 1% lidocaine without epinephrine commercial preparations are stocked for liposuction surgery.[10]

TUMESCENT INFUSION

Tumescent anesthesia fluid is delivered by a peristaltic pump using 15.2-cm to 30.4-cm (6-inch–12-inch) blunt-tipped infusion microcannulae (12-gauge–16-gauge). These cannulae are less

traumatic than sharp-tipped needles, with less risk of penetrating deeper vital structures.[10] Eighteen-gauge to 20-gauge spinal needles are acceptable in skilled hands.[49] There is an argument that there is less potential for infection with these disposable needles. Straight blunt tip 15.2-cm nerve block needles, available in 20 gauge, are a consideration.

IV FLUIDS

In true tumescent liposuction, fluid loss is entirely compensated for by hypodermoclysis. Because of the risk of intravascular fluid overload and pulmonary edema, significant volumes of IV fluids should be used with extreme caution in any tumescent liposuction procedure.[8–10,35]

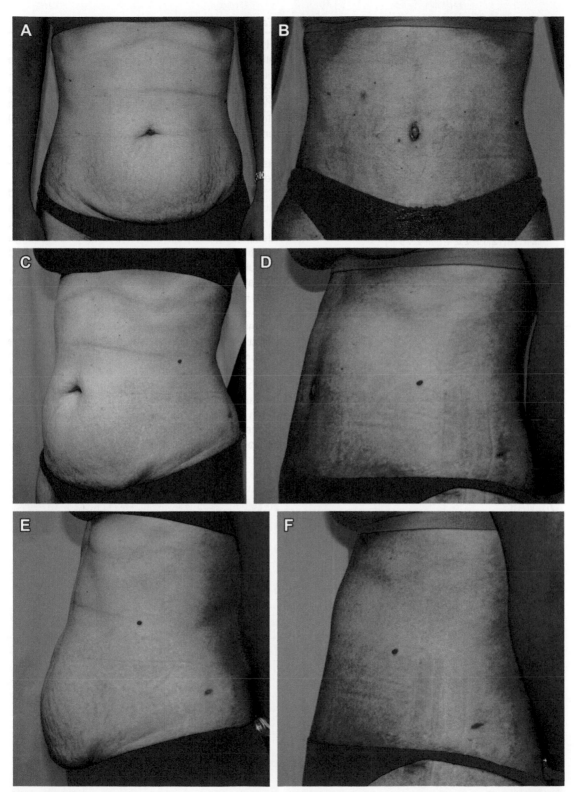

Fig. 3. (*A*) Preoperative frontal view of a 38-year-old woman complaining of abdominal wall laxity. (*B*) Postoperative frontal view at 3 months after lipoabdominoplasty with no general or spinal anesthesia. (*C*) Preoperative oblique view. (*D*) Postoperative oblique view. (*E*) Preoperative lateral view. (*F*) Postoperative lateral view.

CANNULA SIZE

Microcannulae (internal diameter [ID] $\leq$2.2 mm; **Table 11**) are necessary for optimal results with tumescent liposuction.

Table 11
Cannula specifications

	ID (mm)	Outer Diameter (mm)
Gauge		
10	2.7	3.4
Microcannulae		
12	2.15–2.2	2.75
14	1.6	2.1
16	1.2	1.6

ADVANTAGES OF TUMESCENCE AND MICROCANNULAE
Less Pain

When anesthesia is entirely local with (at most) minimal sedation, microcannulae are mandatory, because larger cannulae are not well tolerated.

Easier Penetration/Accuracy

Hydrodissection takes place as the pressure of infiltrated tumescent fluid splays apart fibrous tissue bundles. The advancing microcannula then encounters less resistance. This situation facilitates treatment of more fibrous territory such as the dorsal-lateral fat pads below the bra line (**Fig. 4**) and the glandular tissue of male breasts.

A cannula that can be advanced through target tissue easily is less likely to deviate from its intended path into danger zones.

Because microcannulae penetrate tumesced fibrous tissue with minimum force, there is less articular wear and tear for the liposuction surgeon, decreasing the potential for osteoarthritic change (particularly trapeziometacarpal, elbow, and shoulder joints). It might be argued that power-assisted liposuction affords the same benefit, but this is at the expense of greater tissue trauma and longer incisions associated with larger cannulae.

Tumescing the fat layer magnifies its volume and defects such that desired fat sculpting can be accomplished with greater accuracy and better feathering of edges. This situation is of particular advantage where there is little room for error such as medial thighs and jowls. These advantages lessen the likelihood of requiring a secondary procedure (**Fig. 5**).

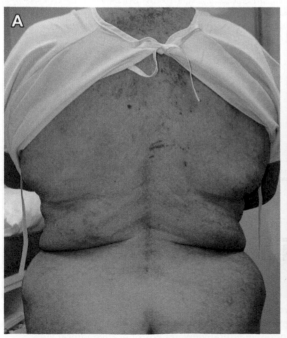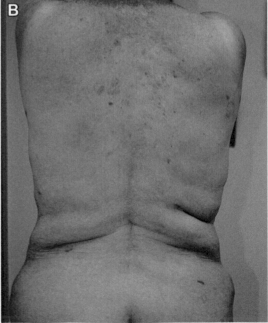

Fig. 4. (*A*) Preoperative view of 68-year-old patient complaining of fat rolls on her back in the area of her bra. (*B*) Postoperative view after liposuction with local anesthesia of the upper back and arms.

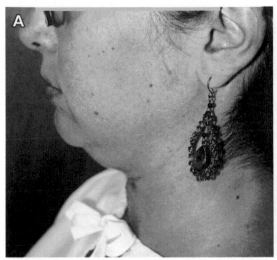
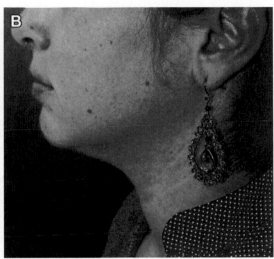

Fig. 5. (*A*) Preoperative view of 32-year-old patient complaining of submental fat. (*B*) Postoperative view after liposuction of the neck. There was no other suturing or suspension.

Expanding the fat layer can also create a safety cushion, elevating the target work area away from underlying vital structures. This situation is of particular benefit in NMSC (or thin melanoma) excision over facial nerve and artery danger zones.

More Complete Fat Removal

More fat can be removed using microcannulae than with larger cannulae.

Smaller Incisions/Accelerated Healing

Microcannulae require only 2-mm to 4-mm incisions, which allows greater latitude regarding incision placement. Multiple incisions without sutures accelerate drainage, which reduces ecchymoses, edema, and tenderness. Wounds within fat created by microcannulae are narrow tunnels that heal more rapidly than larger tunnels. The greater net surface area of the walls of these cylindrical microtunnels promotes more rapid absorption of residual fluid within the subcutaneous space. The net effect is accelerated healing.[10]

Conversely, larger cannulae produce a proportionally smaller wound as cannula diameter increases. For a cylindric tunnel, surface area (A) = 2 p r h and volume (V) = p r2 h. The relation of A to V is

A = 2V/r

such that the surface area is inversely proportional to the radius. If we did a split body comparison using a 10 gauge cannula on one thigh and 14 gauge on the other (extracting the same volume from both thighs), there would be more blood vessels transected using the smaller cannula. Thus, earlier liposuction techniques did not permit the use of

microcannulae given that, in the absence of profound hemostasis, smaller cannulae result in more bleeding. The key differences are epinephrine-induced vasoconstriction and sufficiently

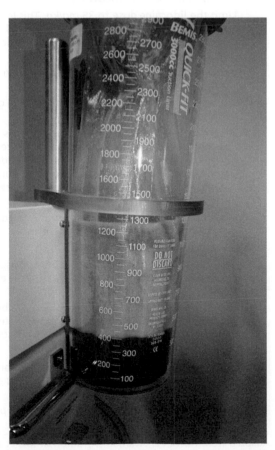

Fig. 6. Effluent waste is collected and examined for fat and water quantities.

Table 12
Plastic and Reconstructive Surgery 2009 liposuction recommendations summary

	Level of Evidence Grade
Liposuction Technique	
No one single liposuction technique is best suited for all patients in all circumstances. Factors such as the patient's overall health, the patient's body mass index, the estimated volume of aspirate to be removed, the number of sites to be addressed, and any other concomitant procedures to be performed should be considered.	B
Because of the amount of blood loss associated with the dry technique, use is not recommended except in limited applications with a total aspirate volume ≤100 mL.	D
Anesthetic Infiltrate Solutions	
Small-volume liposuction, infiltrate solutions containing local anesthetic agents may be sufficient to provide adequate pain relief without the need for additional anesthesia measures	B
Insufficient data are available to support the use of bupivacaine or prilocaine in addition to or as a substitute for lidocaine. These agents should be used cautiously if included in infiltrate solutions because of their potential for severe side effects.	D
Lidocaine wetting solutions have the potential to cause systemic toxicity when administered to large or multiple regions of the body. Preventive measures include the following:	
Limit the lidocaine dose to 35 mg/kg. This level may not be safe in patients with low protein levels and other medical conditions, in whom the metabolic byproducts of lidocaine breakdown may reach problematic levels.	B
Reduce the concentration of lidocaine when necessary (eg, depending on the site of infiltration).	D
Consider avoiding the use of lidocaine when general or regional anesthesia is used.	D
Epinephrine use should be avoided in patients who present with pheochromocytoma, hyperthyroidism, severe hypertension, cardiac disease, or peripheral vascular disease. In addition, cardiac arrhythmias can occur in predisposed individuals or when epinephrine is used with halothane anesthesia. The surgeon must carefully evaluate these types of patients before performing liposuction.	D
Consider staging the infiltration of multiple anatomic sites to reduce the possibility of an excess epinephrine effect.	D
Liposuction Volume	
Large-volume liposuction (>5000 mL of total aspirate) should be performed in an acute care hospital or in a facility that is either accredited or licensed, regardless of the anesthetic method.	D
Under certain circumstances, it may be in the best interest of the patient to perform large-volume procedures as separate serial procedures and to avoid combining them with additional procedures.	D
Multiple Procedures	
Large-volume liposuction combined with certain other procedures (eg, abdominoplasty) has resulted in serious complications, and such combinations **should be avoided.**	D
Individual patient circumstances may warrant performing liposuction as a separate procedure.	D

Adapted from Haeck PC, Swanson JA, Gutowski KA, et al. Evidence-based patient safety advisory: liposuction. Plast Reconstr Surg 2009;124(4 Suppl):28S-44S; with permission.

even, thorough and complete tumescence to exert significant hydrostatic pressure on adipose tissue vasculature. Both are mandatory for microcannula use.

ADDITIONAL BENEFITS

An alert patient is able to assist with positioning. Their mobility is not compromised such that anti-embolism stockings or sequential compression pumping are required to prevent deep vein thrombosis.

Postoperative recovery is negligible if they have had no general anesthetic or MAC and only mild sedation.

On the other hand, an alternative skill set is required to deal with a patient who is alert throughout surgery.

STERILE VERSUS CLEAN

In 3240 consecutive cases using true tumescent liposuction, Habbema[49] noted only 2 low-grade postoperative infections. Although gloves and instruments were initially sterile and a preoperative chlorhexidine scrub was used, conditions were described as *clean*. All patients were given a course of oral prophylactic antibiotics, and the postoperative infections resolved with additional antibiotics.

MAXIMUM TOTAL VOLUME FAT ASPIRATE

The AAD, in its guidelines of care for liposuction, recommends that the volume of fat removed be in proportion to the weight/size/% body fat of the patient, generally limited to less than 4500 mL in a single session (**Fig. 6**).[8]

ASDS guidelines of care for liposuction recommend that if the anticipated volume of supernatant fat is greater than 4 L, liposuction should be divided into more than 1 operative session (serial liposuction).[9]

Table 12 is adapted from the 2009 executive summary of liposuction recommendations in plastic and reconstructive surgery.

SUMMARY

The innovation of tumescent liposuction was the result of dermatology's preference for local anesthesia. The dermatology literature has documented that true tumescent liposuction is performed more safely, patients experience quicker recovery and, arguably, better aesthetic results. It has not yet reached a tipping point in specialties outside dermatology; however, Gladwell[69] describes this situation as the peak rate of diffusion, when a practice is adopted by 10% to 20% of the community.

Acceptance of true tumescent anesthesia has been hampered by a reluctance to adhere to true tumescent standards. Nomenclature has been an issue as well. There has been much confusion regarding the meaning of true tumescent liposuction, and it may be that this term is considered awkward, suggestive of a religious connotation. Some have managed this concern by the use of an alternative term, *pure tumescent liposuction*.[11] Perhaps an eponym, such as Klein tumescent liposuction, would more clearly designate the narrow meaning of this term.

True tumescent liposuction, as defined by Klein, is

- Not modified by the use of general anesthesia (IV or inhalational).
- Permits only minimal sedation (anxiolysis, ie, 1–2 mg lorazepam)

The addition of MAC constitutes semitumescent rather than true tumescent technique. It is no longer true tumescent liposuction if sedatives/dissociative agents (propofol, ketamine, etomidate, midazolam), or analgesics that result in moderate or deep sedation (fentanyl, morphine, ketamine) are used.

Primum Non Nocere

In the pursuit of safer surgical outcomes, all specialties that practice liposuction should pool outcome information via mandatory provincial or state adverse event reporting.[70] These data should then be analyzed and shared for everyone's benefit.

VIDEOS ONLINE

Supplementary data in the form of video related to this article can be found online at http://dx.doi.org/10.1016/j.cps.2013.07.006.

REFERENCES

1. Glicenstein J. Dujarier's case. Ann Chir Plast Esthet 1989;34(3):290–2 [in French].
2. Lewis C. Early history of lipoplasty in the United States. Aesthetic Plast Surg 1990;14(2):123–6.
3. Field L. Liposuction surgery: a review. J Dermatol Surg Oncol 1984;10(7):530–8.
4. Flynn TC, Coleman WP III, Field LM, et al. History of liposuction. Dermatol Surg 2000;26:515–20.
5. Hanke CW, Sattler G. History of liposuction. In: Hanke CW, Sattler G, editors. Procedures in

cosmetic dermatology series–liposuction. London: Elsevier Saunders; 2005. p. 1–2.

6. Yagiela JA. Local anesthetics. Anesth Prog 1991; 38:128–41.

7. Liljestrand G. The historical development of local anesthesia. In: Lechat P, editor. International encyclopedia of pharmacology and therapeutics, Sect. 8, local anesthetics, vol. 1. New York: Pergamon; 1971. p. 1–38.

8. Coleman WP III, Glogau RG, Klein JA, et al, American Academy of Dermatology Guidelines/Outcomes Committee. Guidelines of care for liposuction. J Am Acad Dermatol 2001;45:438–47.

9. Coldiron B, Coleman WP III, Cox SE, et al. ASDS guidelines of care for tumescent liposuction. Dermatol Surg 2006;32(5):709–16.

10. Klein JA. Tumescent technique: tumescent anesthesia & microcannular liposuction. St Louis (MO): Mosby; 2000.

11. Jacob CI, Kaminer MS. Tumescent liposuction. In: Kaminer MS, Arndt KA, Dover JS, et al, editors. Atlas of cosmetic surgery. 2nd edition. Philadelphia: Saunders Elsevier; 2009. p. 323–64.

12. Miller R. Anaesthesia. 7th edition. Philadelphia: Churchill Livingstone; 2009.

13. Melton JL, Hanke CW, Sattler G. Tumescent local anesthesia technique. In: Hanke CW, Sattler G, editors. Procedures in cosmetic dermatology series–liposuction. London: Elsevier Saunders; 2005. p. 21–32.

14. Kucera IJ, Lambert TJ, Klein JA, et al. Liposuction: contemporary issues for the anesthesiologist. J Clin Anesth 2006;18(5):379–87.

15. Klein JA. Tumescent technique for regional anesthesia permits lidocaine doses of 35 mg/kg for liposuction. J Dermatol Surg Oncol 1990;16(3):248–63.

16. Klein JA. The tumescent technique. Anesthesia and modified liposuction technique. Dermatol Clin 1990;8(3):425–37.

17. Klein JA. Tumescent technique chronicles. Local anesthesia, liposuction, and beyond. Dermatol Surg 1995;21(5):449–57.

18. Klein JA. Tumescent technique for local anesthesia improves safety in large-volume liposuction. Plast Reconstr Surg 1993;92(6):1085–98 [discussion: 1099–100].

19. Klein JA. Anesthesia for dermatologic cosmetic surgery. In: Coleman WP III, Hanke CW, Alt TH, et al, editors. Cosmetic surgery of the skin: principles and techniques. Philadelphia: BC Decker; 1991. p. 39–45.

20. Kaplan B, Moy RL. Comparison of room temperature and warmed local anesthestic solution for tumescent liposuction: a randomized double-blind study. Dermatol Surg 1996;22:707–9.

21. Butterwick KJ, Goldman MP, Sriprachya-Anunt S. Lidocaine levels during the first two hours of infiltration of dilute anesthetic solution for tumescent liposuction: rapid versus slow delivery. Dermatol Surg 1999;25(9):681–5.

22. Ostad A, Kageyama N, Moy RL. Tumescent anesthesia with a lidocaine dose of 55 mg/kg is safe for liposuction. Dermatol Surg 1996;22:921–7.

23. Ling KH, Leeson GA, Burmaster SD, et al. Metabolism of terfenadine associated with CYP3A(4) activity in human hepatic microsomes. Drug Metab Dispos 1995;23(6):631–6.

24. Wendel C, Becker R, Behrer H, et al. Midazolam is metabolized by at least three different cytochrome P450 enzymes. Br J Anaesth 1994;73:658–61.

25. Zhou S, Chan E, Lim LY, et al. Therapeutic drugs that behave as mechanism-based inhibitors of cytochrome P450 3A4. Curr Drug Metab 2004;5(5): 415–42.

26. Igra H, Lanzer D. Avoiding complications. In: Hanke CW, Sattler G, editors. Procedures in cosmetic dermatology series–liposuction. London: Elsevier Saunders; 2005. p. 131–40.

27. Klein JA. Antibacterial effects of tumescent lidocaine. Plast Reconstr Surg 1999;104(6):1934–6.

28. Stratford AF, Zoutman DE, Davidson JS. Effect of lidocaine and epinephrine on *Staphylococcus aureus* in a guinea pig model of surgical wound infection. Plast Reconstr Surg 2002;110(5):1275–9.

29. Johnson SM, Saint John BE, Dine AP. Local anesthetics as antimicrobial agents: a review. Surg Infect (Larchmt) 2008;9(2):205–13.

30. Craig SB, Concannon M, McDonald GA, et al. The antibacterial effects of tumescent liposuction fluid. Plast Reconstr Surg 1999;104:1934.

31. Peterson LR, Shanholtzer CJ. Tests for bactericidal effects of antimicrobial agents: technical performance and clinical relevance. Clin Microbiol Rev 1992;5(4):420–32.

32. Gajraj RJ, Hodson MJ, Gillespie JA, et al. Antibacterial activity of lidocaine in mixtures with Diprivan. Br J Anaesth 1988;81:444–8.

33. Trescot AM. Local anesthetic "resistance". Pain Physician 2003;6(3):291–3.

34. Kavlock R, Ting PH. Local anesthetic resistance in a pregnant patient with lumbosacral plexopathy. BMC Anesthesiol 2004;4(1):1.

35. Trott SA, Beran SJ, Rohrich RJ, et al. Safety considerations and fluid resuscitation in liposuction: an analysis of 53 consecutive patients. Plast Reconstr Surg 1998;102(6):2220–9.

36. Rossi AM, Mariwalla K. Prophylactic and empiric use of antibiotics in dermatologic surgery: a review of the literature and practical considerations. Dermatol Surg 2012;38(12):1898–921.

37. Lillis PJ. Liposuction surgery under local anesthesia: limited blood loss and minimal lidocaine absorption. J Dermatol Surg Oncol 1988;14(10): 1145–8.

38. Butterwick KJ, Goldman MP. Safety of lidocaine during tumescent anesthesia for liposuction. In: Hanke CW, Sattler G, editors. Procedures in cosmetic dermatology series–liposuction. London: Elsevier Saunders; 2005. p. 33–7.

39. Bernstein G, Hanke CW. Safety of liposuction: a review of 9478 cases performed by dermatologists. J Dermatol Surg Oncol 1988;14(10):1112–4.

40. Teimourian B, Rogers WB. A national survey of complications associated with suction lipectomy: a comparative study. Plast Reconstr Surg 1989; 84:628–31.

41. Dillerud E. Suction lipoplasty: a report on complications, undesired results and patient satisfaction based on 3511 procedures. Plast Reconstr Surg 1991;88:239–46.

42. Hanke CW, Bernstein G, Bullock S. Safety of tumescent liposuction in 15,336 patients. National survey results. Dermatol Surg 1995;21(5):459–62.

43. ASPRS Task Force on Lipoplasty, Bruner JG (Chair). 1997 Survey Summary Report. Arlington Heights, Ill.: American Society of Plastic and Reconstructive Surgeons; 1998.

44. Grazer FM, de Jong RH. Fatal outcomes from liposuction: census survey of cosmetic surgeons. Plast Reconstr Surg 2000;105:436–46.

45. Hughes CE. Reduction of lipoplasty risks and mortality: an ASAPS survey. Aesthet Surg J 2001;21:120–5.

46. Housman TS, Lawrence N, Mellen BG, et al. The safety of liposuction: results of a national survey. Dermatol Surg 2002;28:971–8.

47. Hanke CW, Cox SE, Kuznets N, et al. Tumescent liposuction report performance measurement initiative: national survey results. Dermatol Surg 2004; 30:967–78.

48. Habbema L. Safety of liposuction using exclusively tumescent local anesthesia in 3420 consecutive patients. Dermatol Surg 2009;35:1728–35.

49. Coleman WP III, Hanke CW, Lillis P, et al. Does the location of the surgery or the specialty of the physician affect malpractice claims in liposuction? Dermatol Surg 1999;25:343–7.

50. Coldiron B. Office surgical incidents: 19 months of Florida data. Dermatol Surg 2002;28:710–3.

51. Coldiron B, Schreve E, Balkrishnan R. Patient injuries from surgical procedures performed in medical offices: three years of Florida data. Dermatol Surg 2004;30:1435–43.

52. Geerts WH, Bergqvist D, Pineo GF, et al. Prevention of venous thromboembolism: American College of Chest Physicians evidence-based clinical practice guidelines (8th edition). Chest 2008;133(Suppl 6): 381S–453S.

53. Haeck PC, Swanson JA, Gutowski KA, et al. ASPS Patient Safety Committee evidence-based patient safety advisory: liposuction. Plast Reconstr Surg 2009;124(Suppl 4):28S–44S.

54. Braga LH, Farrokhvar F, Bhandari M. Practical tips for surgical research–confounding: what is it and how do we deal with it? Can J Surg 2012;55(2):132–8.

55. Rao RB, Ely SF, Hoffman RS. Deaths related to liposuction. N Engl J Med 1999;340:1471–5.

56. Hanke CW, Sterling JB, Melton JL, et al. Review of liposuction safety studies. In: Hanke CW, Sattler G, editors. Procedures in cosmetic dermatology series–liposuction. London: Elsevier Saunders; 2005. p. 141–8.

57. Martinez MA, Ballesteros S, Segura LJ, et al. Reporting a fatality during tumescent liposuction. Forensic Sci Int 2008;178:e11–6.

58. Memetoglu ME, Kurtcan S, Kalkan A, et al. Combination technique of tumescent anesthesia during endovenous laser therapy of saphenous vein insufficiency. Interact Cardiovasc Thorac Surg 2010;11(6):774–7.

59. Yoho RA, Romaine JJ, O'Neil D. Review of the liposuction, abdominoplasty, and face-lift mortality and morbidity risk literature. Dermatol Surg 2005;31: 733–43.

60. Narita S, Sakano S, Okamoto S, et al. Tumescent local anesthesia in inguinal herniorrhaphy with a PROLENE hernia system: original technique and results. Am J Surg 2009;198(2):e27–31.

61. Kayaalp C, Olmez A, Aydin C, et al. Tumescent local anesthesia for excision and flap procedures in treatment of pilonidal disease. Dis Colon Rectum 2009;52(10):1780–3.

62. Bertelson CA. Cleft-lift operation for pilonidal sinuses under tumescent local anesthesia: a prospective cohort study of peri- and postoperative pain. Dis Colon Rectum 2011;54(7):895–900.

63. Mizukami T, Hanamoto M. Tumescent local anesthesia for a revascularization of a coronary subclavian steal syndrome. Ann Thorac Cardiovasc Surg 2007;13(5):352–4.

64. Mago V, Prasad M. Tumescent local anesthesia for release of postburn neck contractures. J Burn Care Res 2009;30(6):1049.

65. Kryger ZB, Fine NA, Mustoe TA. The outcome of abdominoplasty performed under conscious sedation: six-year experience in 153 consecutive cases. Plast Reconstr Surg 2004;113(6):1807–17.

66. Hunstad JP, Jones SR. Abdominoplasty with thorough concurrent circumferential abdominal tumescent liposuction. Aesthet Surg J 2011;31(5):572–90.

67. Brauman D, Capocci J. Liposuction abdominoplasty: an advanced body contouring technique. Plast Reconstr Surg 2009;124(5):1685–95.

68. Field LM. Adjunctive liposurgical debulking and flap dissection in neck reconstruction. J Dermatol Surg Oncol 1986;12(9):917–20.

69. Gladwell MT. The tipping point. Boston: Little Brown; 2000.

70. Hanke CW. Advocating for mandatory adverse event reporting. Dermatol Surg 2012;38:178–9.

Hair Transplant and Local Anesthetics

Samuel M. Lam, MD, FACS

KEYWORDS

- Hair transplant • Local anesthesia • Platelet-rich plasma • Robotic follicular-unit extraction
- Hairline design • Hair restoration

KEY POINTS

- The surgeon should understand the natural Norwood hair-loss patterns so as to recreate natural patterns.
- The surgeon should have thorough knowledge of dermatologic conditions that preclude surgery, such as scarring alopecia, and also be well versed in the medical management aspects of hair restoration, such as the use of finasteride and minoxidil.
- The surgeon should understand the principles of good hairline design and the objective of framing the face for aesthetic purposes.
- The surgeon should be technically well versed in recreating the natural angle and direction of recipient sites according to the specific region of the scalp.
- The team should be excellent at both graft preparation and graft placement, and be aware that inferior performance leads to devastating outcomes.
- The surgeon should be a lifetime student, learning new techniques by attending workshops and major conferences as well as reading and analyzing his own work.

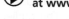 Video of technique for donor and recipient tumescence for hair transplant accompanies this article at www.plasticsurgery.theclinics.com

INTRODUCTION

Hair restoration has advanced remarkably since the bygone era of unnatural "plug" grafting.[1,2] Nevertheless, despite the use of follicular-unit grafting, bad results persist because of technical errors, lack of judgment, and poor artistry. Many plastic and cosmetic surgeons look askance at hair transplantation because it is thought of as an easy procedure to master, which is absolutely not the case, or that it can be taxingly boring and tedious, which is an erroneous perception. Hair restoration, when mastered, can be an extremely rewarding procedure for both the patient and surgeon alike. In this author's opinion hair transplantation is thoroughly enjoyable because artistically designed patterns can be created that fit a patient naturally, will age well for him, and have been created in such a way that provides optimal visual density for the number of grafts transplanted. Besides outlining the fundamentals of what every surgeon should know when performing a hair-transplant procedure, this article also discusses some of the major advances in the past several years in hair restoration, including regenerative medicine (the use of platelet-rich plasma [PRP] and ACell [Acell Inc, Columbia, MD]), and follicular-unit extraction (FUE) methods that obviate a linear scar. Hair transplantation can be undertaken with any level of anesthesia, but because it is essentially a skin-based surgery it can be easily performed from start to finish under local anesthesia only.

Willow Bend Wellness Center, 6101 Chapel Hill Boulevard, Suite 101, Plano, TX 75093, USA
E-mail address: drlam@lamfacialplastics.com

Clin Plastic Surg 40 (2013) 615–625
http://dx.doi.org/10.1016/j.cps.2013.08.006
0094-1298/13/$ – see front matter © 2013 Elsevier Inc. All rights reserved.

plasticsurgery.theclinics.com

TREATMENT GOALS AND PLANNED OUTCOMES

Before outlining what is surgically necessary, the larger scope of understanding the nature of male pattern baldness (MPB) is critical. Discussing every type of hair loss lies beyond the scope of this article, so the focus here is on the principal type of hair loss, MPB. Many surgeons are over-zealous to begin their career in hair restoration without this prerequisite knowledge, and this can be a great disservice to the patient who may encounter a serious problem perhaps not today but in a decade, when the hair-transplant result that originally looked natural now cannot be fixed as a consequence of poor or absent judgment.

The best way to explain the nature of MPB is that hairs transition from thick "terminal" hairs slowly over time into thin, wispy, "vellus" hairs that in turn ultimately disappear altogether to leave a bald pate. Medications such as oral finasteride and topical minoxidil, along with laser technology, are useful if not in fact particularly important in slowing down this process, and any male patient who is in the early process of hair loss should be counseled vigorously on the importance of medi-cal management to slow down and partially re-verse hair loss, and perhaps avoid the need for surgical intervention, at least for the present. Finasteride and minoxidil are synergistic in their benefit and should be considered better together than either alone; they work toward slowing down the conversion of terminal hairs to vellus hairs and also retard the conversion of vellus hairs to absence of hairs, and finally help reconvert hairs from vellus hairs back, at least partly, to thick ter-minal hairs. Their biggest drawback is that once patients stop taking these medications, they lose all the hairs that were preserved during the time they were taking them. Despite this limitation, it is important to counsel every man who is expe-riencing hair loss about how potent these medica-tions are, and also on the patient's suitability as safe candidates for surgery, something that demands further explanation.

The reason that young men (eg, early to mid-twenties) may be unsafe as candidates for hair transplantation is that they may lose more hair over time and not have a sufficient supply of donor hair in the occipital region to cover further hair loss over the longer term. It is a losing battle of in-creasing demand for hair and an ever dwindling supply of donor hair, owing to either further bald-ing or use of the donor hair for transplantation. Taking a step back to explain the preciousness of donor hair may be important here. Norman Orentreich discovered in the 1950s that hair taken from the baldest man (think of a horseshoe config-uration in the occiput) and transplanted to the front of the scalp retains the genetic characteristics of the native donor region; that is, it will not be lost after being moved to the front of the head. How-ever, for young men who are losing hair one cannot predict with absolute accuracy how much donor hair is actually safe to transplant and how their hair loss will progress. At this point the surgeon with experience use considered judgment to prognosticate if there will most likely be enough donor hair to address both present hair loss and additional demands for future transplants going forward. Furthermore, it is important that every budding hair-transplant surgeon also takes the time to review dermatologic conditions that can mimic MPB but that may in fact represent nontransplantable conditions such as scarring alopecia, especially if the physician is not a derma-tologist by training.

PREOPERATIVE PLANNING AND PREPARATION

When planning to perform a hair-transplant proce-dure, the surgeon should keep in mind the afore-mentioned tenets of whether the patient has the proper hair density, usable donor hair, and degree and area of baldness, along with the age of the patient. In addition, it is important to look at how much hair is on the verge of being lost (ie, are mini-aturized or vellus in nature) and may need surgical correction to avoid a problem in the near future of progression of hair loss in that area. The curlier and thicker the hair, the greater the impact the hair-transplant result will be. Furthermore, if the color-to-contrast ratio of scalp to hair is minimal (eg, dark scalp and dark hair or light hair and light scalp), the patient will also potentially have a much improved outcome of visual density because the underlying bald scalp will be less apparent. These factors will all be evaluated by an expert physician when determining the successful outcome of a procedure. Every prospective surgeon should re-view the Norwood-Hamilton (N-H) scale of MPB because these patterns represent the majority of how men lose their hair. When designing a pattern for hair transplantation, it is imperative that the physician follows the rules prescribed by the N-H scale so that the result will mimic nature.

The primary goal in most first cases of hair trans-plantation is to "frame the face"; that is, to provide hair along the frontal region of the scalp so that the person has a more attractive face when hair is there to frame the face. Many men who are thinning throughout may become focused on their crown, which is an important area for transplantation.

Nevertheless, the surgeon in most cases should steer a man toward the importance of framing the front of his scalp first, so that there is a frontal aesthetic benefit. This observation brings up an important corollary point, namely that there typically is not enough hair to transplant both the front of the scalp and the crown in a single session of hair restoration when performing a standard linear harvest from the back of the head. Typically a minimum of 1 year should pass before performing a second donor harvest to ensure that the donor scar is sufficiently healed and relaxed, and also so that most of the hair-transplant result can be observed growing in, thus to determine if a few extra grafts would be beneficial in the previously transplanted zone.

PATIENT POSITIONING

Patient positioning for the procedure is important, and will vary depending on the part of the procedure being undertaken, all of which are detailed in the respective subsections herein.

PROCEDURAL APPROACH
Hairline Design

Hairline design is very important because it represents one of the most tell-tale signs of the artistry and judgment of a surgeon, and will be the most conspicuous and lasting testament to his work. A hairline must not only look natural for today's patients; but with predictive capacity accumulated from experience, a surgeon must also ensure that the hairline will not become incongruous for an individual as he further ages. The lowest acceptable, midline point for the hairline is drawn first with a colored eyebrow pencil and typically represents the 45° intersection of the vertical plane of the scalp (the forehead), and the horizontal plane of the scalp (the hair-bearing scalp) (**Fig. 1**). It must be emphasized that this is the lowest point, but the physician may decide to be more conservative with the design and start higher up. However, if the starting point is too high the physician may fail to frame the face properly. The surgeon then should draw the lateral termini of the hairline where, at a point lateral to this terminus, the temporal hair begins. The lateral terminus of the hairline is situated at a vertical line drawn upward through the lateral canthus of the eye. After drawing this lateral point, the surgeon tilts the head downward to ensure that both lateral points are situated symmetrically both in the anterior-posterior direction and laterally from the midline. The surgeon then should gently connect these dots using a rounded arc with the option to suppress the arc more

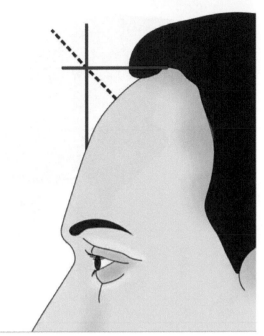

Fig. 1. The lowest acceptable midline, anterior point of a hairline marked at the 45° intersection of the vertical forehead with the horizontal scalp. (*From* Lam SM. Hair transplant 360. vol. 1. Delhi (India): Jaypee Brothers Medical Publishers; 2010.)

concave lateral to the midpupillary line, based on the patient's head shape and other artistic criteria. Once these points are connected, the physician should walk to the side of the patient and ensure that the hairline is either flat along the Frankfort horizontal plane or slopes upward (**Fig. 2**). If the hairline slopes downward from the lateral view, this is not a natural configuration that exists in nature. Finally, the physician should close one eye and use a mirror to evaluate the hairline so that the hairline is observed in a 2-dimensional, flat aspect. Doing so provides rapid feedback as to whether the hairline is reasonably straight, although it may look tilted even though it looks straight 3-dimensionally with both eyes open. The reason for this discrepancy is that the asymmetric topography of bony scalp can throw off the shape of the hairline more on one side than the other. Accordingly, it is important for the physician to marry the best 2-dimensional and 3-dimensional evaluations of a planned hairline. Once the hairline has been confirmed by the patient and the surgeon to be appropriate, the surgeon can then reinforce the initial tentative eyebrow marking with a more tenacious Sharpie permanent marker, but slightly irregularizing the line when drawing it in to ensure that the hairline will be more irregular (ie, natural) than a straight line.

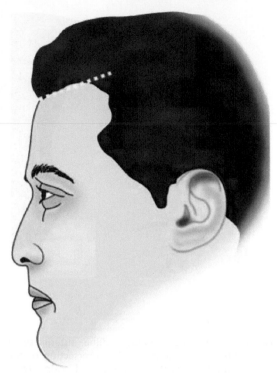

Fig. 2. Side view of the hairline, which should either slope upward or be relatively flat but should never slope downward on the profile view. (*From* Lam SM. Hair transplant 360. vol. 1. Delhi (India): Jaypee Brothers Medical Publishers; 2010.)

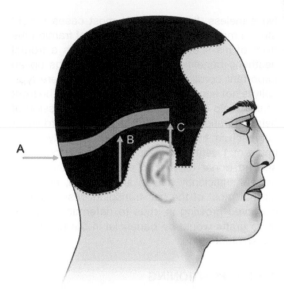

Fig. 3. The parameters of the safe donor hair, starting at the occipital protuberance (A) in the midline, arching upward over the mastoid protuberance (B), and ending approximately 2 fingerbreadths above the superior helix (C). The donor hair can be removed above this point, depending on how sure the surgeon is that advancing recession of hair loss will not encroach on the proposed harvest area. (*From* Lam SM. Hair transplant 360. vol. 1. Delhi (India): Jaypee Brothers Medical Publishers; 2010.)

Donor Planning

Once the area of baldness has been outlined, the surgeon should now plan how many hair grafts will be needed to fill the proposed circumscribed region. One can accomplish this task by first determining how many follicular units (FU) exist per cm^2 in the donor area. For example, if there is observed to be on average 100 FU/cm^2 the donor area and there are 100 cm^2 of area to be transplanted in the recipient area with the desire for approximately 25 FU transplanted per cm^2 in the recipient area, then one will need 25 FU/cm^2 × 100 cm^2 = 2500 FU. If the donor density again is 100 FU/cm^2, one will need to harvest an area of approximately 25 cm long × 1 cm wide to attain the requisite number of grafts to cover the proposed area for transplantation. There will undoubtedly be some transection of hairs during harvesting, so the surgeon should factor 5% to 10% loss when planning the donor area.

The so-called safe donor area is roughly situated around the occipital protuberance in the midline occiput and arches upward to approximately 2 fingerbreadths above the superior helix of the ear (**Fig. 3**). This area is then shaved with a short guard (leaving approximately 1 to 2 mm of hair left) for 2 to 3 cm around the proposed area of harvesting, with the long hair above the incision taped upward to keep it out of the way for donor harvesting. Of note, the patient is sitting upright for the entire period of hairline design, donor planning, and donor harvesting.

Donor Harvesting and Closure

Conscious sedation

See author's video on preparation of donor and recipient tumescence. In his practice the author prefers intravenous level-2 conscious sedation for performing hair-transplant procedures. However, most clinics rely on simple oral narcotics and anxiolytics to perform their procedures, with minimal discomfort. The first goal is to anesthetize the donor and recipient area by performing a ring block around the head that anesthetizes the entire area superior to the ring block. Before the ring block is administered, the author prefers to start with a supraorbital nerve block using 0.25% bupivacaine with 1:100,000 epinephrine for a total of 0.5 mL per side. The physician palpates the supraorbital notch with his nondominant thumb and then injects below the notch using a 30-gauge needle, withdrawing first to ensure that it is not intra-arterial. Injecting the patient with this anesthetic first truly makes the anterior half of the ring block significantly less uncomfortable and also tends to allow the anesthesia of the anterior half of the scalp to be more uniformly long lasting, to the completion of the procedure in most cases, whereas not doing so many lead to more irregular longevity of the anterior ring block.

Ring block

After the supraorbital block is administered, the ring block can now be performed. During the injection of the circumferential ring block of anesthesia, if the patient is not receiving intravenous sedation a vibration anesthesia device (Blaine Labs, Santa Fe Springs, CA) can be used to further mitigate the pain. Ten milliliters of 1% lidocaine with 1:100,000 epinephrine is infiltrated into the subcutaneous plane along the inferior border of the planned donor area, and an additional 10 mL of 1% lidocaine with 1:100,000 epinephrine is infiltrated to complete the anterior half of the ring block, ensuring that the block circumscribes the area below the planned hairline and area for transplantation. The anesthetic is slowly infiltrated, which can truly minimize the pain, and a buffered solution is avoided because it has been shown to possibly increase the postoperative edema along the forehead. Current opinion states that the speed of anesthesia delivery has more bearing on the level of perceived discomfort than does rendering the anesthetic more alkaline in nature.

Once the ring-block anesthetic has been administered, it is imperative that the donor area be adequately tumesced with fluid (consisting of 250 mL 0.9% sodium chloride, 1.25 mL epinephrine 1:1000, and 12.5 mL plain lidocaine 2%) to minimize transection of underlying neurovascular structures and of the individual hairs planned for harvesting. Approximately 100 to 250 mL tumescent fluid is rapidly injected into the subcutaneous plane until the tissue feels rigid and appears flat and blanched. At this time, the physician may begin to undertake the donor harvest. The injector developed by Cole Instruments (Atlanta, GA) allows for rapid infusion of tumescent anesthesia; it involves a 3-mL syringe outfitted to a spring-loaded trigger that siphons from a 250-mL intravenous bag hanging superior to it. The author prefers to use a multiblade instrument that houses 2 blades, to ensure that the donor width will be uniformly 1 cm. However, a multiblade device increases the risk of transection in inexperienced hands, and the surgeon may elect to use a single-blade device. If he does so, he should mark the 1-cm width using a Sharpie permanent marker to ensure that too narrow or too wide a strip would not be inadvertently removed, which would lead to inadequate grafts or too much closing tension, respectively. A No. 10 Personna blade is used as the harvesting instrument of choice, whether a single-blade or double-blade approach is used.

Donor harvesting should progress very slowly, ensuring that the blades are not transecting the hair shafts, adjusting the blades upward or downward when transection is evident. In addition, as mentioned previously, care should be taken to avoid cutting beyond the base of the hair follicles where the nerve and blood supply could be compromised. The neophyte surgeon must be aware that it is imperative to stay far above the galea and not to ever go through it, as this will destroy the nerve and blood supply and also exponentially increase closing tension. A pair of Metzenbaum scissors is used to remove the donor strip, which is in turn placed immediately into a chilled saline bath in preparation for graft dissection (see later discussion). To reduce closing tension exacerbated by the recently applied tumescent fluid, the surgeon should use towel clamps placed across the wound to aid with dispersion of the remaining fluid before donor closure commences. Once the donor strip has been removed, the surgeon can then close the donor incision with a running, nonlocking 3-0 nylon suture with the needle passing approximately through the mid-follicular depth. After the donor incision is closed, 10 mL of 0.25% bupivacaine with 1:200,000 epinephrine mixed with 0.1 mL of triamcinolone 40 mg/mL is infiltrated along the posterior half of the ring block to reinforce it, and 10 mL of 0.25% bupivacaine with 1:200,000 epinephrine without triamcinolone is infiltrated along the anterior half of the ring block. The plane of infiltration is in the subcutaneous plane. The patient is then placed into a supine position in preparation for recipient-site creation.

Recipient-Site Creation

Recipient-site creation is one of the highest expressions of a surgeon's artistic ability, making hair-transplant work satisfying and enjoyable. It is important that the recipient sites be created in such a way that the angle (the anterior-posterior direction of a recipient site) and the direction (the radial pointing either forward or laterally to one side of the recipient site) are done to mimic how hair naturally grows on the head (**Fig. 4**) and for maximal visual density. It lies beyond the scope

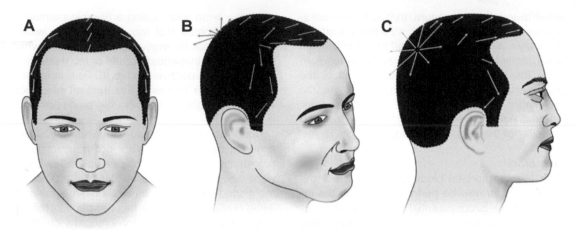

Fig. 4. (*A–C*) How hair grows differently in the various regions of the scalp, which will dictate how recipient sites are created to ensure natural results. (*From* Lam SM. Hair transplant 360. vol. 1. Delhi (India): Jaypee Brothers Medical Publishers; 2010.)

of this article to detail how hair grows on every region of the scalp, so the focus here is on the male hairline and the central area of density behind it known as the central forelock. There are many ways to create recipient sites, including needles and micro punches; also, if a needle is used there is variation as to whether the direction of the slit runs in the anterior-posterior direction (known as a sagittal or parallel site) or side-to-side (known as a coronal or perpendicular site). For the sake of simplicity, only parallel (sagittal) sites made by needles are discussed here. In general, standard needles bent twice to match the length of a dissected graft (**Fig. 5**) are made, with 20-gauge (which generally accommodates 1-hair grafts), 19-gauge (for 2-hair grafts), and 18-gauge (for 3- and 4-hair grafts) needles. It is important that the

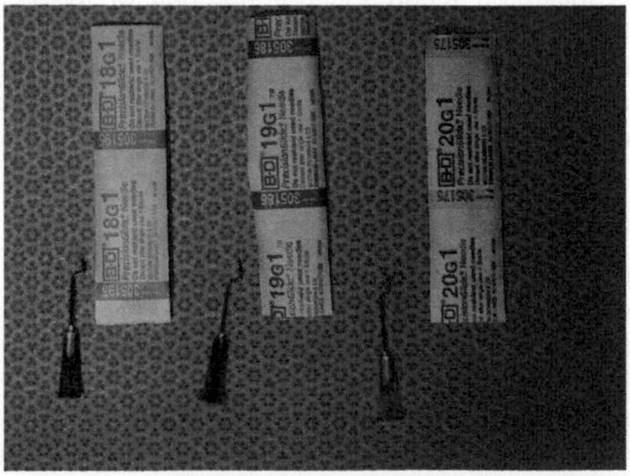

physician tests placing the dissected grafts into 2 to 3 test sites for each size of needle to ensure that the depth and width of each site will fit the dissected graft. Once confirmed, the surgeon can create all of the recipient sites feeling certain that the grafts should fit his sites. Recipient tumescent fluid (100 mL of 0.9% sodium chloride, 0.5 mL epinephrine 1:1000, 5.0 mL 2% plain lidocaine, and 1.0 mL triamcinolone 40 mg/mL) is injected subcutaneously in a sequential fashion into the subcutaneous plane in each area where the surgeon is making recipient sites, to minimize trauma to the underlying neurovascular supply. Typically a total of 50 to 100 mL of recipient tumescent fluid is infiltrated in total into the recipient area over a period of from 1 to 2 hours that is required to make recipient sites, typically in boluses of 5 to 15 mL at a time.

The first order of business is to create a natural and sufficiently dense hairline. It is important that all hairline and midscalp recipient sites have a direction that faces forward and does not splay radially outward. In addition, all of the recipient sites must have a very low angle (ie, low anteriorly). The surgeon can ensure that he keeps a low angle by having the patient in a fully supine position, which will help his hand to naturally fall into a very low anterior angle for site creation. The low angle is important because the hairs will shingle over the scalp like an awning, and thereby create a more favorable shadow over the naked scalp. Also, the low-angled grafts will appear more natural because one cannot see their point of insertion into the scalp as well, an area that can look unnatural because of imperfect graft placement (see later discussion). The

Fig. 5. Three bent needles used to make recipient sites. The 18-gauge generally accommodates 3-hair grafts; the 19-gauge, 2-hair grafts; and the 20-gauge, 1-hair grafts.

reason that the grafts cannot splay open radially on the scalp is that this method will lead to an uncombable result and also reduce visual density where it counts, which is in the central forelock and anterior hairline. If anything, the recipient sites can slightly converge medially to improve visual density in the midline of the scalp, where the central forelock is situated. Furthermore, the recipient sites should be tightly interlocked and not arranged in a parallel fashion; that is, each successive row of recipient sites should be staggered from the one in front of it. By doing so, the grafts will create more visual density and also be able to be more tightly arranged. The author begins by creating the irregularly irregular hairline using a 19-gauge needle along the anterior hairline that will accommodate 2-hair grafts and continue backward for 2 to 3 cm to complete the main hairline zone (**Fig. 6**A, B), before creating 1 to 2 rows of recipient sites using the 20-gauge needle to accommodate 1-hair

grafts and to frame the 2-hair grafts. In addition, occasionally floating "sentinel" 1-hair grafts are placed to further blur the linearity of the hairline (see **Fig. 6**C). Finally, the author builds the wall of central density behind the hairline zone with recipient sites made with an 18-gauge needle to accommodate 3-hair and the less frequently encountered 4-hair grafts (see **Fig. 6**D). Discussion of how to build temporal hairline, temporal points, crown, female hairlines, and so forth lie beyond this introductory article, and the reader is encouraged not to perform any of these advanced recipient-site techniques until the basic hairline and midscalp density design has been sufficiently mastered.

Graft Preparation (Slivering and Graft Dissection)

Typically the surgeon is not responsible for graft preparation, but as the team leader he should

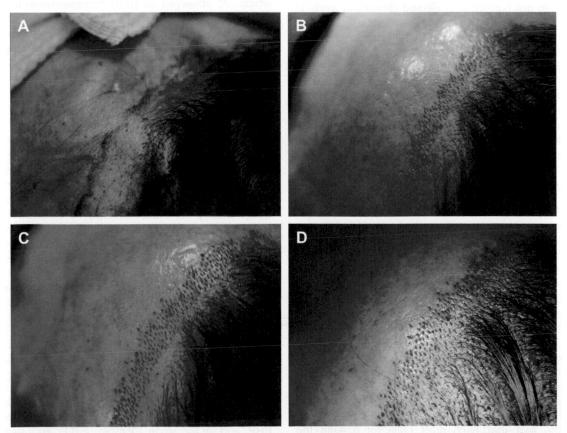

Fig. 6. (*A*) Close-up view shows a hairline drawn in preparation for creation of the recipient sites. (*B*) The first step in recipient-site creation, whereby a 19-gauge needle is used to create sites for the hairline zone to accommodate 2-hair grafts. (*C*) Next, 1 to 2 rows of 20-gauge sites are made to accommodate 1-hair grafts in addition to free-floating "sentinel" single hairs that stand in front and separate from the hairline to further blur the linearity of the hairline appearance. (*D*) Finally, an 18-gauge needle is used to make the rows behind the hairline to accommodate 3- and 4-hair grafts, to further support the visual density of the anterior hairline.

understand the dynamics of what constitutes good graft preparation to ensure that his results are of excellent quality. Without a properly trained and dedicated team, no matter how beautiful the surgeon's work is, the ultimate result will fall far short of the desired aesthetic mark.

Graft preparation involves 2 steps:

1. Slivering
2. Graft dissection

The linear strip of the harvested donor tissue must be first sliced across the short axis of the donor strip in an act known as slivering. Slivering involves cutting a single row of follicular units with the aid of microscopic magnification and illumination. It is analogous to cutting a slice of bread from a loaf. Once the sliver is created, the grafts can be dissected into individual 1-, 2-, 3-, and 4-hair grafts in a process known as graft dissection. Minimal manipulation and transection of the grafts along with maintaining uniform size (based on the cuff of fat that surrounds each follicular unit) are hallmarks of elegant dissection work. In addition, graft preparation would ideally be undertaken in a timely fashion to minimize ex vivo graft time, but quality should trump quantity and speed in the early phases of team development. Keeping hair-transplant sessions to very low numbers, in the 100s of grafts rather than thousands, may be a good start for any new surgeon and team. One can even split the sessions into multiple days to limit ex vivo time and team fatigue when the staff and physician are in the nascent training phase.

Graft Placement

After the recipient sites are completed and the grafts have been properly dissected (keeping them hydrated throughout in a chilled saline bath), the grafts must be placed into the recipient sites based on their respective size. A drawing may be made on the electronic medical record indicating the distribution of recipient-site sizes so that staff has a better understanding of how to place the grafts into the proper-sized sites (**Fig. 7**). Just as with optimal graft preparation, grafts must be minimally manipulated during insertion and also must be well hydrated. Besides putting grafts into the right-sized site, the grafts must be angled correctly so that the natural curl of the hair faces forward and down. The curl refers to the fact that each graft curls as it exits the epidermis. Also, the grafts must be placed at the right depth, typically about 1 to 2 mm above the surrounding native tissue, because they will sink with resolution of edema. It is important that the grafts do not sit flush to the skin because they

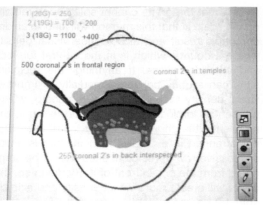

Fig. 7. Schematic in the electronic medical record to document the number, orientation, and sizes of recipient sites for future reference, and also to be used as a guide to help the assistant team place grafts more effectively and accurately into the premade recipient sites.

will sink inward and potentially cause pitting, which are observed as small depressions in the skin at the insertion site. If they sit more than 2 mm above the surrounding skin they can cause a cobblestoned appearance, or the graft may desiccate and die. To minimize graft trauma, the graft should be tucked into the site in 2 strokes:

Stroke 1: to push the graft halfway inward
Stroke 2: to push the graft all the way in

By doing this, the graft has less chance of folding over or popping out.

Another potentially devastating mistake is to "piggy-back" one graft over another, which can cause buried grafts underneath and engender cysts. Clearly there are many points of concern in performing excellent graft preparation and graft placement, and this section has only brushed the surface of technical competency required to ensure consistently superior results and avoid surgical misadventures. There is no substitute for proper training and experience to facilitate excellent outcomes.

Advances in Hair Transplantation

There is no doubt that the most significant development in the last decade with regard to hair restoration is the advent of regenerative medicine to support graft growth. The author has been using PRP and ACell since October 2011, and has witnessed a remarkable improvement in hair-transplant results, not in terms of shortening the recovery period but in terms of more uniform graft growth, higher percentage of grafts growing, finer appearing grafts, and faster onset to graft growth (typically as early as 4 months when noticeable growth was observed, rather than prior to this era at around 6 months). The author believes that both PRP and ACell are required to achieve such results. Without ACell, the grafts do not appear as fine as when enlisting both products. A method is used to integrate the products whereby the PRP drawn at the outset of the case (it is important to draw it before any physical trauma to the patient) is mixed with 100 mg of fine-powdered ACell. The majority of the mixture is injected immediately after the ring block into the subcutaneous tissue of the recipient bed. The remainder is placed into the donor incision after closure, and the rest bathed around the grafts before graft placement.

Another advance over the past decade has been the use of FUE, whereby no linear scar is present. The author has found the ARTAS robotic FUE system (Restoration Robotics, Mountain View, CA) to be a reliable device with which to perform FUE. There are many competing companies offering a version of this technique. To debate and discuss the pros and cons of FUE lie beyond the scope of this article. At present, about two-thirds of the author's cases still use linear harvesting, with one-third being FUE based.

POTENTIAL COMPLICATIONS AND MANAGEMENT

Complications can occur at every stage of a hair-transplant procedure, and caution should be exercised throughout every phase. Starting with good judgment about who is a proper candidate as outlined in the preoperative section, the physician should know on whom to operate and on whom not to operate. Sometimes complications do not arise until further down the road when the patient runs out of donor hair and is left with an unnatural result. As mentioned earlier, the art of estimating how much usable donor hair is available must be acquired over time so that patients are not left as "hair cripples." Proper hairline design that fits a patient's age, ethnicity, gender, facial shape, and degree of hair loss, and that will age well for that person over time, are important considerations. If a hairline is too low it is difficult to repair, but if it is too high it may lack the aesthetic raison d'être of a hairline: to frame the face properly.

During the surgical procedure, improper donor harvesting may lead to a high transection rate, nerve damage, and widened scarring. These conditions are hard to repair, and widened scarring typically is not as easily amenable to excision but often needs targeted FUE grafting into it for partial success. Recently, the trend has been to micropigment the scar with punctate tattoos, to simulate

hair and mask the area where graft take of revision FUE grafts may be poor. As mentioned earlier, recipient-site creation must follow the angle and direction outlined in **Fig. 4**. If a surgeon does not understand how hairs naturally grow on a scalp, he will be unable to create natural results. If the unnatural sites sparsely cover the head and reside above a desired and proposed new hairline, the surgeon can correct these errors by overpowering the grafts with better grafting. When the grafts, or worse yet, plugs, are too strong or too low, they will most likely need to be punch excised and recycled in smaller and better ways. Again micropigmentation may be enlisted as needed to salvage the problem. Unfortunately, because hair takes between 6 months and a year to grow, bad results performed months previously will not be evident for some time. This delay further impedes a surgeon's ability to review his work on a timely basis, and may lead to multiple poor surgical cases before the error or change of technique can be rectified.

Graft preparation and graft placement offer a wide spectrum of opportunity for additional failure. Excessive graft manipulation can lead to kinky hair growth. If grafts are poorly trimmed, they may not fit the sites, may desiccate and die, may be transected and lost, and so forth. There is a host of problems that can arise from poor graft handling, which may lead to many errors that reinforce the tenet that a team is of commensurate importance to the surgeon leading the team (**Figs. 8–10**). Quality must be ensured at every phase by every team member to achieve superiorly consistent outcomes.

POSTPROCEDURE CARE

At the end of the case, the patient's head is blow dried at a cool setting to seal in the grafts. The author prefers not to use any emollients or occlusive dressings, but some surgeons do advocate these supplemental measures. If temple hair is transplanted, the patient is asked not to wear a baseball cap for 24 hours, as these hairs are very susceptible to being displaced with the abrasion of donning or doffing a hat. Otherwise wearing a hat is absolutely acceptable. Showering should not be resumed for 24 hours from the time of concluding the operative case. Thereafter, the patient is encouraged to shower twice daily with nonirritating baby shampoo at a very low shower pressure. The patient is also warned that the back incision can feel tight, numb, uncomfortable, pruritic, or some combination of these sensations, especially until sutures are removed on the 10th postoperative day. The patient is warned that

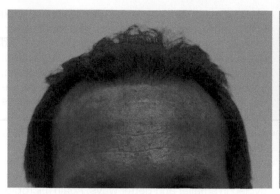 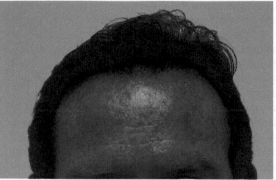

Fig. 8. (*Left*) Male patient after an unnatural hair transplant. The hairline is too straight, the grafts are too large for the hairline, and the grafts do not fit the sites and are too large, being compressed into a doll's-head appearance. (*Right*) The same patient after correction of the transplant. There is a more natural-appearing hairline shape, with proper graft sizes for the various points of the hairline and behind the hairline zone.

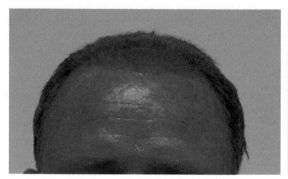 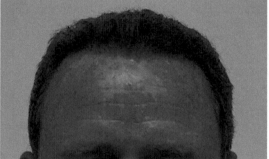

Fig. 9. (*Left*) Male patient after an unnatural hair transplant. The hairline is too straight, the hair grafts appear too kinky because of excessive manipulation during graft placement, and the hair has sparse density. (*Right*) The same patient after correction of his hairline. The hair is far more natural and denser.

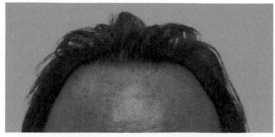 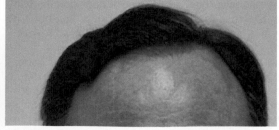

Fig. 10. (*Left*) Male patient after an unnatural hair transplant. The hairline is too straight, the grafts are too large for the hairline, and they sit too perpendicularly (high angle) to the scalp. (*Right*) The same patient after correction of his hairline. The hair is far more natural and denser.

exuberant edema can be evident along the brow and midface for the first 2 to 5 days, sometimes lasting up to a week, and that he should not be concerned. The patient may be encouraged to use hand manipulation to sweep the edema around the orbital rim down into the face to expedite the resolution of the unsightly edema. Scabs that remain after a week should be vigorously scrubbed to be removed after that time (a process that can be facilitated by using a topical emollient hair conditioner to soften them for a few minutes) or they may interfere with graft growth. The patient should avoid submersing his head in water of any kind (as most water is a source of infection) for a minimum of 6 weeks. The patient can resume exercise early on, with care taken not to overtly traumatize the grafts and especially not to injure the newly sealed donor region.

SUMMARY

The comprehensive art and science of hair transplantation cannot be effectively communicated in a brief article. However, the pertinent overview of facts and philosophy can be underscored so that a prospective surgeon who is looking to enter the field can understand the requisite knowledge required by himself and his team, so that patients may enjoy the great reward that hair restoration offers when done properly, and so that the surgeon and his team can also reap the same reward in providing the solution to their patient.

VIDEOS ONLINE

Supplementary data in the form of video related to this article can be found online at http://dx.doi.org/10.1016/j.cps.2013.08.006.

REFERENCES

1. Lam SM. Hair transplant 360, vol. 1. Delhi (India): Jaypee Brothers Medical Publishers; 2010.
2. Karamanovski E. Hair transplant 360, vol. 2. Delhi (India): Jaypee Brothers Medical Publishers; 2010.

Rhinoplasty with Intravenous and Local Anesthesia

Michael Sklar, BSc, MD[a], Jerod Golant, BSc, MD, FRCPC[b],
Philip Solomon, BSc, MD, FRCSC[c],*

KEYWORDS

• Anesthesia • Rhinoplasty • Sedation • Open technique

KEY POINTS

• Procedural sedation for rhinoplasty is best achieved with combination local anesthesia and systemic pharmacology.
• In our practice, 80% of rhinoplasty is performed via a closed technique with a cartilage delivery approach to address the nasal tip.
• General anesthesia is used at the patient's request and for long and difficult cases.

 Videos of Local Anesthesia; Cartilage Delivery; Dorsal Exposure; Dorsal Reduction; Osteotomies; Caudal Septoplasty; and Retrograde Cephalic Trim accompany this article at http://www.plasticsurgery.theclinics.com/

SEDATION FOR RHINOPLASTY

Procedural sedation for a rhinoplasty, like any procedure, relies on careful patient selection and patient and surgeon compliance (**Fig. 1**).[1,2,3,4,5,6] Patients should have an American Society of Anesthesia (ASA) score of 1 or 2, with a possibly well-controlled 3 also acceptable, and should be devoid of certain comorbidities, including obstructive sleep apnea, gastroesophageal reflux disease, and obesity (body mass index ≥35).

Before the procedure begins, clinicians must explicitly communicate to patients that they will feel no pain; however, because they are being sedated, they may know what is occurring at the time of surgery. A common misconception about sedation is that it involves general anesthesia without an airway. Clinicians must reassure patients that the anesthetist will be with them the entire time, and any discomfort can be dealt with immediately and the anesthesia titrated to an acceptable level.

ANESTHETIC TECHNIQUE

For the actual anesthetic technique, given that this is an anesthetic for airway surgery with a shared airway with the surgeon, certain goals must be maintained at all times.

• Immediate access to the airway is not always accessible, thus the level of sedation must be on a plane of anesthesia that allows the patient to maintain their oxygen saturation, hemodynamics, and airway reflexes to prevent aspiration of blood and gastric contents.
• Like any anesthetic, nothing-by-mouth guidelines as per the ASA must be met before the procedure is started.

Anesthesia can be administered in multiple ways. This article provides insight into the authors' technique; however, each anesthetic must be tapered to the individual needs of the surgeon, patient, and anesthesiologist.

[a] Department of Otolaryngology - Head & Neck Surgery, University of Toronto, St. George Campus, 190 Elizabeth Street, Rm 3S438, RFE Building, Toronto, Ontario M5G 2N2, Canada; [b] Department of Anesthesia, Mackenzie Health, 10 Trench Street, Richmond Hill, Ontario L4C 4Z3, Canada; [c] Division of Facial Plastic and Reconstructive Surgery, Department of Otolaryngology - Head & Neck Surgery, Mackenzie Health, St. Michael's Hospital, University of Toronto, 30 Bond Street, Toronto, Ontario M5B 1W8, Canada
* Corresponding author.
E-mail address: cpsolomon@rogers.com

Clin Plastic Surg 40 (2013) 627–629
http://dx.doi.org/10.1016/j.cps.2013.08.002

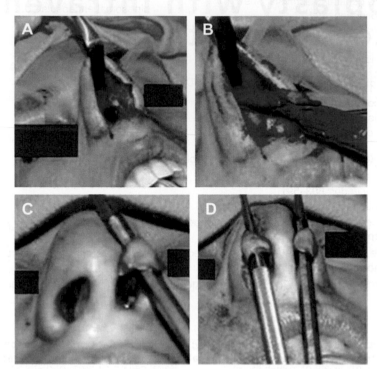

Fig. 1. Demonstration of open rhinoplasty technique. (*A, B*) Dorsal cartilage reduction. (*C, D*) Cartilage delivery technique.

1. The procedure begins with preoxygenation through a facemask delivering a minimum of 8 liters per minute of oxygen. The standard monitors are applied to the patient (eg, noninvasive blood pressure amplifier, electrocardiogram, pulse oximeter).
2. Through a free-flowing intravenous tube connected to saline or lactated Ringer solution, a cocktail is injected consisting of the following:
   - Anxiolytic medication, such as a benzodiazepine (2–3 mg of midazolam)
   - Short-acting narcotic (50–100 μg of fentanyl)
   - An antinausea medication with sedative properties (diphenhydramine, 50 mg)

This injection provides the baseline sedation for the procedure. Subsequently, every 30 to 60 minutes, depending on the level of the patient's sedation, the authors "top-up" with 1 mg of midazolam and 50 μg of fentanyl for the duration of the case.

SURGICAL INFILTRATION

Surgical infiltration is achieved with lidocaine 1% diluted to 1:100,000 with epinephrine. For maximal vasoconstrictive effects, the authors recommend allowing 10 to 15 minutes between the initial incision and the final injection of local anesthetic.

- The authors begin their local infiltration technique of the upper lateral cartilage with a long 27-gauge needle, and it is continued along the lateral wall of the dorsum between perichondrium and the periosteum of the nasal bones.
- They then perform columellar anesthesia through introducing the needle at the columellar-nostril junction and infiltrating to the contralateral alar facial junction.
- The opposite side is then infiltrated.
- The vestibular skin on the inferior surface of the lower lateral cartilages is then infiltrated to target the nasal tip.
- Finally, injection along the plane of the lateral osteotomies is performed, as described later.

To further decongest and reduce bleeding throughout the procedure and decrease nasopharyngeal pooling, nasal pledgets soaked in 1:1000 epinephrine are placed in the nose bilaterally, and these stay in for the duration of the procedure (Video 1). The pledgets are moist but not oversaturated in epinephrine.

PROCEDURAL TECHNIQUE

In the authors' clinic, approximately 80% of the rhinoplasties are performed via a closed technique. Most of these procedures involve a cartilage delivery technique to address the nasal tip. In certain situations a retrograde tip-plasty is performed. Of the cases, 15% to 20% are performed with an open technique using a transcolumellar incision. Indications for the open technique include severely twisted noses requiring mid-third reconstruction, and this is the preferred technique in certain revision procedures.

The delivery approach is believed to be highly versatile and allows suture techniques, cartilage incision, excision, and tip cartilage grafting.

Cartilage delivery is described here and in Video 2:

- The upper lateral cartilage is identified and an intercartilaginous incision is made in the projecting rim of the upper lateral cartilage.
- The skin and soft tissue structure is then manipulated and elevated free from the underlying cartilaginous skeleton (Video 3).
- At the inferior margin of the lower lateral cartilage, a curved incision is made in the vestibular skin.
- The lateral crural and dome cartilage is dissected and made mobile for delivery through the nostril, where cartilage reduction and reshaping can occur (Videos 4–6).

Retrograde dissection is chosen when only subtle reductions of the nasal tip are required to achieve the desired cosmetic goal. Retrograde dissection is performed through an intercartilaginous incision. The cephalic edge of the lower lateral cartilage is exposed and trimmed (Video 7).

Open technique rhinoplasty allows for direct visualization of the skeletal and cartilaginous framework. In the open technique, the overlying skin and soft tissue is reflected off of the underlying cartilaginous and boney framework. Optimum visualization allows for precise calculated reduction and augmentation techniques. Debate continues regarding the pros, cons, and indications for open versus closed rhinoplasty techniques. Generally, both procedures can produce excellent results. Rhinoplasty surgeons must pick the technique they feel most comfortable with to achieve the desired surgical outcome.

ADJUNCT TECHNIQUES FOR PATIENT COMFORT DURING RHINOPLASTY

The authors have adopted several adjunct techniques to aid in patient comfort. Vibratory stimulation is successful in some patients. Using commercially available vibration tools, the activation of larger myelinated sensory fibers and dampening of pain-transmitting C fibers has helped with patient comfort. Additionally, soft music, nature sounds, running water, or patient-requested music can be played during infiltration and induction. Some clinics use acupuncture needles in the neck; however, this technique is not used in the authors' practice.

The choice of anesthetic protocol depends on both patient and surgical factors. When the choice is made to proceed with local anesthetic alone, intramuscular antiemetic, oral analgesia, and full anesthetic monitoring are used. Cases typically chosen for this approach include caudal septal deflections for nostril asymmetry, caudal septal shortening, and alar base reduction alone. Intravenous and local sedation is generally chosen for patients who do not desire general anesthetic, procedures that can be performed in less than 80 minutes, and isolated dorsal hump reductions with or without osteotomies or dorsal hump reductions combined with a straightforward nasal tip-plasty, including cephalic trim and domal sutures.

The authors offer general anesthetic in the following situations:

- If requested by the patient
- When cases are expected to take longer than 80 minutes
- When cases are intuited to be complex in nature

The aforementioned are general principles. In every case, the authors consider the patient and the comorbidities and anatomy, and then choose the best anesthetic and surgical approach.

VIDEOS ONLINE

Supplementary data in the form of videos related to this article can be found online at http://dx.doi.org/10.1016/j.cps.2013.08.002.

REFERENCES

1. Adams WP Jr, Rohrich RJ, Hollier LH, et al. Anatomic basis and clinical implications for nasal tip support in open versus closed rhinoplasty. Plast Reconstr Surg 1999;103:255–61.
2. Bailey BJ, Johnson JT, Newlands SD. Head & neck surgery: otolaryngology. Baltimore MD: Lippincott Williams & Wilkins; 2006.
3. Behmand RA, Ghavami A, Guyuron B. Nasal tip sutures part I: the evolution. Plast Reconstr Surg 2003;112:1125–9.
4. Cummings CW, Flint PW, Phelps T, et al. Cummings otolaryngology: head & neck surgery. Philadelphia PA: Mosby/Elsevier; 2010.
5. Kamer FM, Pieper PG. Nasal tip surgery: a 30-year experience. Facial Plast Surg Clin North Am 2004; 12:81–92.
6. Metzinger SE, Bailey DJ, Boyce RG, et al. Local anesthesia in rhinoplasty: a new twist? Ear Nose Throat J 1992;71:405.

Oculoplastic Surgery

Sonul Mehta, MD, Michel J. Belliveau, MD, FRCSC,
James H. Oestreicher, MD, FRCSC*

KEYWORDS

- Blepharoplasty • Ptosis • Levator palpebrae advancement
- Tarso-mullers muscle-conjunctival resection • Lateral tarsal strip • Punctoplasty
- Full-thickness excision of marginal eyelid lesion • Eyelid retraction

KEY POINTS

- By manually lifting a ptotic eyelid to a normal anatomic position, a ptosis of the contralateral upper lid can often be unmasked (Hering effect).
- Laxity of the lower lid causes ectropion or entropion. The lateral tarsal strip procedure is an effective way to restore tension.
- Punctal stenosis can cause excessive tearing. Three-snip punctoplasty increases tear flow into the canaliculus.
- When excising a marginal eyelid lesion with a full-thickness resection, it is important to reapproximate the tarsus and eyelid margin accurately to prevent lid notching.
- When removing orbital fat in blepharoplasty surgery, meticulous attention to hemostasis can reduce the risk of immediate and delayed post-septal hemorrhage.

INTRODUCTION

Esthetic and functional surgery in the periocular region falls into the domain of oculoplastic surgeons, as well as plastic surgeons and otorhinolaryngologists with training in facial plastic surgery. The presence of the eye in the vicinity of the surgically targeted tissues requires careful attention. Inadvertent touching of the ocular surface by instruments, suture material, or cautery can easily lead to corneal and/or conjunctival damage. Disastrous consequences, such as ocular penetration by a needle during administration of local anesthetic or postseptal hemorrhage, can lead to blindness. Disruption of the eyelid protective function, caused in particular by excessive upper lid tissue removal or ptosis overcorrection, can lead to exposure of the cornea. This requires aggressive lubrication with artificial tears and gels to prevent epithelial compromise and risk of corneal ulceration, which can be vision threatening.

This article provides a description of 8 common eyelid procedures that are routinely performed under local anesthesia, with or without mild intravenous sedation. It is important to tell the patient that a needle is being injected close to the eye, that he or she will feel a pinch as the needle is being injected, and that it is imperative that he or she not move. When injecting near the eye, it is important for the surgeon to stabilize his or her hand on the patient's face, so that if there is any surprise movement, the hand will follow, and any undesired complication is avoided. We instill a drop of 0.5% proparacaine or 0.5–1% tetracaine into each eye before injection of local anesthesia and add additional drops during the procedure as an adjunct as required. We prefer a 50:50 mix of lidocaine 2% with epinephrine (1:100,000) and bupivacaine 0.5% as the local anesthetic for the procedures discussed. Small-gauge (25 to 30 G) needles are used.

Postoperative care includes ophthalmic antibiotic ointment applied 3 to 4 times daily for 2 weeks. This causes temporary blurring of vision, so patients are advised to time application with activities, such as driving and reading, accordingly. We recommend acetaminophen, with or without codeine, for pain control. Patients are instructed to apply ice-cold water compresses at all times

Department of Ophthalmology and Vision Sciences, University of Toronto, Suite 309, 1033 Bay Street, Toronto, Ontario M5S 3A5, Canada
* Corresponding author.
E-mail address: james.oestreicher@gmail.com

Clin Plastic Surg 40 (2013) 631–651
http://dx.doi.org/10.1016/j.cps.2013.08.005

while awake for the first 72 hours to minimize bruising and swelling. We suggest that they place ice and water in a large bowl and alternate between 2 facecloths every 5 minutes to maximize the effect. We recommend that patients sleep on their back with their head elevated for the first couple of weeks following surgery to minimize swelling and reduce the risk of wound dehiscence.

Serious complications are rare. The rate of postoperative infection in the highly vascularized eyelid tissues is less than 1% in our experience. We reserve routine oral antibiotic use for hard palate mucosal grafting to the eyelid where infection in the oral cavity is the principal concern, and following lateral tarsal strip where infection, albeit rare, can lead to dehiscence of the strip and failure. Postseptal hemorrhage is an uncommon but vision-threatening complication and may occur in any procedure in which the orbital septum is violated. The incidence following blepharoplasty has been estimated at 1/2000 to 1/25,000.[1] Orbital fat removal increases the risk, as vessels are directly severed. Cutting of clamped fat pedicles followed by bipolar cautery before release and subsequent retraction posteriorly into the orbit, or use of a CO_2 laser for cutting are 2 commonly used techniques that are believed to reduce the risk. Blepharoplasty is associated with a multitude of complications. We have comprehensively reviewed the prevention and management of many of the complications of blepharoplasty in a freely accessible article available in PubMed Central.[2]

PROCEDURE 1: LEVATOR PALPEBRAE ADVANCEMENT PTOSIS REPAIR

Synopsis–Description of the anterior approach to upper lid ptosis repair by levator palpebrae advancement.

Introduction

This is the classic approach to upper lid ptosis repair involving an external incision into the eyelid skin crease. It can be performed under local anesthesia without intravenous (IV) sedation. The upper lid is infiltrated subcutaneously with 3 mL of local anesthetic ensuring distribution throughout the upper lid, including the lid margin. Our preferred delivery is by serial puncture (3–4) with a short needle rather than a single puncture with a longer needle. This minimizes inadvertent loss of the desired plane.

Treatment Goals and Planned Outcomes

1. To raise the upper eyelid to match the lid height of the contralateral eyelid, or to return both to the original anatomic position if the ptosis is bilateral.

2. To maintain lid contour.
3. To hide the incision within the existing lid crease, or to create a new lid crease in a more desirable location.

Preoperative Planning and Preparation

It is important to assess the position of the contralateral upper lid. By the lifting the ptotic lid to a normal anatomic position, a ptosis of the contralateral upper lid can often be unmasked (Hering effect).

Patient Positioning

1. Supine.
2. Lid position checked with patient upright before levator suture secured.

Procedural Approach

1. The lid crease is identified and marked with the patient upright before sterile draping.
2. A #15 blade is used to incise skin to the level of orbicularis oculi.
3. Blunt dissection is used to clear the orbicularis exposing the orbital septum.
4. Attention is next directed to the tarsus. Orbicularis is removed from the superior one-half to one-third of the tarsus to ensure that the levator will be directly attached.
5. The septum is then breached by sharp dissection exposing the preaponeurotic orbital fat. The fat is teased aside using fine forceps or moistened cotton swabs bringing the levator aponeurosis into view.
6. The distal end of the levator aponeurosis is then engaged with a 6-0 monofilament polypropylene suture. The suture is then passed partial thickness through the upper one-third of the tarsus. The lid is immediately everted to confirm that the suture is not visible on the conjunctival surface. The distal end of the levator aponeurosis is engaged again, creating a horizontal mattress configuration straddling the pupil. The location of the engagement and amount of tightening are determined by the amount of ptosis present. The lid is observed for immediate effect as the suture is tightened. Once a satisfactory position is achieved, a single throw of the suture is performed.
7. The patient is seated upright to confirm the position. When the desired height is reached, the suture is secured in a standard 3-1-1-1 fashion with the patient supine. Additional sutures may be placed to refine the height and contour, and can be removed if the desired effect is not achieved. Care should be taken, however, to not repeatedly pass sutures through the tarsus, which is damaged with each pass.

8. The skin is then approximated using the same 6-0 monofilament polypropylene suture in a running fashion. Very superficial engagement of the levator between the wound edges is performed on several passes of the running suture. This aids is reformation of the lid crease.

Postprocedural Care

1. Ophthalmic antibiotic ointment.
2. Follow-up at 1 week.
   a. Remove skin suture.

b. Examine the eyelid for lagophthalmos.
c. Examine the cornea for signs of exposure.

Outcomes

1. Correction of lid height and contour.
2. Position of eyelid crease.

Summary

Blepharoptosis repair by levator advancement is an effective method and generally allows a greater range of correction than posterior approaches to ptosis repair.

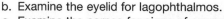

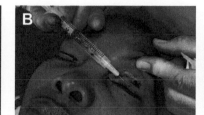

Figure 1A. The lid crease is identified and marked with the patient upright before sterile draping.

Figure 1B. The upper lid is infiltrated subcutaneously with 3 mL of local anesthetic ensuring distribution throughout the upper lid including the lid margin. Our preferred delivery method is by serial puncture (3–4) with a short needle rather than a single puncture with a longer needle.

Figure 1C. A #15 blade is used to incise skin to the level of orbicularis oculi.

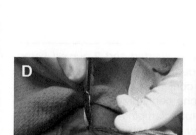

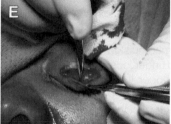

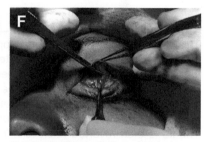

Figure 1D. Blunt dissection is used to clear the orbicularis exposing the orbital septum.

Figure 1E. Orbicularis is removed from the superior one-half to one-third of the tarsus to ensure that the levator will be directly attached.

Figure 1F. Fibers of the orbital septum are transected.

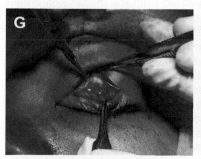

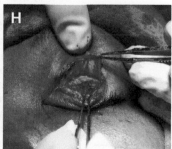

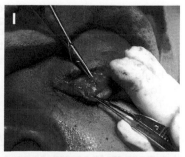

Figure 1G. The septum is then breached by sharp dissection exposing the pre-aponeurotic orbital fat.

Figure 1H. The fat is teased aside using fine forceps or moistened cotton swabs bringing the underlying levator aponeurosis into view.

Figure 1I. The distal end of the levator aponeurosis is engaged with a 6-0 monofilament polypropylene suture. The suture is then passed partial thickness through the upper one-third of the tarsus.

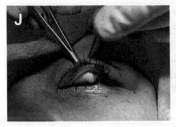

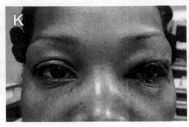

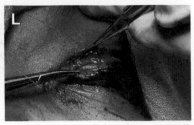

Figure 1J. The lid is immediately everted to confirm that the suture is not visible on the conjunctival surface. The distal end of the levator aponeurosis is engaged again creating a horizontal mattress configuration straddling the pupil. The location of the engagement and amount of tightening are determined by the amount of ptosis present. The lid is observed for immediate effect as the suture is tightened. Once a satisfactory position is achieved, a single throw of the suture is performed.

Figure 1K. The patient is seated upright to confirm the position. When the desired height is reached, the suture is secured in a standard 3-1-1-1 fashion with the patient supine.

Figure 1L. Very superficial engagement of the levator between the wound edges is performed on several passes of the running suture. This aids in reformation of the lid crease.

PROCEDURE 2: TARSO-MULLERS MUSCLE-CONJUNCTIVAL RESECTION PTOSIS REPAIR

Synopsis–Description of a posterior approach to upper lid ptosis repair using tarso-Mullers muscle-conjunctival resection.

Introduction

This is an alternative approach to upper lid ptosis repair that does not involve an external incision into the eyelid skin. It can be performed under local anesthesia without IV sedation. The upper lid is everted, and 1.5 mL of local anesthetic is injected above the tarsal margin in a subconjunctival plane. The lid is then reverted back to normal position, and another 1.5 mL of local anesthetic is injected into the upper eyelid skin across the entire length of the eyelid.

Treatment Goals and Planned Outcomes

1. To raise the upper eyelid to match the lid height of the contralateral eyelid, or to return both to the original anatomic position if the ptosis is bilateral.
2. To maintain lid contour.
3. To avoid an external incision.

Preoperative Planning and Preparation

It is important to assess the position of the contralateral upper lid. By lifting the ptotic lid to a normal anatomic position, a ptosis of the contralateral upper lid can often be unmasked (Hering effect).

Patient Positioning

Supine

Procedural Approach

1. The upper lid is everted and 2 curved hemostats are placed across the upper edge of the tarsal plate, conjunctiva, and Muller's muscle in a moustache configuration. It is imperative to avoid simply clamping straight across, as that will allow too much tissue to be excised centrally, resulting in a central peak in the lid contour that can be very difficult to repair. The amount of tissue to be resected depends on the amount of ptosis present.
2. A 6-0 plain gut fast-absorbing suture is passed through the skin of the upper lid crease medially and tied to itself in a 2-1-1 fashion.
3. It is then passed from the medial skin crease out onto the medial tarsal plate above the medial snap.
4. This suture is then woven in a running fashion above the snaps to exit laterally.
5. It is then passed from the lateral tarsal plate out onto the lateral skin crease.
6. The suture is passed once more through the skin crease, and tied to itself in 2-1-1 fashion.
7. The snaps are removed. The excess tarsal plate, Muller's muscle, and conjunctiva are removed with scissors in the previously snapped area to avoid cutting the suture.
8. The lid is reverted into normal position. Eyelid contour and height are examined.

9. A bandage contact lens and antibiotic ointment are placed into the eye. The eye is patched with a double-patch dressing.

Postprocedural Care

1. Remove patch after 24 hours.

2. Examine the cornea for abrasion, remove contact lens if no abrasion.
3. Ophthalmic antibiotic ointment.

Outcomes

1. Correction of lid height.
2. Maintenance of lid contour.

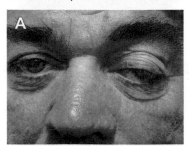

Figure 2A. Ptosis of the left upper lid.

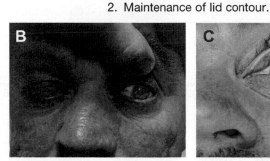

Figure 2B. Demonstration of Hering's law.

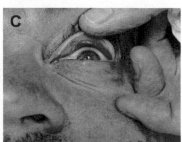

Figure 2C. Eversion of the left upper lid for administration of local anesthetic.

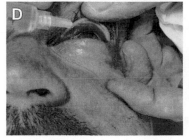

Figure 2D. Initial subconjunctival injection of local anesthetic.

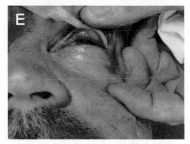

Figure 2E. Serial subconjunctival injection of local anesthetic.

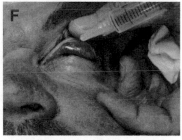

Figure 2F. Continuing serial subconjunctival injection of local anesthetic.

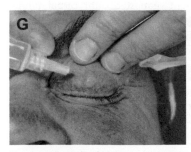

Figure 2G. Subcutaneous injection of local anesthetic.

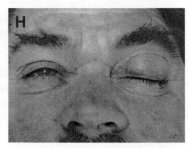

Figure 2H. After local anesthetic has been injected.

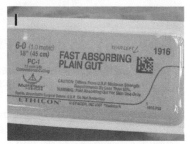

Figure 2I. 6-0 fast absorbing plain gut suture.

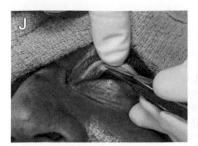

Figure 2J. Eversion of upper lid.

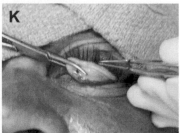

Figure 2K. Curved hemostat placed medially with the desired amount of tarsus-Mullers muscle-conjunctiva to be resected.

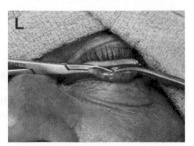

Figure 2L. Curved hemostat positioned laterally.

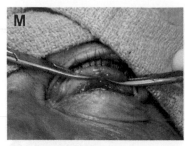

Figure 2M. Posterior view: note moustache configuration of clamps. This is to avoid peaking of the lid.

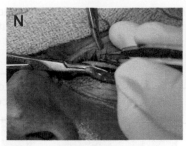

Figure 2N. Securing the suture in the medial lid crease.

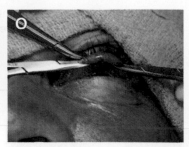

Figure 2O. Running the suture medial to lateral proximal to the clamped area.

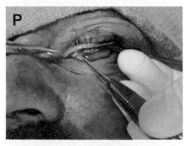

Figure 2P. Removing the medial clamp.

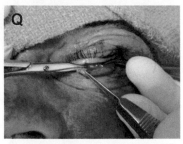

Figure 2Q. Cutting the previously snapped area.

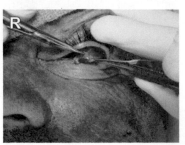

Figure 2R. Removing the lateral snap and cutting the previously snapped area.

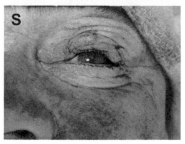

Figure 2S. Reverting eyelid.

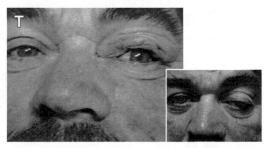

Figure 2T. Position of the eyelid at the end of the procedure, inset comparing ptosis prior to procedure.

PROCEDURE 3: LATERAL TARSAL STRIP

Synopsis–Description of the lateral tarsal strip approach to correcting involutional ectropion or entropion.

Introduction

One major cause of excessive tearing is lower lid laxity. The lateral tarsal strip is a well-known procedure that is used to correct this condition. This operation can be tailored to the degree of horizontal laxity present (ie, the more severe the laxity, more tightening can be achieved). There are many subtle variations to the lateral tarsal strip procedure. We describe our basic technique in this article. This procedure is done under local anesthetic without sedation. Distracting the eyelid away from the globe and directing the needle away from the globe, 1 mL of local anesthetic is in-filtrated into the middle lamella of the lateral eyelid. Everting the lower lid and directing the needle away from the globe, 1 mL of local anesthetic is in-filtrated inferior to the tarsal margin in the lateral corner of the lid. An additional 0.5 mL of local anesthetic is also placed subcutaneously in the upper lateral eyelid region just above the eyelid margin. Finally, 1 mL is infiltrated deep in the lateral canthal angle toward the periosteum of the lateral orbital rim. The best way to do this is to palpate for the lateral orbital rim in the lateral canthal angle, gently pushing and protecting the globe with your finger, directing the needle away from the globe and aiming toward the lateral orbital rim.

Treatment Goals and Planned Outcomes

1. Restore lateral canthal anatomy by reattaching the lateral edge of tarsus to the lateral orbital tubercle.
2. Tighten the lower lid by decreasing horizontal lower lid laxity.
3. Improve symptoms of tearing and ocular irritation.

Preoperative Planning and Preparation

1. The degree of laxity is assessed to plan appropriate correction.
2. Lateral distraction of the eyelid is useful to determine whether medial ectropion will be corrected with a lateral tarsal strip alone, or whether an additional procedure, such as medial conjunctival spindle, will be required.

Patient Positioning

Supine

Procedural Approach

1. Using Steven scissors, a lateral canthotomy is performed angling 15° superiorly to achieve the best cosmetic result.
2. Hemostasis is achieved with bipolar cautery.
3. An inferior cantholysis is then performed.
4. Again, hemostasis is achieved with bipolar cautery.
5. The lower lid is then overlapped on the upper lid laterally, and the amount of shortening required to correct the ectropion/entropion is marked with a #15 blade.
6. The skin, lid margin, conjunctiva, and lower lid retractors are removed from the excess lid creating a new lateral tarsal strip.

7. Bipolar cautery is used to achieve hemostasis along the newly fashioned lateral tarsal strip.
8. A 5-0 monofilament polypropylene suture is passed horizontally obliquely upward to the periosteum just inside the lateral orbital rim twice. It is then passed posteriorly to anteriorly then anteriorly to posteriorly through the tarsal strip. It is tied in a 3-1-1-1 fashion and cut short.
9. An additional interrupted 5-0 monofilament polypropylene suture is placed through the attached lateral tarsal strip and the periosteum of the lateral orbital rim, and tied and cut short.
10. The lateral canthal angle is reformed a 6-0 chromic gut suture by placing the suture in the wound of the lateral canthal angle exiting out of the gray line of the upper lid margin, then placed equidistant in the gray line of the lower lid margin and out through the wound. It is then tied in 2-1-1 fashion and the knot is buried in the wound (as opposed to the conjunctival surface decreasing the risk of postoperative ocular irritation).
11. The canthotomy wound is closed with interrupted 6-0 chromic gut sutures.

Potential Complications

1. Wound dehiscence: requires surgical debridement of wound edges and repair of dehisced wound.
2. Infection: place on oral antibiotics for skin flora coverage.
3. Injury to the lateral rectus if not careful during the anesthetic procedure/technique.

Postprocedural Care

1. Oral antibiotics for 10 days.
2. Ophthalmic antibiotic ointment.
3. Follow-up at 1 week.

Outcomes

1. Tightening of lower lid.
2. Restored eyelid in normal anatomic position.
3. Decreased symptoms of ocular irritation and excessive tearing.

Summary

The lateral tarsal strip is an effective procedure to address excessive tearing due to horizontal lower lid laxity that results in involutional ectropion or entropion.

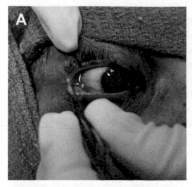

Figure 3A. Expose lateral canthus.

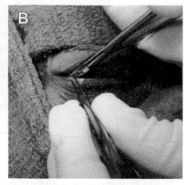

Figure 3B. Lateral canthotomy.

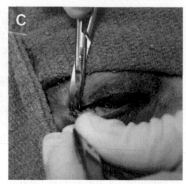

Figure 3C. Inferior cantholysis.

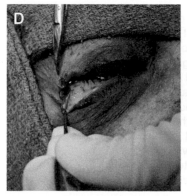

Figure 3D. Completed inferior can-thotomy and cantholysis.

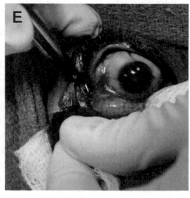

Figure 3E. Bipolar cautery to achieve hemostasis.

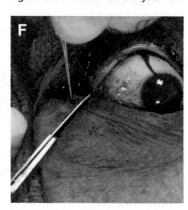

Figure 3F. Marking to approximate amount of horizontal tightening.

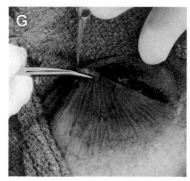

Figure 3G. Separating anterior lamella from the lateral tarsal strip.

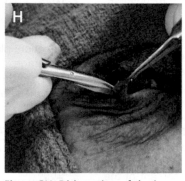

Figure 3H. Disinsertion of the lower lid retractors.

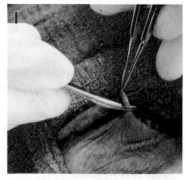

Figure 3I. Removal of lid margin.

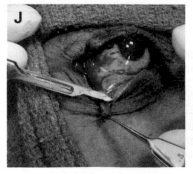

Figure 3J. Scraping of conjunctiva from tarsal strip.

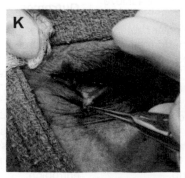

Figure 3K. Lateral tarsal strip.

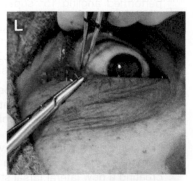

Figure 3L. A 5-0 monofilament poly-propylene suture passed through the periosteum at the lateral tubercle.

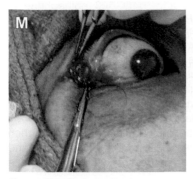

Figure 3M. Periosteal suture.

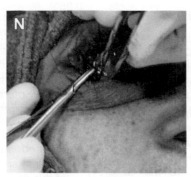

Figure 3N. Second pass of same 5-0 monofilament polypropylene suture through the periosteum.

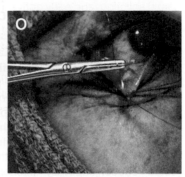

Figure 3O. First pass through the tarsal strip: posterior to anterior.

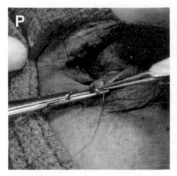

Figure 3P. Second pass through the tarsal strip: anterior to posterior.

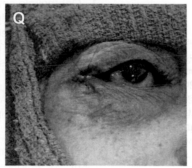

Figure 3Q. Secure lateral tarsal strip to periosteum.

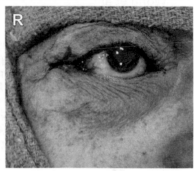

Figure 3R. Position of lower lid after periosteal suture secured.

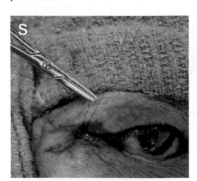

Figure 3S. Second periosteal suture.

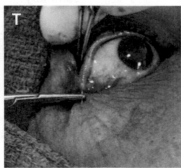

Figure 3T. Reformation of canthal angle.

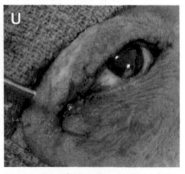

Figure 3U. After reformation of the lateral canthal angle.

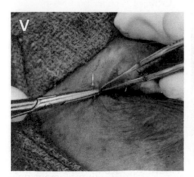

Figure 3V. Skin closure.

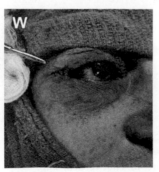

Figure 3W. Completed skin closure.

PROCEDURE 4: 3-SNIP PUNCTOPLASTY FOR PUNCTAL STENOSIS

Introduction

Punctal stenosis can be a contributing factor to excessive tearing. Three-snip punctoplasty is done to enlarge the punctal opening and help increase tear flow and decrease epiphora. Approximately 0.5 mL of local anesthetic is injected subcutaneously near each punctum. In the lower punctum, additional local anesthetic can be injected subconjunctivally inferior to the tarsal margin.

Treatment Goals and Planned Outcomes

1. Increase tear flow.
2. Decrease epiphora.

Preoperative Planning and Preparation

To be effective at tear drainage, the punctum must lie in the tear lake. Punctal position should be assessed to determine whether additional procedures, such as lateral tarsal strip and/or medial conjunctival spindle, will be required to correct punctal position.

Patient Positioning

Supine

Procedural Approach

1. Stabilize the eyelid margin with Bishop forceps lateral to the punctum, 1 blade of the Vannas scissors is placed vertically into the punctum and 1 blade posteriorly against the conjunctival surface, 1 vertical snip is made.
2. This is followed by a horizontal snip, where 1 blade of the Vannas scissors is placed into the canaliculus and the other blade outside the canaliculus angled slightly posteriorly to create a triangle. This will expose the underlying canalicular tissue.
3. The triangular flap of tissue created is then grasped with the Bishop or 0.5 forceps, and the final snip is made horizontally at the base of this flap.

Postprocedural Care

1. Ophthalmic antibiotic ointment.
2. There is usually minimal bruising and swelling with this procedure if performed in isolation so ice cold water compresses for 24 hours is sufficient. Patients may resume their normal activities the next day and do not need special instructions for sleep position.

Outcomes

The major outcome of this procedure is improvement in epiphora by alleviating the punctal stenosis.

Summary

This relatively low-risk procedure can be done alone or in conjunction with an eyelid tightening procedure, depending on the degree of epiphora and the presence or absence of lid laxity.

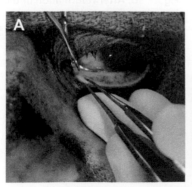
Figure 4A. View of left lower lid punctum and Vannas scissors.

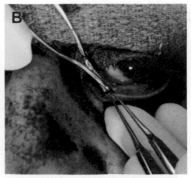
Figure 4B. First vertical snip.

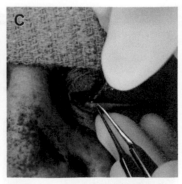
Figure 4C. Second horizontal snip.

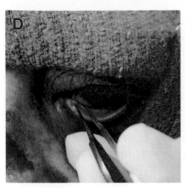

Figure 4D. Triangular flap.

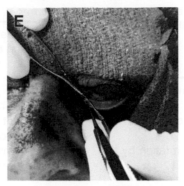

Figure 4E. Cutting across the base of the triangular flap (third snip).

PROCEDURE 5: EXCISION OF MARGINAL EYELID LESION AND RECONSTRUCTION OF A FULL-THICKNESS MARGINAL EYELID DEFECT
Introduction

A full-thickness defect in the eyelid margin, whether following trauma or resection of suspicious lesion, requires appropriate closure. After everting the eyelid, perform a series of subconjunctival injections of 1 mL of local anesthetic at the proximal border of tarsus. After the first injection, the surgeon will notice the conjunctiva balloon. Continue serial injections using the raised areas of conjunctiva as a point of insertion for the next injection across the lid. One should be able to visualize the needle tip at all times. Also, instruct the patient to look away from the direction of the needle. Do not to inject into the tarsus, which is ineffective and painful. After the posterior lamella is injected, revert the eyelid back into normal position and inject subcutaneously near the lid margin.

Treatment Goals and Planned Outcomes

1. Excision of a marginal eyelid lesion.
2. Reconstruction of the full-thickness defect in the eyelid margin.

Preoperative Planning and Preparation

The lid lesion is marked and outlined in a pentagonal fashion. The anticipated size of the defect should be determined so that reconstruction will be successful. If too large to close primarily, cantholysis or a local flap may be required.

Patient Positioning

Supine

Procedural Approach

1. Using a #15 blade, a vertical incision is made through the eyelid margin.
2. The resection is completed in the premarked pentagonal fashion with curved Steven scissors.
3. Bipolar cautery is used to achieve hemostasis.
4. Reconstruction of the full-thickness defect is then carried out. A 5-0 polyglactin 910 suture is passed in mattress fashion through the tarsus partial thickness to prevent corneal irritation and abrasion. It is very important at this point to check the alignment of the tarsus and make sure it is exactly aligned to prevent lid notching.
5. Additional 5-0 polyglactin 910 sutures are passed in a similar fashion superiorly to this for the length of the tarsus to be reapproximated.
6. The 6-0 chromic gut suture or 6-0 silk can be used to repair the lid margin. The first suture is passed through the gray line on the medial aspect of eyelid margin defect to the gray line of the lateral aspect of the eyelid margin. Again, in a mattress fashion, staying equidepth and equidistant on both sides. It is important to check that the eyelid margin is well-approximated at this point to prevent lid notching as well. Tie the suture in a 2-1-1 fashion. This suture will be kept long in order to imbricate the sutures on the skin.
7. Another 6-0 chromic gut or 6-0 silk is passed through the lash line in a similar manner to the suture passed through the gray line.
8. An optional final suture in the eyelid margin may be placed through the mucocutaneous junction just posterior to the gray line.
9. The skin defect is then closed with the same 6-0 chromic gut or 6-0 silk. Imbricate the long ends of the suture used in the closure of the

eyelid margin into one of the skin sutures to avoid corneal abrasion and irritation from the sutures.

Postprocedural Care

1. Ophthalmic antibiotic ointment immediately postoperatively.
2. If nonabsorbable sutures are used, remove at 10–14 days postoperatively.
3. Check the cornea for signs of irritation by the sutures.

Outcomes

Closure of the eyelid margin defect without eyelid notching and corneal irritation.

Summary

It is important to ensure that the tarsus and eyelid margin are correctly approximated to prevent eyelid notching when reconstructing a full-thickness eyelid margin defect.

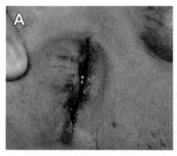

Figure 5A. Pentagonal marking around the lesion.

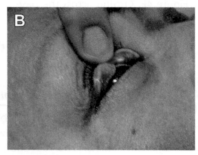

Figure 5B. Eversion of upper eyelid.

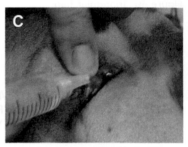

Figure 5C. Initial subconjunctival injection with local anesthetic.

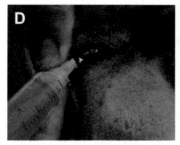

Figure 5D. Serial subconjunctival injection.

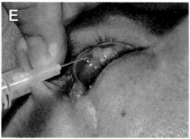

Figure 5E. Continuing serial injections.

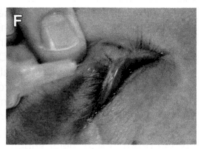

Figure 5F. Subcutaneous injection of local anesthetic.

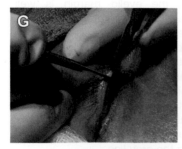

Figure 5G. Using a #15 blade to make vertical incisions through the margin of the eyelid in pre-marked areas.

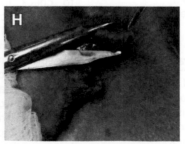

Figure 5H. Complete resection of lesion with curved Steven scissors.

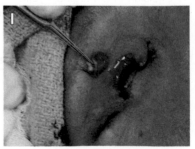

Figure 5I. Completed resection of the marginal lid lesion.

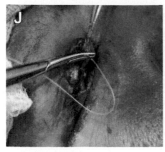

Figure 5J. Initial partial thickness tarsal pass with 5-0 polyglactin 910 suture.

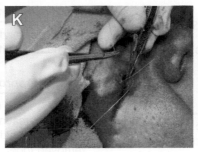

Figure 5K. Second tarsal pass in a mattress fashion.

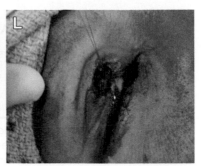

Figure 5L. Note exact approximation of tarsal edges.

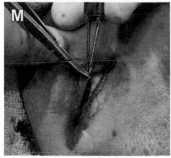

Figure 5M. Reapproximation of gray line.

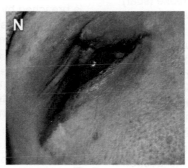

Figure 5N. Exact approximation of gray line.

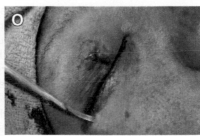

Figure 5O. Closure of skin.

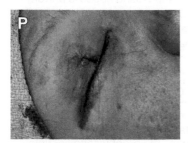

Figure 5P. Before imbrication of marginal eyelid sutures.

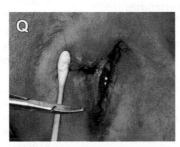

Figure 5Q. Imbrication of marginal eyelid sutures into skin sutures.

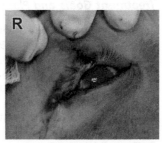

Figure 5R. Immediate postoperative result, inset comparing lesion preoperatively.

PROCEDURE 6: UPPER EYELID BLEPHAROPLASTY WITH CO_2 LASER

Synopsis–Description of our authors' approach to upper eyelid blepharoplasty.

Introduction

This is a modification of the classic approach to upper lid blepharoplasty designed to remove excess skin and in most cases some orbital fat. A CO_2 laser is used for the skin incisions and fat removal rather than a blade. Careful preoperative marking is key, as this will determine the final location of the eyelid skin crease (scar) and serve as a guide to limit excessive tissue removal. It can be performed under local anesthesia without IV sedation. The upper lid is infiltrated subcutaneously with 3 mL of local anesthetic, ensuring distribution throughout the upper lid, including the medial aspect overlying the medial orbital fat pad, which is a consistently sensitive area. Our preferred delivery is by serial puncture (3–4) with a short needle rather than a single puncture with a longer needle. This minimizes inadvertent loss of the desired plane.

Treatment Goals and Planned Outcomes

1. To remove excess tissue from the upper eyelid to restore a more youthful appearance.
2. In severe cases, to clear the visual axis and reduce mechanical ptosis.
3. To create a lid crease in desirable location.
4. To maintain lid contour.
5. To hide the incision within the existing lid crease.
6. To limit iatrogenic lagophthalmos.

Preoperative Planning and Preparation

It is important to mark the patient in an upright, seated position so that the effect of gravity is not lost. The position of the brow should be carefully noted. If the brow is to be lifted, it should be manually splinted in the desired location to avoid excessive tissue removal. The position of the lid crease is marked and if a new crease position is preferred, this is appropriately marked. With the patient supine, confirm that at least 20 mm total of eyelid tissue will remain inferior to the brow and superior to the lid margin once skin removal is completed. A corneal protector is used in both eyes during the procedure.

Patient Positioning

1. Upright for marking.
2. Supine for additional marking and procedure.

Procedural Approach

1. The CO_2 laser used to superficially incise the skin demarcating the area to be removed.
2. The strip of skin and orbicularis oculi is then removed together.
3. Hemostasis with bipolar cautery is achieved.
4. In some cases, the medial and/or central fat pads may already be exposed through an attenuated orbital septum. If not, the septum is breached by sharp dissection with Westcott spring scissors to adequately expose the fat.
5. Judicious fat removal is carried out by draping the fat over a cotton swab and excising with the CO_2 laser. The draping creates a barrier limiting the penetration of laser energy beyond the desired tissue depth. Ballottement of the globe can assist in prolapsing the fat anteriorly.
6. Hemostasis is again confirmed before wound closure.
7. The skin is approximated using 6-0 monofilament polypropylene suture in a running fashion. Very superficial engagement of the levator between the wound edges is performed on several passes of the running suture. This aids is reformation of the lid crease. Additional interrupted sutures are placed to perfect apposition.

Postprocedural Care

1. Ophthalmic antibiotic ointment.
2. Follow-up 1 day.
   a. Visual acuity.
   b. Extraocular movement.
3. Follow-up 1 week.
   a. Remove skin sutures.
   b. Examine the eyelid for lagophthalmos.
   c. Examine the cornea for signs of exposure.

Rehabilitation and Recovery

1. No heavy lifting or strenuous activity for 2 weeks.
2. Ice cold water compresses, as outlined in the article Introduction, are critical.

Outcomes

1. Reduction of excessive upper eyelid skin and esthetic appearance of upper eyelid.
2. Position of eyelid crease.

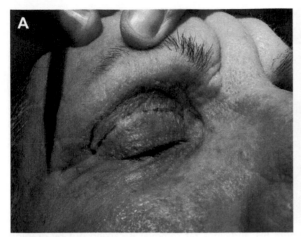

Figure 6A. Upper eyelid marked.

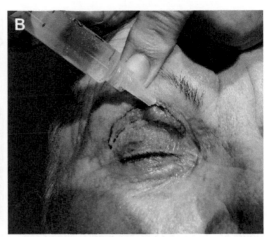

Figure 6B. Infiltration of local anesthetic.

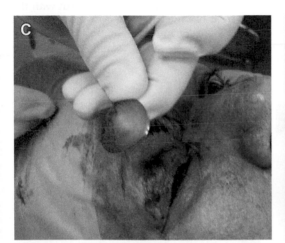

Figure 6C. Corneal protector.

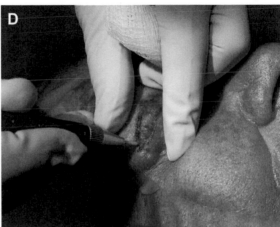

Figure 6D. The CO_2 laser is used to superficially incise the skin demarcating the area to be removed.

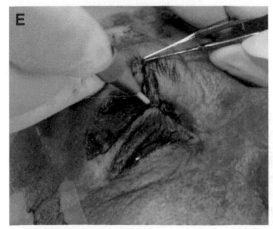

Figure 6E. The strip of skin and orbicularis oculi is then removed together.

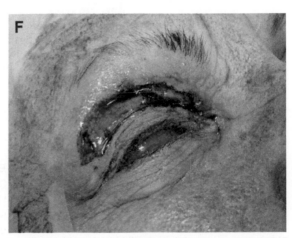

Figure 6F. Hemostasis with bipolar cautery is achieved.

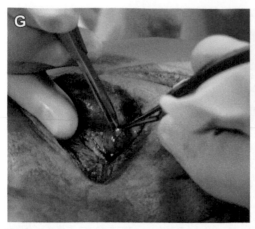

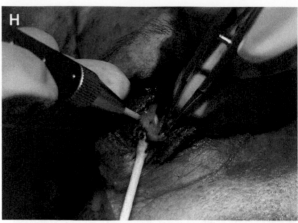

Figure 6G. In some cases, the medial and/or central fat pads may already be exposed through an attenuated orbital septum. If not, the septum is breached by sharp dissection with Westcott spring scissors to adequately expose the fat.

Figure 6H. Judicious fat removal is carried out by draping the fat over a cotton swab and excising with the CO_2 laser. The draping creates a barrier, limiting the penetration of laser energy beyond the desired tissue depth. Note how there is less bleeding where the fat has been cut with the laser than where it has not; this is due to the hemostatic effects of the CO2 laser. Ballottement of the globe can assist in prolapsing the fat anteriorly. Hemostasis is again confirmed prior to wound closure.

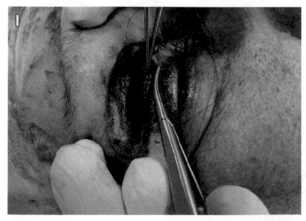

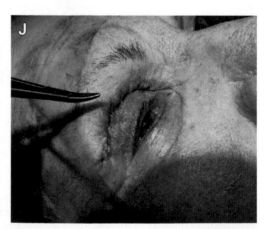

Figure 6I. The skin is approximated using 6-0 monofilament polypropylene suture in a running fashion. Very superficial engagement of the levator between the wound edges is performed on several passes of the running suture. This aids is reformation of the lid crease.

Figure 6J. Additional interrupted sutures are placed to perfect apposition.

PROCEDURE 7: LOWER EYELID BLEPHAROPLASTY WITH CO₂ LASER

Synopsis–Description of authors' approach to lower eyelid blepharoplasty.

Introduction

This is our approach to lower lid blepharoplasty using a CO_2 laser via a transconjunctival incision. It is most readily performed under local anesthesia with IV sedation. Midazolam with fentanyl is our standard sedative. The inferior conjunctival fornix is infiltrated with 3 mL of local anesthesic while the patient directs his or her gaze superiorly.

Treatment Goals and Planned Outcomes

1. To remove excess subcutaneous soft tissue (fat) from the area beneath the lower eyelid

(so-called tear trough) to restore a more youthful appearance.

2. Avoid hollowing of the area above the orbitomalar sulcus.

Preoperative Planning and Preparation

1. The extent of orbital fat prolapse into the area above the orbitomalar sulcus is carefully assessed to ensure that fat removal by blepharoplasty is the best approach. Other considerations include the use of filler in the sulcus and alternative procedures, such as orbital fat repositioning with release of the orbitomalar retaining ligament.

2. A corneal protector is used in both eyes during the procedure.

Patient Positioning

Supine

Procedural Approach

1. The CO_2 laser is used to incise the palpebral conjunctiva overlying the anterior aspect of the inferior orbital rim.

2. The incision is extended inferiorly in the retro-orbicularis plane until fat is encountered.

3. The inferior oblique muscle must be identified before fat removal so that it is not inadvertently injured.

4. Orbital fat removal is carried out by draping the fat over a cotton swab and excising with the CO_2 laser. The draping creates a barrier limiting the penetration of laser energy beyond the desired tissue depth. Proactive bipolar cautery to vessels on the surface of fat pedicles reduces bleeding and it is recommended before cutting. Ballottement of the globe can assist in prolapsing the fat anteriorly.

5. Removal proceeds from all 3 fat compartments to a variable extent depending on the preoperative assessment.

6. Hemostasis is achieved by direct effect of the CO_2 laser and additional bipolar cautery as needed.

7. No wound closure is required.

Postprocedural Care

1. Ophthalmic antibiotic ointment.
2. Follow-up 1 day.
   a. Visual acuity.
   b. Extraocular movement.
3. Follow-up 1 week.

Rehabilitation and Recovery

1. No heavy lifting or strenuous activity for 2 weeks.
2. Ice cold water compresses, as outlined in the article Introduction, are critical.

Outcomes

1. Reduction of excessive lower eyelid fat.
2. Esthetic appearance of lower eyelid and upper cheek junction.

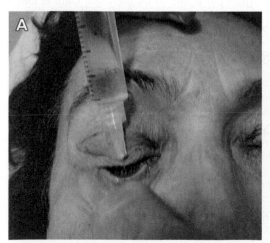

Figure 7A. Infiltration of local anesthetic into the lower conjunctival fornix.

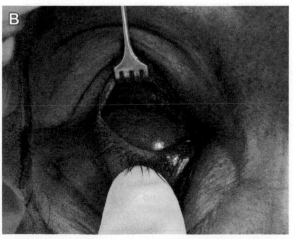

Figure 7B. Retraction of the lower eyelid exposing the conjunctiva (surgeon's view). Corneal protector in place.

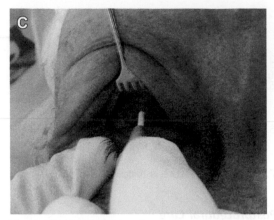

Figure 7C. The CO_2 laser is used to incise the palpebral conjunctiva overlying the anterior aspect of the inferior orbital rim. The incision is extended inferiorly in the retro-orbicularis plane until fat is encountered.

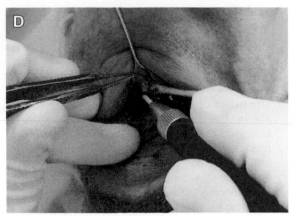

Figure 7D. Orbital fat removal is carried out by draping the fat over a cotton swab and excising with the CO_2 laser. The draping creates a barrier limiting the penetration of laser energy beyond the desired tissue depth. Hemostasis is achieved by direct effect of the CO_2 laser and additional bipolar cautery as needed.

PROCEDURE 8: LOWER EYELID ELEVATION WITH HARD PALATE MUCOSAL GRAFT

Synopsis–This is a description of the correction of lower eyelid retraction using a mucosal graft from the hard palate. This is primarily used in patients with lid retraction associated with thyroid eye disease, as well as postblepharoplasty retraction and in seventh nerve palsy.

Introduction

This procedure can be performed using local anesthesia, and we prefer adding IV midazolam with fentanyl for mild sedation. The local anesthetic is delivered in 2 stages. Injection into the hard palate is sensitive but generally well tolerated. Most patients will have experienced the sensation previously during dental procedures and know what to expect. The graft is harvested while wearing a sterile gown and gloves and with the patient draped. Because of the contamination risk associated with working in the oral cavity, we routinely reglove and add an additional new sterile drape following the harvest. At this point, we perform the infiltration of local anesthesia to the lower eyelid conjunctival fornix and skin.

Treatment Goals and Planned Outcomes

1. Raise the lower eyelid to the level of the limbus or slightly above.
2. Maintain lid contour and apposition.

Preoperative Planning and Preparation

1. The patient obtains a custom oral appliance (mouthguard) from his or her dentist before the day of the procedure.

2. A headlight is advantageous for viewing into the oral cavity.
3. Following graft harvest from the palate, new gloves are donned and a new body drape is placed over the patient. The instruments used in the harvest are isolated from the sterile set up.

Patient Positioning

1. Supine with neck in exaggerated extension for the graft harvest.
2. Supine for the eyelid portion.

Procedural Approach

1. The hard palate is marked before sterile draping and before injection of anesthetic, typically in a pointed oval configuration, one graft per eyelid to be elevated. Care is taken to avoid the midline and the soft palate.
2. A #15 blade is used to incise the edges of the mucosa to be removed.
3. Fine-toothed forceps are used to lift a corner of the graft and sharp dissection proceeds with Westcott scissors. A third hand is very helpful in providing constant suction to this vascularized area.
4. Bipolar cautery is used to achieve hemostasis in the donor bed. Caution is used to not touch any area of the mouth not anesthetized. Cyanoacrylate glue can be applied at this point to aid hemostasis. The custom oral appliance is inserted.
5. Attention is next shifted to the lower eyelid where two 5-0 silk traction sutures are placed through the lid margin and secured to the drape.
6. The conjunctiva is incised at the inferior border of the lower eyelid tarsus.

7. The lower eyelid retractors and septum are then freed from the inferior tarsal border and dissected off the overlying orbicularis. In cases of severe scarring, the retractors are also dissected off the underlying conjunctiva and resected.
8. Using the silk traction sutures, the lid is pulled superiorly to ensure that it has been freed adequately.
9. The graft is thinned using Westcott scissors before placement.
10. Securing of the graft inferior to the tarsus is performed using interrupted 7-0 chromic gut sutures. We position the graft with the mucosal surface on the lid conjunctiva so that the edges of the future superior border of the graft are adjacent. The suture is passed partial thickness from the underside of the graft exiting superiorly and then through the inferior tarsal border. We typically place 5 interrupted sutures along the superior border ensuring that the medial and lateral ends are well anchored.
11. The graft is then flipped into its proper orientation.
12. Suture passes are then performed analogously for the inferior border. We typically require 3 interrupted sutures. Care is taken to ensure all the 7-0 chromic sutures are buried.
13. The final lid position is assessed and a lateral tightening procedure, such as lateral tarsal strip (in cases of laxity) or Elschnig tarsorrhaphy (in cases with pure retraction), should be added.
14. A bandage contact lens is placed into the eye.
15. The lower eyelid traction sutures are secured tightly to the forehead with adhesive tape.

Postprocedural Care

1. Release the traction sutures on postoperative day 1.
2. Examine the cornea on postoperative day 1and remove the bandage contact lens if the cornea shows no abrasion.
3. Wear the oral appliance at all times for 3 weeks and perform daily chlorhexidine rinsing.
4. Oral antibiotics for 10 to 20 days.
5. Ophthalmic antibiotic ointment.
6. Follow-up 1 week.

Outcomes

1. Correction of lid height.
2. Proper lid-globe apposition.

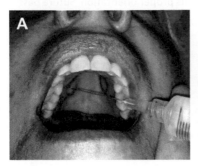

Figure 8A. Injection of local anesthesia into the hard palate is sensitive but generally well tolerated.

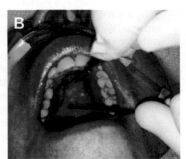

Figure 8B. A #15 blade is used to incise the mucosa to be removed.

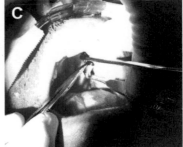

Figure 8C. Fine-toothed forceps are used to lift a corner of the graft and sharp dissection proceeds with Westcott scissors. A third hand is very helpful in providing constant suction to this vascularized area.

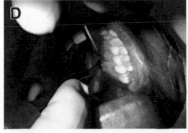

Figure 8D. Bipolar cautery is used to achieve hemostasis in the donor bed. Caution is used to not touch any area of the mouth not anesthetized.

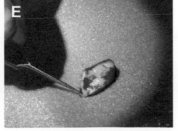

Figure 8E. Hard palate mucosal graft.

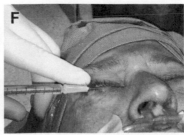

Figure 8F. Infiltration of local anesthesia into the lower eyelid after regloving and redraping.

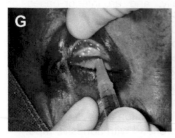

Figure 8G. Infiltration of local anesthetic into the inferior conjunctival fornix (surgeon's view). Note that this patient has a previous hard palate mucosal graft above the area of infiltration that was successful in correcting retraction for almost 10 years.

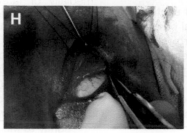

Figure 8H. Conjunctiva, lid retractors, and orbital septum dissected from the orbicularis and inferior tarsal border. In cases of severe scarring, the retractors are also dissected off the underlying conjunctiva and resected.

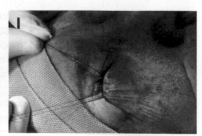

Figure 8I. The lid is pulled superiorly to ensure that it has been freed adequately.

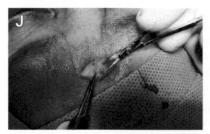

Figure 8J. Thinning of the hard palate graft.

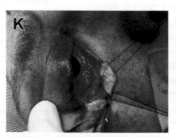

Figure 8K. Securing of the graft inferior to the tarsus is performed using interrupted 7-0 chromic gut sutures. We position the graft with the mucosal surface on the lid conjunctiva so that the edges of the future superior border of the graft are adjacent. The suture is passed partial thickness from the underside of the graft exiting superiorly and then through the inferior tarsal border. We typically place 5 interrupted sutures along the superior border ensuring that the medial and lateral ends are well anchored. In this patient, there is a preexisting hard palate graft so the sutures are anchored to submucosal tissue.

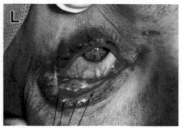

Figure 8L. The graft is flipped into its proper orientation. Suture passes are then performed analogously for the inferior border anchoring to submucosal tissue. We typically require 3 interrupted sutures.

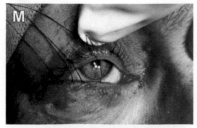

Figure 8M. The final lid position is assessed and a lateral tightening procedure, such as lateral tarsal strip or Elschnig tarsorrhaphy, is added as needed.

REFERENCES

1. Hass AN, Penne RB, Stefanyszyn MA, et al. Incidence of postblepharoplasty orbital hemorrhage and associated visual loss. Ophthal Plast Reconstr Surg 2004; 20:426–32.

2. Oestreicher J, Mehta S. Complications of blepharoplasty: prevention and management. Plast Surg Int 2012;2012:252368. http://dx.doi.org/10.1155/2012/252368 Article ID 252368.

FURTHER READINGS

LEVATOR PALPEBRAE ADVANCEMENT PTOSIS REPAIR

Anderson RL, Dixon RS. Aponeurotic ptosis surgery. Arch Ophthalmol 1979;97:1123–8.

Cetinkaya A, Kersten RC. Surgical outcomes in patients with bilateral ptosis and Hering's dependence. Ophthalmology 2012;119:376–81.

Kratky V, Harvey JT. Tests for contralateral pseudoretraction in blepharoptosis. Ophthal Plast Reconstr Surg 1992;8:22–5.

TARSO-MULLERS MUSCLE-CONJUNCTIVAL RESECTION PTOSIS REPAIR

Fasanella RM. Surgery for minimal ptosis: the Fasanella-Servat operation, 1973. Trans Ophthalmol Soc U K 1973;93:425–38.

Pang NK, Newsom RW, Oestreicher JH, et al. Fasanella-Servat procedure: indications, efficacy, and complications. Can J Ophthalmol 2008;43:84–8.

Skibell BC, Harvey JT, Oestreicher JH, et al. Adrenergic receptors in the ptotic human eyelid: correlation with phenylephrine testing and surgical success in ptosis repair. Ophthal Plast Reconstr Surg 2007; 23:367–71.

LATERAL TARSAL STRIP

Hsuan J, Selva D. The use of a polyglactin suture in the lateral tarsal strip procedure. Am J Ophthalmol 2004;138:588–91.

Jordan DR, Anderson RL. The lateral tarsal strip revisited. The enhanced tarsal strip. Arch Ophthalmol 1989;107:604–6.

Nowinski TS, Anderson RL. The medial spindle procedure for involutional medial ectropion. Arch Ophthalmol 1985;103:1750–3.

3-SNIP PUNCTOPLASTY FOR PUNCTAL STENOSIS

Caesar RH, McNab AA. A brief history of punctoplasty: the 3-snip revisited. Eye (Lond) 2005;19:16–8.

UPPER EYELID AND LOWER EYELID BLEPHAROPLASTY WITH CO2 LASER

Oestreicher J, Mehta S. Complications of blepharoplasty: prevention and management. Plast Surg Int 2012;2012:252368. http://dx.doi.org/10.1155/2012/252368 Article ID 252368.

LOWER EYELID ELEVATION WITH HARD-PALATE MUCOSAL GRAFT

Kersten RC, Kulwin DR, Levartovsky S, et al. Management of lower-lid retraction with hard-palate mucosa grafting. Arch Ophthalmol 1990;108:1339–43.

McAlister CN, Oestreicher JH. Repeat posterior lamellar grafting for recalcitrant lower eyelid retraction is effective. Orbit 2012;31:307–12.

Oestreicher JH, Pang NK, Liao W. Treatment of lower eyelid retraction by retractor release and posterior lamellar grafting: an analysis of 659 eyelids in 400 patients. Ophthal Plast Reconstr Surg 2008;24: 207–12.

Cosmetic Face, Neck, and Brow Lifts with Local Anesthesia

Nasim S. Huq, MD, FRCSC, MSc, FACS, CAQHS, DABPS*,
Tariq I. Nakhooda, MD, BSc

KEYWORDS

- Rhytidectomy • SMAS • Optimum mini lift • Office lift • Cervicomental angle • Platysma muscle
- Platysmaplasty • Coronal incision

KEY POINTS

- Full and limited or mini facelifts and neck lifts can easily be performed entirely with local anesthesia without IV sedation or general anesthesia.
- Open brow lifts can be combined with face and neck lifts all with local anesthesia, and with appropriate patient selection.
- The brow is often an under-appreciated but important area for facial rejuvenation.
- The neck is a very sensual area in the overall facial appearance.
- Eyelid surgery is one of the most delicate and unforgiving areas of facial rejuvenation.

THE FACE

Key Points in Facelift
1. Skin incisions
2. SMAS manipulation
3. Anesthesia options

Introduction

Cosmetic facial surgery can have a profound effect on the psychological well-being and many other areas of a person's life (**Figs. 1** and **2**).

Over the last several decades there have been many approaches to facial rejuvenation. Some of the approaches have included skin only, a loop suspension,[1] a MACS-lift,[2] the lateral SMA-Sectomy,[3] SMAS-lift,[4] and the FAME[5] technique. People have tried different approaches with skin incisions including the S lift,[6] as well as the quick-lift.[7]

There have also been various approaches to the levels of anesthesia involved in facial rejuvenation. Some people have consistently used general anesthesia with controlled hypotension,[8] as well as conscious sedation.[9] Total intravenous anesthesia,[9] as well as simple local anesthesia, is an alternative method of delivering anesthesia.

Michael Jackson did not die from any of his multiple cosmetic surgeries. He died of a poorly administered general anesthetic, by someone who was not adequately trained to do so. Clearly, mistakes can happen and to "keep it simple" may leave less room for human error. There may be some value to minimizing sedation and avoiding general anesthesia in procedures of the face, neck, and brow if the local anesthesia is properly administered.

Facial Anatomy

Although there may be as many different types of facial procedures as there are faces, the basic principles still remain the same. Some factors to

The authors have nothing to disclose.
Niagara Plastic Surgery Centre, McMaster University, 5668 Main Street, Suite 1, Niagara Falls, Ontario L2G 5Z4, Canada
* Corresponding author.
E-mail address: Niagaraplasticsurgery@gmail.com

Clin Plastic Surg 40 (2013) 653–670
http://dx.doi.org/10.1016/j.cps.2013.08.007

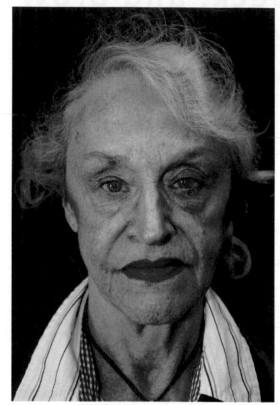

Fig. 1. Patient preoperatively who underwent rhytidectomy and upper and lower blepharoplasties.

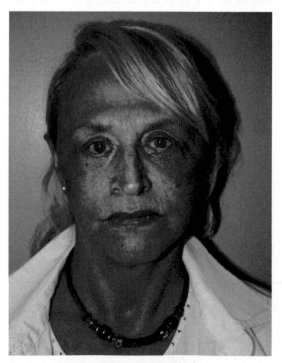

Fig. 2. Patient 2 weeks postoperatively.

consider in facial rejuvenation include the following:

1. Skin type[10]
2. Facial structure including cheek bones, jaw, and chin shape[11]
3. Skin laxity as well as the anterior hairline and sideburn
4. Nasolabial fold formation
5. Jowls
6. The submental fat
7. Cervical bands
8. Skin laxity, as well as many other factors.[12]

Although the combination of techniques may be used to target the areas in need of improvement, the surgeon must also direct the procedure toward the potential complications, anesthesia type, as well as the patient's own desires.[13]

As the youthful face ages, there is some consistency that is often found. There is often an increase in the laxity of cutaneous ligaments as well as a descent in well-known fat pads. This descent particularly occurs around the lower lid (preseptal space of fat pads), the malar fat pads (prezygomatic space), the nasolabial folds (vestibule of the oral cavity), jowls (premasseter space), and the labial mandibular folds (masticator space).[14]

It is the understanding of the facial anatomy that allows the surgeon to determine the layer of the face in which the dissection is best performed and used for redraping.

The 2 key factors in facial rejuvenation include appropriate release and appropriate repositioning or suspension.

It is the senior author's opinion that barbed threads do not produce long-term results that are even comparable to traditional surgical lifting techniques. It is also thought that the face that is less aged may require a less aggressive approach with less dissection and possibly smaller incisions.[15] The authors have completely stopped using barbed threads in 2006, for the poor performance at the time.

Local Anesthesia

Although there are many approaches to the anesthesia to be used in facial rejuvenation, the senior author has had the opportunity and the experience to evaluate most of the commonly described facelift techniques, as well as the different anesthetic techniques used. After performing hundreds of facelifts with different approaches in the last 6 years, it has been found that most patients can in fact tolerate a local anesthetic facelift without the need for any intravenous sedation or general anesthesia. Although some authors use a local anesthetic of 100 mL or 0.25% Lidocaine with 100,000 and 200,000 units epinephrine,[16] there are other authors such as Aston[17] who recommend a different combination of local anesthetic solution. The MACS lift uses a standard anesthetic solution of 100 mL sodium chloride 0.9%, 20 mL Lidocaine 2%, 10 mL Ropivacaine at 10 mg/mL, 2 mL sodium bicarbonate 8.4%, 0.2 mL Levorenin at 1 mg/mL, and 10 mg Triamcinolone.[18] The anesthetic solution of choice is really up to the experience and preference of the surgeon.

Some authors use a tumescent approach similar to the amount of infiltration used in liposuction cases.[19] It is the senior author's opinion that the tissue does not mobilize as well when too much infiltration has been used.

The authors have found it useful to maintain a consistency in all infiltration and all procedures to help eliminate human error (**Fig. 3**). The authors routinely start on the left side of the face and infiltrate it in a similar fashion, starting from above and behind the left ear, and moving in a sequential fashion anteriorly along the areas of marking where the local anesthetic will end in the subcutaneous plane (**Fig. 4**). It is helpful to first infiltrate the area of the infraorbital nerve and the great auricular nerve, as this may decrease the sensation of the needle around the ear (**Fig. 5**).

Although mild oral sedation with Tylenol-Codeine, oral Gravol® or sublingual lorazepam (Ativan™) has routinely been used, the authors have never used intravenous sedation in an office setting (**Fig. 6**). Mild intravenous sedation can be administered by a surgeon; however, heavy sedation should probably be monitored by a separate person.[20] It is noted that oral sedation with Ativan alone may have unpredictable absorption and will often have late onset, and a relatively, unnecessarily long, half-life.[21]

Treatment Goals and Planned Outcomes

The goal of facial rejuvenation procedures is to gain harmony of the upper and lower parts of the face with the desired replenished look.[22]

Preoperative Planning and Preparation

The surgeon should evaluate and document the following areas, which include the bone structure of the entire face, the skin quality and laxity, location of particular fat deposits as well as the mid face thickness, laxity and mobility, the deepness in mobility of the nasolabial folds, the neck shape, size, and platysmal muscle anatomy.[23] Furthermore, the malar areas and lower lids should be noted and other areas outside of the actual face

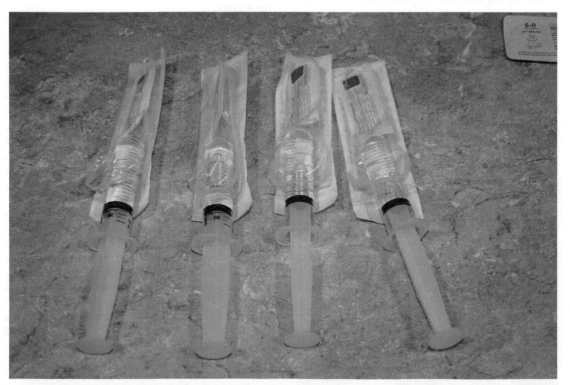

Fig. 3. Routinely for rhytidectomy, 4 syringes of local anesthetic are prepared to help ensure the established threshold is never exceeded.

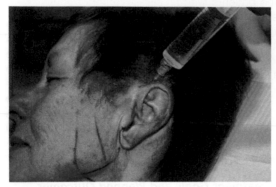

Fig. 4. The anterior ear and cheek and neck are infiltrated first.

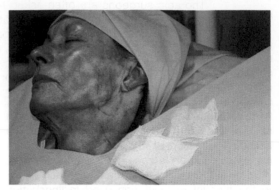

Fig. 6. The face is prepared and there is no need for supplemental oxygen.

and neck lift area, including the brow and location of the posterior auricular hair skin. The surgeon must determine the patient's main areas of concern and motivation for surgery and note detailed photographs.[24]

Patient Positioning

It is the senior author's opinion to keep the head in a neutral position and not turn the head from left to right during the surgery. It is also recommended to avoid hyperextending the neck. It is best to keep a headrest and possibly a donut-type pillow to allow access to the face with minimal turning or repositioning of the head. Minimal turning will allow for the maximal amount of SMAS and platysmal repositioning and tension, as well as a natural position to compare the left and right sides of the face for appropriate symmetry and contouring.[25]

Procedural Approach

For most rhytidectomies, the face should be marked on both sides for the incision pattern, as well as the area for the infiltration. Areas requiring attention to elevation and key landmarks for movement and redraping should also be marked.[26]

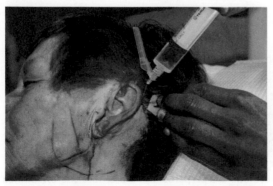

Fig. 5. The posterior ear and neck are then infiltrated.

The pretragal and retrotragal incisions have been well described and this is primarily a surgeon's preference.[27] The senior author prefers the retrotragal incision for both male and female patients, and the hair follicles are simply trimmed out of the skin flap for male patients.[28]

If the patient seeks a "ponytail friendly" incision, it is best to end the incision at the area of the earlobe.[29] It may depend on the amount of laxity on the tissue around the face and the neck regarding how far anterior to the ear the incision has to go. If there is considerable laxity in the neck, then a posterior auricular incision may be necessary.

The posterior auricular incision only needs to cross over the posterior concha for a few millimeters to allow some space for possible scar migration. The point where the hairline meets the ear at the superior aspect of the posterior ear should be noted, and the incision can be curved in this direction.[30] It is noted that the amount of skin and neck movement over the mastoid may vary and this may change the posterior hairline position. The scar may go into the posterior scalp to hide the scar, or come down in an inferior fashion to keep the hairline in a similar position; however, the scar may still be present.[31]

A W-plasty-type incision is made in the hair in front of the ear no higher than the level of the takeoff of the helix anteriorly. A second incision is made superior to the helix in a more posterior fashion. After the skin is elevated, the skin is rotated posteriorly, which decreases the large temporal dog ear, and the scar rarely goes anterior to the sideburn and never elevates the hair above the takeoff of the helix.[32] This approach was used in a comparative study of 4 different, popular facelifts by Alpert and colleagues.[33]

After the flaps were elevated appropriately, according to the techniques of Baker, the surgeon has the ability to reposition the SMAS in the appropriate vector in a primarily vertical fashion. The senior author generally start from an inferior portion of platysma, tacking this in a posterior but more superior direction toward the mastoid using a figure-of-8 cruciate stitch. The cruciate stitch produces a 4-strand type of repair over the area and is fairly quick and efficient as used in flexor tendons.[34] The SMAS is split at the area of the platysma and the lateral SMASectomy is performed anterior as previously described by other authors.[3] The 3-0 clear PDS™ is used in a similar circuiting fashion anterior to the ear suturing in a direction toward the cartilaginous portion, anterior to the tragus near the external auditory canal. Further plication may be performed more superiorly, if necessary, in the area where one would dissect along tension for a high lateral SMAS or the anterior third loop stitch over the malar prominence. The SMAS may also be plicated up toward the temporalis fascia.[35]

Various types of sutures have been used in the plication and the senior author have seen that Vicryl™ clearly does not suspend sufficiently for long-term results. Mersilene™ sometimes will stick out and will have to be removed through the skin.[36] Nylon is sometimes palpable; however, if not cut too short, it can be less problematic. It is noted on redo or revision facelift surgery and on secondary or even tertiary surgery where the Nylon sutures are identified from previous lifts; that tension seems to be very loose and is not holding tissue at that point. The senior author found 3-0 PDS™ strong enough and large enough to be able to give a lasting resuspension of the tissue, and the authors have not had any problems thus far with the thread protruding from the wound or getting infected. The senior author occasionally augment the PDS™ with a 4-0 clear Nylon for added lasting suspension of the SMAS and platysma.[37]

With the advancement of facial rejuvenations, surgeons have been able to combine the SMAS platysma type of facelift with the FAME technique to help improve the mid face in the nasolabial folds.[5]

It is noted that the dissection of tissue can be performed in many different ways including the finger-assisted technique. It has been found that the spreading of tissue in a superior to inferior direction or with traditional facelift-type scissors or Kaye scissors works very efficiently, and skin flaps can be elevated in a matter of minutes in the appropriate plane, including over the SMAS and platysma (**Fig. 7**).[38]

After the SMAS and platysma have been plicated and/or repositioned in the appropriate positions, the skin is redraped with relatively small amounts of tension, with the face in the neutral

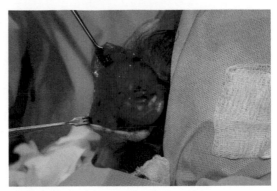

Fig. 7. The skin flaps are elevated and the key suspension sutures are in place.

position. The position of the earlobe is determined first and a buried 3-0 PDS is placed in the subcutaneous plane from the new corner of the new skin, to the new position from where the medial aspect of the earlobe will sit. The 3-0 PDS™ is buried and left behind the ear (**Figs. 8 and 9**). The rest of the skin is trimmed for the appropriate positioning and buried 4-0 Vicryl™ is used for the tacking sutures (**Fig. 10**). The skin is defatted in the area of the tragus, and just in front of the tragus a single buried 4-0 Vicryl™ is used to help prevent distortion of the tragus (**Fig. 11**). To prevent scar migration behind or in front of the ear into the cartilaginous areas, 4-0 Vicryl is also used. Staples can be used in the hair baring scalp area or 3-0 Vicryl Rapide™. For the rest of the skin closures, 5-0 Vicryl Rapide™ has been used.

Potential Complications and Management

The standard complications for any facelift operation include bleeding (hematoma, ecchymosis), edema, infection, pathologic scars, seromas, contour irregularities, asymmetry, alopecia, motor or sensory nerve damage, and skin loss.[39] Fortunately these complications are fairly rare and

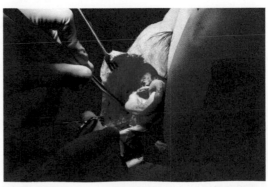

Fig. 8. The skin flaps are elevated and the key suspension sutures are in place.

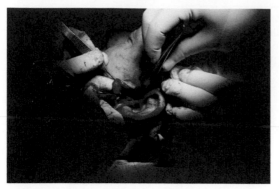

Fig. 9. Skin is trimmed at the level where there is minimal tension.

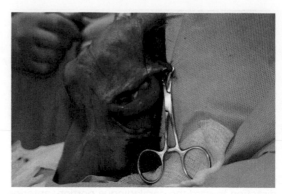

Fig. 11. The skin flaps are elevated and the key suspension sutures are in place.

each complication should be treated on an individual basis according to the surgeon's experience and tailored to that patient.

The use of drains has been compared in previous studies.[40] It is the authors' experience that even trying to place a drain on only one side of the face, the swelling and local anesthesia are removed faster in the area that is drained. It is found by patients and documented by the senior author's experience that the drain itself is inconvenient, and beyond 1 week there is no difference between both sides, whether they are drained or not.

Tisseel™ has been described for the prevention of the use of drains and to decrease hematomas. The authors have not found any significant difference in very small hematoma rates or ecchymosis with the use of Tisseel™.[41]

Postprocedural Care

A light compression bandage is worn for the first 24 to 48 hours and the patients are encouraged to shower. If a small Penrose drain is used, it can be removed in the shower. The patient is to apply a light amount of Polysporin around the incisions and the facelift garment is then worn, if there is

any residual swelling over the next few days. The garment is worn for longer periods if neck or facial liposuction is used.

Rehabilitation and Recovery

The patient may have difficulty in opening the mouth widely for eating. The patient is encouraged to stick with mechanically soft food and small bites, especially simple foods, like soup. Most patients are able to return to work 2 weeks postoperatively.[42]

Outcomes

As described above, infection and bleeding are the major complications; however, with proper surgical techniques and postprocedural care, patients can expect high satisfaction rates. **Figs. 12–19** show preoperative and postoperative photographs of a patient who had rhytidectomy with upper and lower blepharoplasty.[43]

Summary

The SMAS and FAME techniques can be used in combination with one another, to achieve a natural contour and appearance to the upper and lower parts of the face. The procedural approach and skill of the surgeon are major determinants of the procedural outcome. With proper postoperative care, patients will achieve satisfactory results.

THE NECK

Where, you ask, does beauty dwell?

I'll share what I've discovered—

That though the face may draw a crowd,

It's the neck that lures a lover.

—Dr Joel J. Feldman

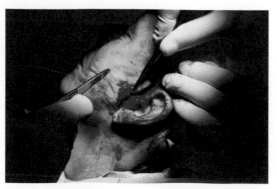

Fig. 10. The tragal suspension suture is placed deep into the dermis.

Key Points for Neck Lift

1. Cervicomental angle: The cervicomental angle is sharp and smooth in the youthful face. This angle often descends and becomes more obtuse with age and muscle laxity.

2. Platysma muscle: This muscle is the most sufficient muscle that often becomes lax and produces platysmal bands.

3. Platysmaplasty: Platysmaplasty is a procedure that repositions the platysma often including an anterior submental incision.

Introduction

Although there are many different types of necks and many different types of neck procedures described, the senior author has found there is much to be learned from the textbook of Dr Joel J. Feldman.[44] One can classify the different types of necks according to the treatment needed, from no treatment needed versus simple elevation, with a limited incision short scar type of MACS lift, to a limited posterior auricular incision or even full

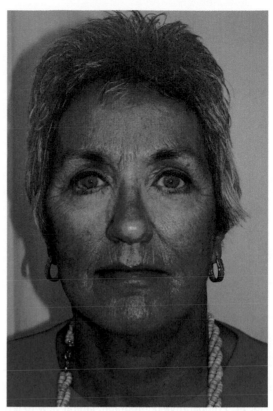

Fig. 13. Postoperative photograph, front view of a patient who underwent rhytidectomy along with upper and lower blepharoplasties.

posterior auricular incision with skin resection as well as redraping.[45] One may also use lateral neck liposuction or a submental incision for liposuction versus a full open submental lipectomy and platysmaplasty.[46]

For most necks, the senior author has found the full submental platysmaplasty is not often required unless specifically requested by the patient. For most facial rejuvenation in patients, there can be considerable improvement with a traditional rhytidectomy approach with lateral and submental liposuction. Platysmal band release may also be performed with a percutaneous release, with an 18-gauge needle along the course of the band and with the muscle being repositioned using the traditional lateral SMASectomy and platysma suspension.[47]

Treatment Goals and Planned Outcomes

The treatment goal is to focus on neck rejuvenation through reconstruction or repositioning of the cervical facial angle, as well as improving the jowls and any platysmal bands or malpositioned cervical fat.[48]

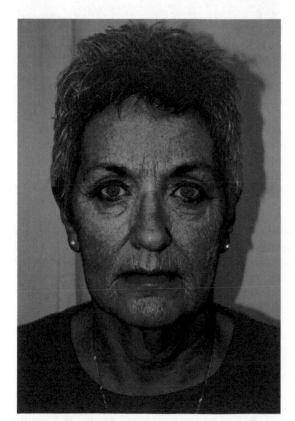

Fig. 12. Preoperative photograph, front view of a patient who underwent rhytidectomy along with upper and lower blepharoplasties.

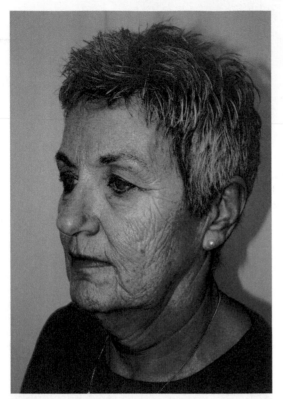

Fig. 14. Preoperative photograph, lateral view to left of a patient who underwent rhytidectomy along with upper and lower blepharoplasties.

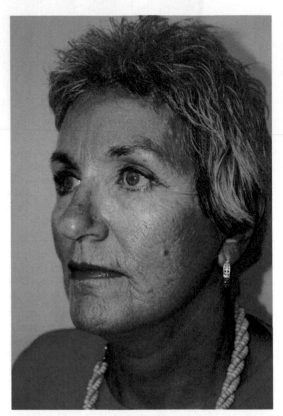

Fig. 15. Postoperative photograph, lateral view to left of a patient who underwent rhytidectomy along with upper and lower blepharoplasties.

Preoperative Planning and Preparation

The first step in the consultation is to visually inspect and palpate the neck. It is important to determine the position of the thyroid cartilage, as well as possibly the size of the thyroid compared with the cervical fat. Skin quality and skin excess are also assessed. One must determine at this point whether liposuction is in fact needed and in what direction, as opposed to simple muscle plication or full open submental fat resection with platysmaplasty.

Patient Positioning

The patient is placed on the operating table with some head elevation and a head drape. The patient is able to hyperextend the neck if necessary; however, for a natural appearance, the head is not turned or extended much beyond normal unless necessary.

Procedural Approach

There are a number of different operative approaches as previously described. For many faces, anterior neck work is not necessary.

For mild necks, simple infiltration marking of the platysmal bands and then infiltration with local anesthetic is used. An 18-gauge needle is used percutaneously to release the platysmal bands between the fingers in 2 or 3 spots for each platysmal band (**Fig. 20**).[49]

The lateral platysmal suspension and SMASectomy are used to reposition the platysma and decrease the recurrence of platysmal band in the postoperative phase.

If necessary, the area of concern with some submental fat can be infiltrated with 20 mL dilute Xylocaine with Adrenaline and bicarbonate with saline. A 5-mm stab incision is placed in the submental crease and the anterior neck liposuction can easily be performed with the handheld liposuction technique. Machine liposuction can also be used; however, only 10 to 20 mL of fat and fluid is removed in a course of only a few minutes and this is often sufficient. There are many simple modified techniques to use the handheld liposuction system with a 60 mL tulip tip syringe and a possible "Johnnie Lock"[46] or even a plastic hub from a 10-mL syringe wedged in the handle of the 60-mL tulip syringe (**Fig. 21**) helps maintain suction.[50]

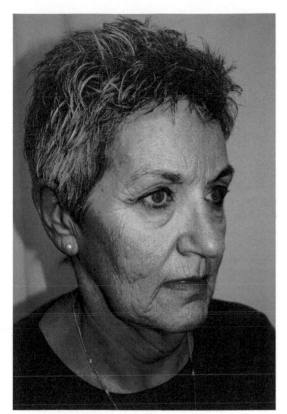

Fig. 16. Preoperative photograph, lateral view to right of a patient who underwent rhytidectomy along with upper and lower blepharoplasties.

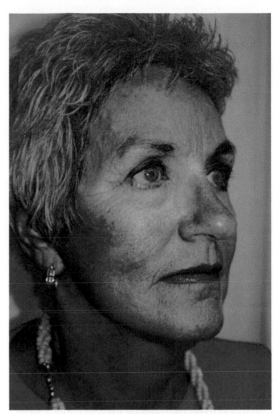

Fig. 17. Postoperative photograph, lateral view to right of a patient who underwent rhytidectomy along with upper and lower blepharoplasties.

For the submental lipectomy and platysmaplasty, an extra 20 mL of diluted Xylocaine solution may be used. The face and neck are still prepared and draped with the head drape, and a longer submental incision is used. It has been found that the incision can in fact be several centimeters long and still heals in a cosmetically acceptable fashion.[51]

The skin flaps are elevated in the subcutaneous plane and the platysma is identified. The authors elevate the subcutaneous plane just above the platysma, isolating the platysma inferiorly and on the neck and this is repeated on each side. The platysma is then elevated on each side, and the submental lipectomy is performed from the inferior floor muscles of the mouth, across the trachea and thyroid cartilages. It is the surgeon or patient's preference and experience that may determine how far inferior the dissection may be warranted. The subplatysmal or deep plane is acquired in a medial-to-lateral approach bilaterally. Many surgeons advocate the resection of the submandibular gland. The extra dissection and potential bleeding are, however, serious drawbacks.

The authors have found no difficulties with running Mersilene™ for the platysmaplasty of the anterior bands. Some may even dip the braided suture in Betadine or Bacitracin solution before the suture to decrease stitch abscesses.[52]

Potential Complications and Management

Hematomas, seromas, nerve injuries, and infection are only a few of the complications that may occur in the neck. The most common complication in the aesthetic procedure of the neck is likely surface contour irregularities and an overzealous reduction of volume leading to the dynamic tethering of the skin onto the underlying platysma.[53]

These complications may require re-elevation and redraping of the skin with fat grafts if necessary.[54]

Postprocedural Care

A standard facelift type of Velcro straps/compression garment is worn for the first week; however, the patient can remove the garment in 1 to 2 days after surgery, as well as remove any

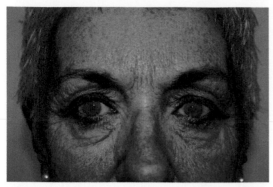

Fig. 18. Preoperative photograph, blepharoplasty of a patient who underwent rhytidectomy along with upper and lower blepharoplasties.

drains. The patient is able to shower. A light layer of antibiotic ointment is also applied to the incisions.

Rehabilitation and Recovery

Patients can expect a recovery time of about 1 week after the procedure and can return to work within 2 weeks. However, patients are advised that resuming normal activities and strenuous exercise must be avoided until 3 weeks after the procedure.

Outcomes

Infection and bleeding are major complications; however, with proper surgical techniques and postprocedural care, patients can expect high satisfactory rates.

Summary

In conclusion, aesthetic surgical procedures involving the structures of the neck are most

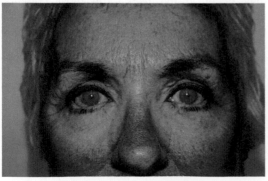

Fig. 19. Postoperative photograph, blepharoplasty of a patient who underwent rhytidectomy along with upper and lower blepharoplasties.

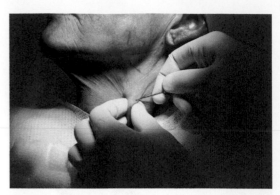

Fig. 20. The platysma is released percutaneously with an 18-guage needle.

effective when used with other rejuvenation efforts in the superficial structures of the neck and face.

THE BROW

Key Points for Brow Lift

1. An understanding of forehead anatomy is fundamental and critical to a successful coronal brow lift.

2. The ideal brow appearance in women and men are different. In women, the medial brow should be above the supraorbital ridge and the apex of the arch lateral to the mid pupil. In men, the brow should lie at the supraorbital rim and is less arched.

3. Every brow lift requires adequate release and adequate fixation.

Introduction

The coronal brow lift targets and corrects brow ptosis. There are 2 specific etiologic factors that contribute the most to brow ptosis: aging and gravity. When the face ages, there is a decrease in the number of elastic fibers, glycosaminoglycans, and collagen in the skin, leading

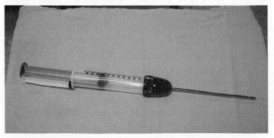

Fig. 21. A simple, inexpensive manual liposuction cannula with a 10-mL syringe stopper can be used very easily in the face and neck.

to a loss of tone. With the loss of muscle support, the effects of gravity result in an increased descent of the lateral brow more than the medial brow.[55]

Temporal and forehead anatomy is essential to the success of brow lift surgery. The scalp is divided into 5 layers: skin, connective tissue, galea aponeurotica, loose areolar connective tissue, and periosteum. The blood supply to the forehead comes from the internal and external carotids and its branches. The nerve supply is the facial nerve and its frontal branch and innervates the forehead muscles. These muscles include frontalis, corrugators, depressor supercilii, and procerus muscles. The supratrochlear and supraorbital nerves are terminal branches of the ophthalmic division of the trigeminal nerve and give sensation to the central and lateral forehead.[56]

The coronal brow lift procedure is usually performed under local anesthesia (1% lidocaine) with hemostasis (epinephrine 1:200,000) and is infiltrated along the incision markings and dissection areas across the supraorbital rim.[57] If the anterior hairline is already too far posterior on the frontal bone, then a "tricophytic lift" is used.[58] An endoscopic brow lift is also frequently used, especially for male or female balding patients and those who object to a coronal incision. The senior author have found a greater and longer lasting lift can be achieved with the open brow lift.

Treatment Goals

The main goal of the coronal brow lift is to treat brow ptosis and to avoid iatrogenic injury that could result in functional impairment.[59] There are 2 essential factors in any brow lift: adequate structural release and adequate fixation.

Preoperative Planning and Preparation

Proper patient selection must be emphasized and is critical for the success of the operation. A complete patient history is obtained with specific focus on eyelid and ocular history, facial surgical history, and forehead trauma. The surgeon must assess visual acuity, hairline position, brow symmetry and position, brow ptosis, and upper eyelid skin. The forehead is examined, focusing on skin quality and rhytid depth, and forehead motor and sensory function.[24] The hairline should not be at or posterior to superior the upper curve of the frontal bone in the forehead. Often greater than 2 cm of scalp is excised and the brow elevates approximately 5 mm. The hairline will move posteriorly and this may seem masculine, like the receding hairline of a man, if there is poor patient selection.

Patient Positioning

All preoperative markings are outlined while the patient is in the seated position, and the patient is placed on the operating table in a supine position with the head in a neutral position (**Fig. 22**).[60] The authors no longer shave the scalp in the area for planned resection because it does not affect the surgery. Some of the hair may be trimmed preoperatively.

Procedural Approach

A coronal incision is made and the flap is elevated in the subgaleal plane between the galea and the periosteum. Although the subperiosteal dissection is commonly used, the authors have found no advantage or improvement of outcomes, and it takes longer.[61] The dissection is made to the superior orbital rim with preservation of the frontal branch of the facial nerve and central forehead neurovascular bundles. Laterally, the dissection is carried down, gently to the zygomatic arches, to preserve the facial nerve area. The medial zygomatic temporal vein (sentinel vein) is identified and preserved in the open technique (**Figs. 23** and **24**). The procerus and corrugator muscles

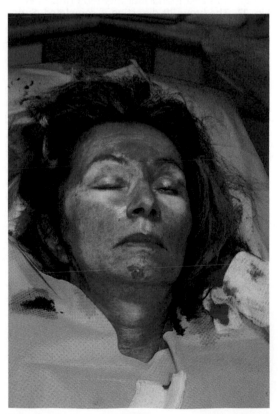

Fig. 22. A patient resting comfortably without sedation.

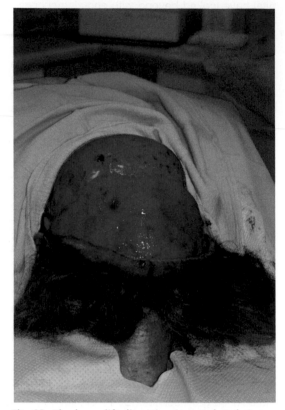

Fig. 23. The brow lift dissection is completed. Supra-orbital nerves are preserved and the glabellar muscles are resected. The airway is protected by the patient on her own without any assistance under her hair and scalp.

are partially excised, releasing the medial brow. The lateral orbicularis oculi is transected as needed to help shape the brow to the desired look, elevation, and arch. This shaping is helpful to restore balance to the asymmetric brow. Buried 3-0 PDS™ or 4-0 Vicryl™ sutures are placed in the galea aponeurosis for brow

suspension after excess scalp is excised in segments and held temporarily with towel clips. The focus is primarily on the lateral elevation with not too much medial elevation to maintain an aesthetically pleasing arch (**Fig. 25**). If the tension is vertical in the temporal scalp, there is less concern for postoperative alopecia. The scalp is stapled or sutured with 3-0 Vicryl Rapide™ and all incisions are closed. Drains are not needed in this procedure.[62]

Potential Complications and Management

There is always numbness posterior to the incision line unless a very large, anteriorly based flap is created but this is not used easily in the local anesthetic brow lift.[63] Complications include alopecia, scar widening, sensory nerve deficit, frontal muscle paralysis, skin necrosis, scar pruritis, infection, hematoma, bleeding, asymmetrical eyebrows, asymmetrical eyelids, chronic pain, overzealous correction, and abnormal soft-tissue contour. Minimal tension along intraoperative incisions helps to reduce scalp alopecia or scar widening. If scalp alopecia or widening occurs, surgical revisions are recommended after a minimum of 6 months postoperatively. Frontalis muscle paralysis can occur when flap dissection at the lateral orbital rim is too superficial and is almost always temporary, taking up to 12 months to regain complete function.[64]

Postprocedural Care

The head is wrapped using Velcro compression bandages or an elastic supportive dressing. The patient's head is kept elevated immediately after surgery. Mild analgesics are prescribed for pain, and the patient must be evaluated for hematoma development. Patients are advised not to shower until postoperative day 2. Ice may be

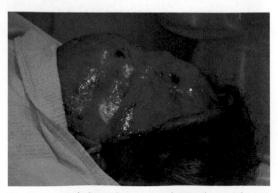

Fig. 24. Lateral view of completed open brow lift with mild oral sedation/1 mg SL lorazepam.

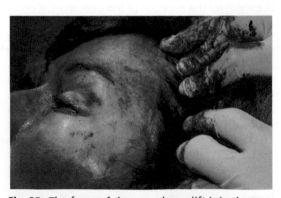

Fig. 25. The focus of the open brow lift is in the temporal area to achieve the desired shape and position of the brow.

placed on the forehead and eyes to help reduce bruising and discomfort. If staples are used, all are removed within 7 to 10 days.[63] The authors have found very acceptable scars with just beveling the incisions, preserving hair follicles, and leaving the 3-0 Vicryl Rapide™ to absorb.

Rehabilitation and Recovery

Recovery time from brow lift surgery is usually 2 weeks in the average patient with no complications.[65] The recovery time is mostly waiting for the bruising to settle. Camouflage makeup can be used to conceal this.

Outcomes

With proper surgical technique and postprocedural care, patients can expect very high satisfaction rates (**Figs. 26** and **27**). For many faces, the best single surgical procedure that can rejuvenate an aging face is the open brow lift, in the senior authors' opinion.

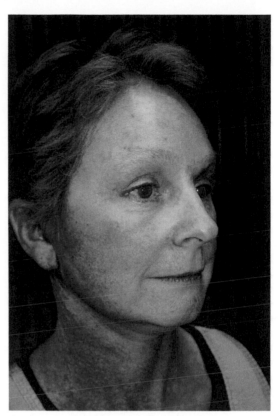

Fig. 27. Postoperative photograph, lateral view, of a patient who underwent rhytidectomy and open brow lift.

Summary

In conclusion, it is critical for the surgeon to follow a proper and thorough preoperative evaluation, patient selection, and surgical plan for a successful outcome and decrease the risk for surgical complications.

APPROACH TO THE MIDFACE LIFT THROUGH THE LOWER LID

Key Points for Midface Lift
1. Appropriate patient selection
2. Adequate lower canthal laxity evaluation
3. Adequate subperiosteal dissection
4. Secure composite flap fixation and suspension

Introduction

The approach in the authors' center is to use local anesthesia for the midface lift, often combined with upper lid blepharoplasty. The preoperative

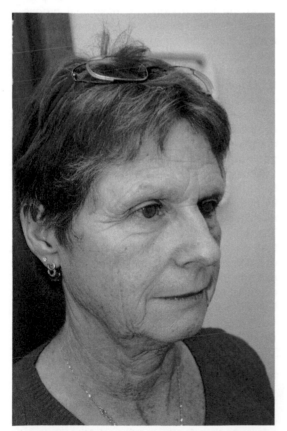

Fig. 26. Preoperative photograph, lateral view, of a patient who underwent rhytidectomy and open brow lift.

markings are noted and the procedure is discussed preoperatively and then reviewed again on the day of surgery. The appropriate nerves to identify for the nerve blocks in midface lift include

- Infraorbital nerve
- Zygomatic facial nerve
- Zygomaticotemporal nerve

Careful attention is taken to preserve these 3 branches as they emerge from their appropriate fascial planes during the dissection.

The authors found adequate anesthesia is obtained with diluted xylocaine with adrenaline, and bicarbonate and saline with the standard facelift solution.

If the patient is particularly anxious, the authors have often found that patients can tolerate a small amount of local anesthetic into the temporal area on each side with a 30-gauge needle just into the subcutaneous area and the authors allow several minutes for this to take effect until further local anesthesia is infiltrated around the area. Too much local anesthesia can make the tissue more difficult to mobilize. The authors have also found just 1 or 2 mg sublingual Ativan™ 1 hour before the surgery may also help, not only with the infiltration, but also during the surgery. Relaxing music is played and the authors can report that patients often fall asleep in the procedure chair.

Treatment Goals

The main goal of the midface lift is to target the loss of facial volume, descent, and laxity of the soft tissues in the midface area.

Preoperative Planning and Preparation

Preoperative planning includes noting the lower lid position including the lower lid laxity and the number of millimeters of distraction of the lower lid as well as the snap retraction test. The position of the descended lid cheek junction may be noted. The severity of the nasojugal trough from mild, moderate, and severe may also be noted, in particular, to define the extent of the dissection. The overall position of the globe itself in relation to the infraorbital rim is very important and would determine if there is a positive, neutral, or negative vector in terms of lid mobilization.[66] A person with some exophthalmos may in fact have a significant lower scleral show with a blepharoplasty if this vector is not taken into appropriate consideration. It is also important to note the descent of the cheek fat pad and the relationship to the orbitomalar ligament. The nasolabial fold is also important to note preoperatively.

Patient Positioning

All preoperative markings are outlined while the patient is in the seated position, and the patient is placed on the operating table in a supine position with the head in a neutral position.

Procedural Approach

The full-thickness lateral triangular wedge of the posterior malar is often resected as a lateral canthoplasty. Lateral canthoplasty may be necessary if there is excess lower eyelid posterior lamella. Often 4-0 Vicryl™ is used in a horizontal fashion with a standard lateral canthoplasty approach. Preoperatively it is important to note if there is greater than 6 mm of anterior displacement of the lower lid and if so a lateral canthoplasty is usually indicated.[67]

The redundant skin can then be cautiously trimmed along the subscleral skin incision after completion of the anchoring of the lateral canthus and suspension of the midface. One should trim only enough skin to have a completely tension-free closure along the lower lid. Before closure, fat may be injected or placed along the tear trough and nasojugal groove if necessary. The orbital septum may also have been opened in conjunction with repositioning and resection of lower lid fat and septal reset may be performed or the redraping of the orbital fat content over the infraorbital rim may also be considered.[66]

The closure, after the very conservative excision of excess skin and muscle along the subciliary margin with sharp curved scissors and closure, is performed often with 5-0 Vicryl Rapide™.[65]

Occasionally a Frost, or temporary lateral tarsorrhaphy suture, is placed for up to a week if there is significant edema. Frost suture has decreased the need for postoperative taping. The patient is often seen in follow-up in less than 1 week to reassess the need for any taping of the lower lid or release of the Frost suture.[65] An example of a patient who underwent this procedure with upper lid blepharoplasty is seen in **Fig. 28** A–D.

Operative Technique

The patient is marked in the sitting position, noting the key features to be addressed with the surgery. The fat pockets and arcus marginalis are marked. The patient rests in a reclined position and the anesthesia is administered after the patient has adequate time for the sublingual Ativan™ to take effect. Calming music is often played in a quiet room. Following local anesthesia, the patient is

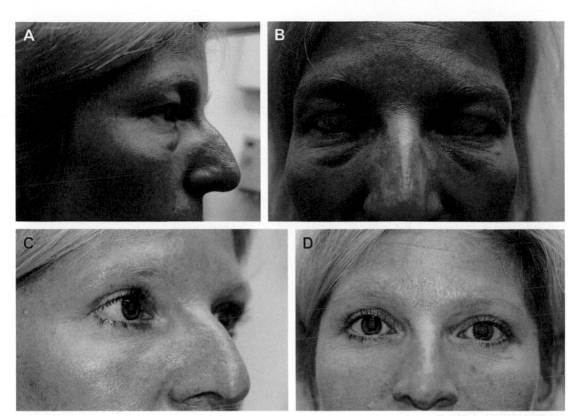

Fig. 28. (*A*) Preoperative view of patient with sunken midface and lower lid festoons. (*B*) A 39-year-old woman complained of her lids and sunken midface. (*C*) Postoperatively at 2 months, the scars are barely visible. (*D*) Two months postoperatively, the lid-cheek junction is well blended; the midface is lifted, and the nasolabial folds are softened.

normally prepared with a betadine solution because chlorhexidine solutions may produce a chemical burn to the cornea. There are diluted forms of chlorhexidine for the aqueous skin preparation solutions.

The subciliary incision is made by tunneling underneath the muscle separating the anterior lamella in a lateral to medial approach. This tunneling is often performed with the elevation going right down to the orbital rim and right across the lower lid all from the lateral portion of the incision. The muscle is then opened with the scissors away from the eyelash follicles. The skin and muscle are then released together as the anterior lamella.[65]

The midface dissection is continued along the orbital rim and in the subperiosteal direction over the maxilla. Attention is focused to identify and preserve the infraorbital nerve and the zygomatic facial nerve.

After the subperiosteal dissection, the cheek flap can then be elevated as a composite flap with the skin muscle and fascia together and not divided. A periosteal elevator can be used to aid

in the dissection and a small, lighted endoscope may also be used. As the dissection is in the subperiosteal plane, the motor branches of the facial nerve should not expose a significant risk of injury.

The composite flap is then elevated along the opposite direction of the nasolabial fold with a posterior and superior vector. Often the authors can obtain over a centimeter of lower lid elevation using this technique. The skin and muscle to be resected can be trimmed; however, the superior lip of the muscle is used as a transposition type of flap in aiding in the fixation of the flap. The muscle is trimmed with a lateral portion remaining intact for the orbicularis oculi. This muscle with its fascia is then tacked to the supraorbital rim and, if necessary, to the temporalis fascia more posteriorly. If necessary, another suture may be used along the medial edge of the lateral orbital rim to help maintain the position of the flap against the globe. The authors have found 4-0 Vicryl™ is sufficient as the suture of choice; however, the authors have also used Mersilene™ as well as PDS™ and 4-0 clear nylon.

Potential Complications and Management

The authors have seen one case of a patient with longstanding persistent chemosis after betadine prep to the eye. It was later identified that the patient in fact did have a shellfish allergy, although she had no known drug allergies. Several months passed while the lower lid swelling gradually subsided; however, the lid position created a cicatrical ectropion with lower lid malposition despite an appropriate placement of the lower lid during surgery.

The incisions do go a few millimeters lateral to the lateral canthus; this is necessary for the suspension. However, it does normally fade and this has not been a problem at the authors' center. Swelling in the area between the lower lid and upper lid incisions has persisted; however, the scar and swelling do blend fairly well in the long run.

Lower lid malposition is a potential problem and in one case in the authors' experience the suspension sutures were inadequate and the entire left side of the face fell, resulting in a greater than 1 cm ectropion. The entire procedure had to be repeated and an adequate result was obtained with good satisfaction after repeat suspension of the midface on a second procedure.

Postprocedural Care

The patient should be informed of the possibility of persistent swelling as chemosis is a significant complication of an extensive periorbital dissection.

Rehabilitation and Recovery

It is advised to patients that it takes at least 2 weeks for the swelling and bruising to resolve and that exercise should be avoided for at least 3 weeks postoperatively.

Outcomes

With proper surgical technique and postprocedural care, patients can expect very high satisfactory results.

Summary

In conclusion, it is important for the surgeon to follow a proper and thorough preoperative and postoperative evaluation, patient selection, and surgical technique for a successful outcome, and decrease the risk for potential complications.

ACKNOWLEDGMENTS

The authors would like to acknowledge the kind assistance of Dr Naweed Ahmed in the preparation of this article.

REFERENCES

1. Ben Simon GJ, Macedo AA, Schwarcz RM, et al. Frontalis suspension for upper eyelid ptosis: evaluation of different surgical designs and suture material. Am J Ophthalmol 2005;140(5):877–85.
2. Jacono AA, Parikh SS. The minimal access deep plane extended vertical facelift. Aesthet Surg J 2011;31(8):874–90.
3. Baker DC. Lateral SMASectomy, plication and short scar facelifts: indications and techniques. Clin Plast Surg 2008;35(4):533–50, vi.
4. Pepper JP, Baker SR. SMAS flap rhytidectomy. Arch Facial Plast Surg 2011;13(2):108.
5. Graf R, Groth AK, Pace D, et al. Facial rejuvenation with SMASectomy and FAME using vertical vectors. Aesthetic Plast Surg 2008;32(4):585–92.
6. Hopping SB, Janjanin S, Tanna N, et al. The S-Plus lift: a short-scar, long-flap rhytidectomy. Ann R Coll Surg Engl 2010;92(7):577–82.
7. Brandy DA. The Quicklift™: a modification of the S-Lift. Amer Soci of Cosm Derm & Aesth Surg 2004;17(6):251–360.
8. Degoute CS. Controlled hypotension: a guide to drug choice. Drugs 2007;67(7):1053–76.
9. Failey C, Aburto J, de la Portilla HG, et al. Office-based outpatient plastic surgery utilizing total intravenous anesthesia. Aesthet Surg J 2013;33(2): 270–4.
10. Roberts WE. Skin type classification systems old and new. Dermatol Clin 2009;27(4):529–33, viii.
11. Mendelson B, Wong CH. Changes in the facial skeleton with aging: implications and clinical applications in facial rejuvenation. Aesthetic Plast Surg 2012;36(4):753–60.
12. Rawlani V, Mustoe TA. The staged face lift: addressing the biomechanical limitations of the primary rhytidectomy. Plast Reconstr Surg 2012; 130(6):1305–14.
13. Chia CY, Almeida MW, Ritter PD, et al. Malar fat pad repositioning in facelifting: a simple technique of suspension and fixation. Aesthet Surg J 2010; 30(6):790–7.
14. Gamboa GM, de La Torre JI, Vasconez LO. Surgical anatomy of the midface as applied to facial rejuvenation. Ann Plast Surg 2004;52(3): 240–5.
15. Rachel JD, Lack EB, Larson B. Incidence of complications and early recurrence in 29 patients after facial rejuvenation with barbed suture lifting. Dermatol Surg 2010;36(3):348–54.
16. Koeppe T, Constantinescu MA, Schneider J, et al. Current trends in local anesthesia in cosmetic plastic surgery of the head and neck: results of a German national survey and observations on the use of ropivacaine. Plast Reconstr Surg 2005; 115(6):1723–30.

17. Aston SJ. Section: facelift; chapter: MACS facelift. Aesthetic Plast Surg 2009;1:137–47.
18. Tonnard P, Verpaele A. The MACS-lift short scar rhytidectomy. Aesthet Surg J 2007;27(2):188–98.
19. Lapid O. Syringe-delivered tumescent anesthesia made easier. Aesthetic Plast Surg 2011;35(4):601–2.
20. Ersek RA. Dissociative anesthesia for safety's sake: ketamine and diazepam—a 35-year personal experience. Plast Reconstr Surg 2004;113(7):1955–9.
21. Gianoutsos MP, Hunter-Smith D, Smith JG, et al. Oral premedication for local anesthesia in plastic surgery: prospective, randomized, blind comparison of lorazepam and temazepam. Plast Reconstr Surg 1994;93(5):901–6.
22. Hazrati A, Izadpanah A, Zadeh T, et al. Ageing midface: the impact of surgeon's experience on the consistency in the assessment and proposed management. J Plast Reconstr Aesthet Surg 2011;64(2):155–9.
23. Sarwer DB, Pruzinsky T, Cash TF, et al. Psychological aspects of reconstructive and cosmetic plastic surgery: clinical, empirical and ethical perspectives. Lippincott, Williams, & Wilkens 2005;13(1).
24. Ho T, Brissett AE. Preoperative assessment of the aging patient. Facial Plast Surg 2006;22(2):85–90.
25. Poore SO, Sillah NM, Mahajan AY, et al. Patient safety in the operating room: preoperative. Plast Reconstr Surg 2012;130(5):1038–47.
26. Aston SJ. Section: facelift; chapter: facelift with SMAS technique and FAME. Aesthetic Plast Surg 2009;1:73–85.
27. Man D. Reducing the incidence of ear deformity in facelift. Aesthet Surg J 2009;29(4):264–71.
28. Rousso DE, Brys AK. Minimal incision face-lifting. Facial Plast Surg 2012;28(1):76–88.
29. Aston SJ. Section: facelift; chapter: short scar facelift. Aesthetic Plast Surg 2009;1:101–14.
30. Ramirez AL, Ende KH, Kabaker SS. Correctin of the high female hairline. Arch Facial Plast Surg 2009;11(2):84–90.
31. Kridel RW, Liu ES. Techniques for creating inconspicuous face-lift scars: avoiding visible incisions and loss of temporal hair. Arch Facial Plast Surg 2003;5(4):325–33.
32. Shockley WW. Scar revision techniques: z-plasty, w-plasty, and geometric broken line closure. Facial Plast Surg Clin North Am 2011;19(3):455–63.
33. Alpert BS, Baker DC, Hamra ST, et al. Identical twin face lifts with differing techniques: a 10-year follow-up. Plast Reconstr Surg 2009;123(3):1025–33 [discussion: 1034–6].
34. Peltz TS, Haddad R, Scougall PJ, et al. Influence of locking stitch size in a four-strand cross-locked cruciate flexor tendon repair. J Hand Surg Am 2011;36(3):450–5.
35. Noone RB. Suture suspension malarplasty with SMAS plication and modified SMASectomy: a simplified approach to midface lifting. Plast Reconstr Surg 2006;117(3):792–803.
36. White JB, Barraja M, Mengesha T, et al. Avoiding early revision rhytidectomy: a biomechanical comparison of tissue plication suture techniques. Laryngoscope 2008;118(12):2107–10.
37. Berry MG, Davies D. Platysma-SMAS plication facelift. J Plast Reconstr Aesthet Surg 2010;63(5):793–800.
38. Ferreira LM, Horibe EK. Understanding the finger-assisted malar elevation technique in face lift. Plast Reconstr Surg 2006;118(3):731–40.
39. Bloom JD, Immerman SB, Rosenberg DB. Face-lift complications. Facial Plast Surg 2012;28(3):260–72.
40. Niamtu J 3rd. Facelift drains and dressings: to be or not to be? Dermatol Surg 2012;38(5):793–6.
41. Zoumalan R, Rizk SS. Hematoma rates in drainless deep-plane face-lift surgery with and without the use of fibrin glue. Arch Facial Plast Surg 2008;10(2):103–7.
42. Zimbler MS, Mashkevich G. Pearls in facelift management. Facial Plast Surg Clin North Am 2009;17(4):625–32, vii.
43. Swanson E. Outcome analysis in 93 facial rejuvenation patients treated with a deep-plane face lift. Plast Reconstr Surg 2011;127(2):823–34.
44. Feldman JJ. Neck lift. Quality Medical Publishing; 2003. Hardcopy edition.
45. Aston SJ. Section: the neck; chapter: deep plane procedures in the neck. Aesthetic Plast Surg 2009;1:231–42.
46. Stebbins WG, Hanke CW. Rejuvenation of the neck with liposuction and ancillary techniques. Dermatol Ther 2011;24(1):28–40.
47. Labbé D, Franco RG, Nicolas J. Platysma suspension and platysmaplasty during neck lift: anatomical study and analysis of 30 cases. Plast Reconstr Surg 2006;117(6):2001–7 [discussion: 2008–10].
48. Ramirez OM, Robertson KM. Comprehensive approach to rejuvenation of the neck. Facial Plast Surg 2001;17(2):129–40.
49. Daher JC. Closed platysmotomy: a new procedure for the treatment of platysma bands without skin dissection. Aesthetic Plast Surg 2011;35(5):866–77.
50. Roland B. Safety of liposuction of the neck using tumescent local anesthesia: experience in 320 cases. Dermatol Surg 2012;38(11):1812–5.
51. Feldman JJ. Corset platysmaplasty. Plast Reconstr Surg 1990;85(3):333–43.
52. Mahabir RC, Christensen B, Blair GK, et al. Avoiding stitch abscesses in subcuticular skin closures: the L-stitch. Can J Surg 2003;46(3):223–4.
53. Daniel M. Review of 500 suture suspension platysmaplasties: complications and potential pitfalls. Plast Reconstr Surg 2012;130(5S-1):88.

54. Guerrerosantos J. Evolution of technique: face and neck lifting and fat injections. Clin Plast Surg 2008; 35(4):663–76, viii.

55. Mühlbauer W, Holm C. Eyebrow asymmetry: ways of correction. Aesthetic Plast Surg 1998;22(5):366–71.

56. Walrath JD, McCord CD. The open brow lift. Clin Plast Surg 2013;40(1):117–24.

57. Bidros RS. Subcutaneous temporal browlift under local anesthesia: a useful technique for periorbital rejuvenation. Aesthet Surg J 2010;30(6):783–8.

58. Owsley TG. Subcutaneous trichophytic forehead browlift: the case for an "open" approach. J Oral Maxillofac Surg 2006;64(7):1133–6.

59. Friedland JA, Jacobsen WM, TerKonda S. Safety and efficacy of combined upper blepharoplasties and open coronal browlift: a consecutive series of 600 patients. Aesthetic Plast Surg 1996;20(6):453–62.

60. Griffin JE Jr, Owsley TG. Management of forehead and brow deformities. Atlas Oral Maxillofac Surg Clin North Am 2004;12(2):235–51.

61. Romo T 3rd, Jacono AA, Sclafani AP. Endoscopic forehead lifting and contouring. Facial Plast Surg 2001;17(1):3–10.

62. Aston SJ. Section:browlift;chapter:coronal browlift. Aesthetic Plast Surg 2009;1:275–9.

63. Connell BF, Lambros VS, Neurohr GH. The forehead lift: techniques to avoid complications and produce optimal results. Aesthetic Plast Surg 1989;13(4):217–37.

64. Byun S, Mukovozov I, Farrohyar F, et al. Complications of browlift techniques: a systematic review. Aesthet Surg J 2013;33(2):189–200.

65. Tonnard PL, Verpaele AM, Zeltzer AA. Augmentation blepharoplasty: a review of 500 consecutive patients. Aesthet Surg J 2013;33(3): 341–52.

66. Codner MA. Midface surgery. Techn & Aesth Plast Surg 2009;9:105–18.

67. Nahai F. Midface rejuvenation. The Art of Aesth Surg: Princ & Techn 2005;36:1362–76.

Local Anesthesia for Otoplasty in Children

Louise Caouette Laberge, MD, FRCSC

KEYWORDS

- Local anesthesia • Otoplasty • Children • Local anesthetics • Ear correction

KEY POINTS

- Children as young as 5 years old can be operated safely under local anesthesia, without premedication or sedation.
- Local anesthetics, either short-acting or a combination of short-acting and long-acting, with adrenalin are used with a very slow infiltration rate.
- Constant attention is directed to the child to explain the procedure and reduce the level of anxiety.
- The anesthesia obtained is appropriate for different otoplasty techniques, either suture-correction or anterior scoring.
- Appropriate doses of local anesthetics in relation to the child's weight and possible complications are reviewed.
- The surgical complications do not differ from surgeries performed under general anesthesia.

Otoplasty is a procedure that can safely and efficiently be performed under local anesthesia in children. Making the decision to undertake the procedure under local rather than general anesthesia is first the surgeon's choice and then the child's and child's parents. The surgeon must be intimately familiar with the surgery because his attention will be partially diverted to chat with the child and reassure him during the procedure. Furthermore, the duration of the procedure should not be excessive because the child becomes restless after 50 to 60 minutes.

Two factors are helpful when performing local anesthesia on the ear:

1. The discrimination of the ear for pain perception is not as good as other areas of the body, such as the nose, the lips, or the fingers.

2. The location of the ear makes it impossible for the child to see what is happening; thus, it is easier to reassure him.

PATIENT SELECTION

Deciding which patient is well suited to have the procedure under local anesthesia depends mainly on the opinion of the child concerning his ears and his motivation for a correction. Placing the child in front of a mirror during the first consultation to show him the change that can be achieved in the shape of his ears is helpful to let him decide whether he likes the new ear shape or not. A child who does not want to change his ears will certainly not accept local anesthesia. The family can then decide to proceed under general anesthesia or

Disclosure: The author has no financial interest in the subject matter or materials discussed in the article.
Department of Surgery, CHU Ste Justine, University of Montreal, 3175 Cote Ste-Catherine O, Room 7907, Montreal, Quebec H3T 1C5, Canada
E-mail address: l.caouette-laberge@umontreal.ca

Clin Plastic Surg 40 (2013) 671–686
http://dx.doi.org/10.1016/j.cps.2013.07.007

wait for the child's collaboration to have the procedure under local anesthesia.

When the child is motivated to have the surgery, the procedure is explained in simple terms avoiding the words "needle" and "cut" but rather "putting the ear to sleep with a pinch," "folding the ear cartilage," and "placing a dressing" for a week. It is important to obtain the child's approval for the plan, insisting on the fact that the only reason to change the ear shape is to please him.

The parents are sometimes surprised with this attitude and the fact that the decision is left to the child, but the majority see this very positively. The parents are asked not to add more details about the anesthesia or the surgery but rather repeat the same explanations. In my practice, more than 95% of otoplasty in children age 5 and older are performed under local anesthesia. The referring physicians are well aware of it and often have informed

His parents have been asked to wash the child's hair the same day or the day before and to feed him normally. No premedication is used; it is easier to control a child who is not sedated and can answer questions, play with words, and keep his mind busy. Topical anesthetic cream before the infiltration is not used routinely: the skin puncture with a 30-gauge needle is not easily detectable by the child. The pain due to tissue distension from the infiltration is unchanged with a topical anesthetic. However, if the family thinks that it is helpful, the author lets them apply the cream 60 minutes before the procedure on the posterior surface of the ear only.

- The child is brought in the operating room (**Fig. 1**A) only when the instruments and the syringe are prepared and covered (see **Fig. 1**B) and the surgeon is ready.

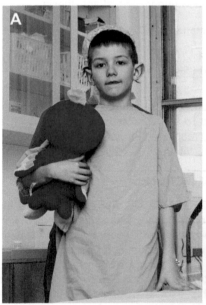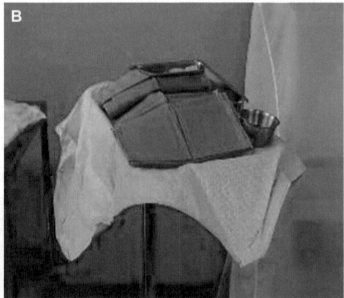

Fig. 1. (*A*) Child walking in the operating room without his parents. (*B*) Instruments and syringe hidden.

the parents so it is unusual for a family to refuse local anesthesia. If, for any reason, a family did refuse, one should not impose local anesthesia.

PATIENT PREPARATION

The child is not admitted to the hospital for the surgery; he comes to the outpatient clinic where the operating room for local anesthesia is located.

- The parents are asked to sit in a waiting area adjacent to the operating room; it is easier for the surgeon to focus his attention on the child and maintain a one-on-one conversation.
- There is no intravenous or monitoring equipment installed and the child is not restrained; he is simply asked to lie on his back with his hands hidden behind his back (**Fig. 2**). No antibiotics are used.

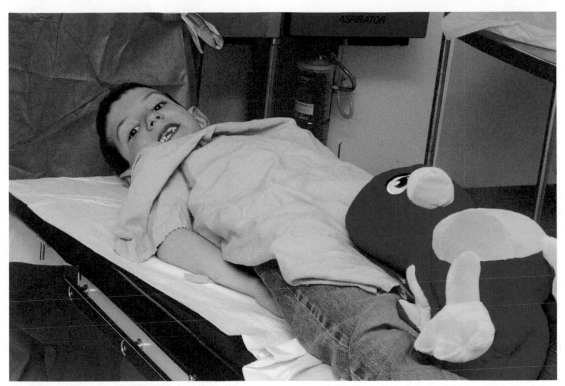

Fig. 2. Child lying down unrestrained hiding his hands behind his back.

- The face, ears, and peri-auricular areas are cleansed with aqueous chlorhexidine solution and a head drape is used, keeping the face completely exposed.

Anesthesia administration note: The author insists on a calm, reassuring, and friendly environment, low voices, no conversation except with the child to explain what is happening and what he may feel. It is important to make the child understand that he is in control: he uses a simple word "gentle" to slow down the infiltration and control the pain. The infiltration is stopped as soon as the child asks for it. He quickly understands his "power" and becomes more tolerant knowing that he can stop the pain anytime: it is a "patient-controlled anesthesia."

- The duration of the procedure including the local anesthesia, the surgery, and the dressing is 1 hour, which is well tolerated by the children.

LOCAL ANESTHESIA TECHNIQUE

The ear is vascularized by branches of the external carotid artery via the superficial temporal and the posterior auricular arteries. The innervation is provided by the greater auricular nerve (anterior and posterior branches) for the lower anterior and posterior regions including the lobule, branches of the auriculotemporal nerve for the anterior upper surface and branches of the lesser occipital nerve for the upper posterior surface. This anatomy makes it less favorable for regional nerve blocks; therefore, local anesthesia infiltration is performed directly in the auricle. This direct infiltration also provides hydrodissection and vasoconstriction of the region. It is well adapted to the anterior scoring technique with direct exposure of the cartilage, or a suture technique.

- The author routinely uses 1% lidocaine with 1/100,000 epinephrine; a total volume of 10 ml or less is used for both ears.
- The infiltration begins with a 30-gauge needle in the subcutaneous tissue on the posterior surface of the ear, where the skin is less adherent to cartilage and more easily distended.
- Pinching the ear very close to the site of needle puncture (**Fig. 3**) distracts the child's attention from the needle.

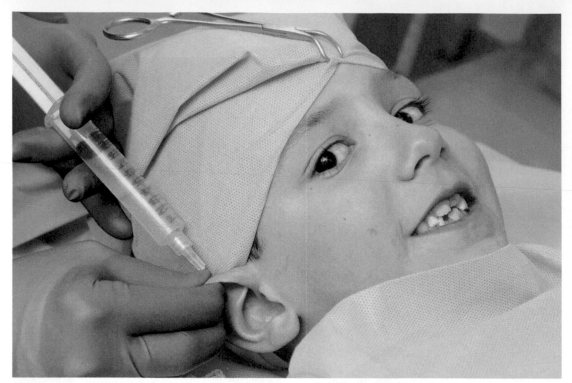

Fig. 3. The ear pinched between 2 fingers adjacent to the 30-gauge needle puncture.

- Only a small volume of fluid is infiltrated when the needle is advanced under the skin (**Fig. 4**); more volume is injected as the needle is withdrawn.

- The anterior surface is accessed with the needle slowly passed from the posterior surface, through the cartilage (**Fig. 5**), to place the anesthetic solution under the perichondrium/skin layer.

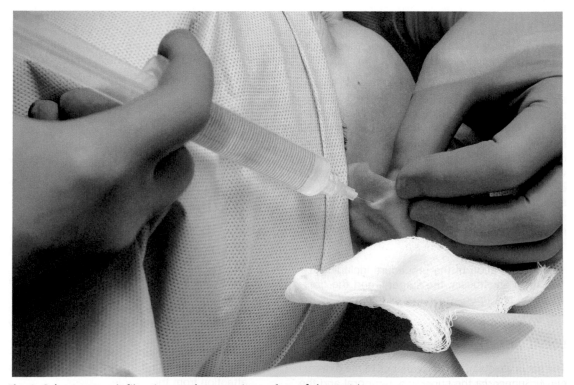

Fig. 4. Subcutaneous infiltration on the posterior surface of the auricle.

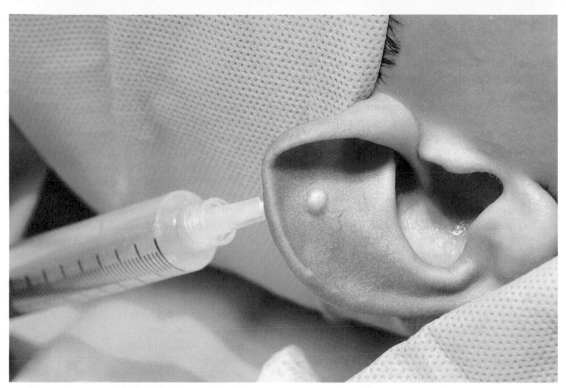

Fig. 5. Transcartilaginous, subperichondral infiltration of the anterior surface of the auricle.

- There is no subcutaneous tissue on the anterior surface and the stretching of the skin and perichondrium must be very slow (**Fig. 6**).

- It is important to keep a constant conversation with the child during this time to focus his attention on any other topic but the ears.

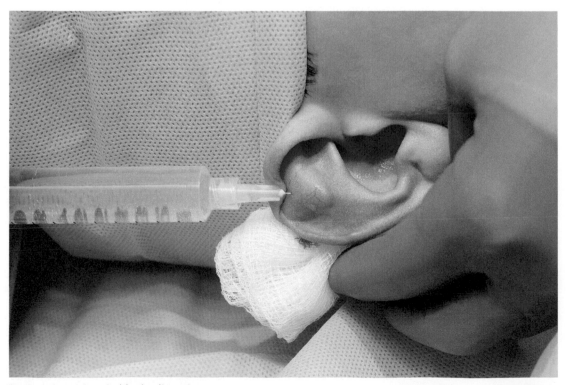

Fig. 6. Subperichondral hydrodissection.

- As the anesthetic infiltration continues, a 1.5-inch 25-gauge needle (**Fig. 7**) is used to replace the initial short 30-gauge needle.
- Care is taken to always reinsert the needle in an area already infiltrated so that the child does not feel repeated needle punctures.
- With this very slow rate of infusion, it takes 10 to 15 minutes to complete the infiltration required for both ears (7–10 ml total). By the time the anesthesia is completed, the epinephrine has provided the adequate vaso-constriction for immediate skin incision.

SURGICAL PROCEDURE

The author's preferred surgical procedure, the anterior scoring otoplasty, is carried on exactly the same way, with the same infiltration whether the patient is awake or under general anesthesia.

- A 3.5-cm posterior auricular incision is located 1 cm from the helical rim (**Fig. 8**) so that it lies in the concavity created by the anti-helical fold and therefore is hidden.
- No skin excision is needed.
- Very little skin undermining is done on the posterior aspect of the ear because the skin incision lies close to the proposed transcarti-laginous incision (**Fig. 9**).

- The cauda helicis and the antitragohelicine fissure are located (**Fig. 10**A) and a transcar-tilaginous incision is made in the scapha (see **Fig. 10**B), parallel to the border of the helical rim superiorly into the upper third of the auricle.
- Access to the anterior surface of the concha and antihelix is then provided by elevation of the anterior skin and perichondrium using a periosteal elevator (**Fig. 11**A) and continued with scissors (see **Fig. 11**B) in the upper portion of the antihelix.
- The incision between the helical rim cartilage and the antihelix cartilage is continued sub-cutaneously with scissors (**Fig. 12**) up to the origin of the helix, maintaining a constant he-lical width.
- The origin of the helix is sectioned (**Fig. 13**A); the skin and perichondral elevation on the anterior surface of the antihelix and triangular fossa is completed, and scarifications con-sisting of partial thickness cartilage incisions (scoring) are then performed with a number 15 blade (see **Fig. 13**B).
- The direction of the scarifications (**Fig. 14**A) is important to have a normal-appearing "fan-shaped" antihelix that curves both superiorly and posteriorly (see **Fig. 14**B).

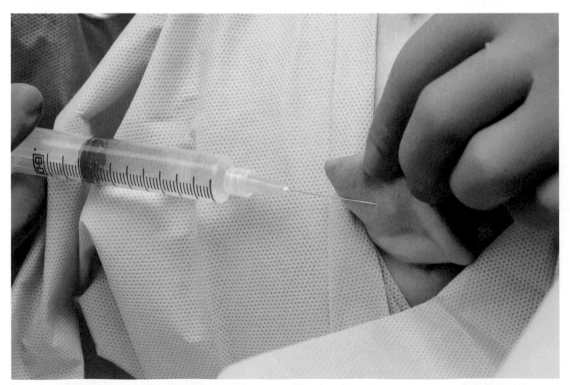

Fig. 7. Infiltration completed with a long, 25-gauge needle.

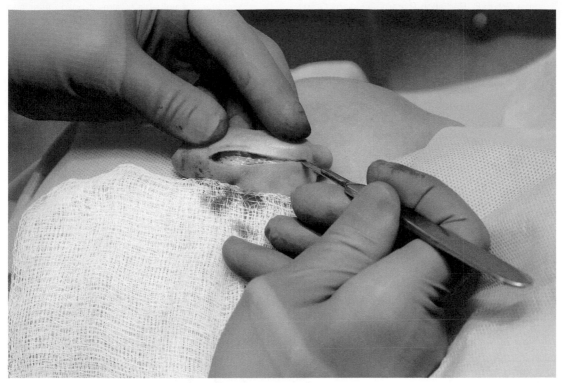

Fig. 8. Posterior auricular incision (3.5 cm) 1 cm from the helical rim.

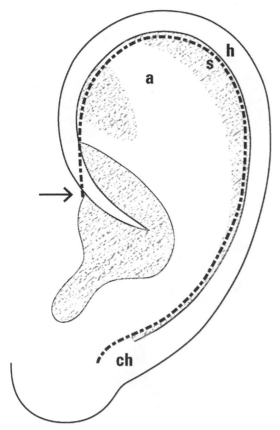

Fig. 9. Transcartilaginous incision (*dotted line*). a, antihelix; arrow, root of helix; ch, cauda helicis; h, helix; s, scapha. (*Modified from* Caouette-Laberge L, Guay N, Bortoluzzi P, et al. Otoplasty: anterior scoring technique and results in 500 cases. Plast Reconstr Surg 2000;105:506; with permission.)

- At the very caudal part of the newly formed antihelix, the incision is full thickness so that the cartilage can be folded sharply upon itself at the appropriately chosen conchal height. The projection of the concha is therefore controlled without the need for an additional concho-mastoid suture. The cartilage should stay in the desired position because its natural elasticity and intrinsic memory have been overcome.
- Two 5-0 plain catgut sutures are used to keep the sharp fold of the caudal end of the new antihelix (**Fig. 15**) and to ensure a smooth cartilage shape in this area where the overlying skin is particularly thin.
- The helical rim and anterior skin flap are then returned to their original position (**Fig. 16**) and the projection of the lobule is examined. The lobule is prominent in most cases. The cartilage of the cauda helicis controls the projection of the lobule: it is mobilized and sutured posteriorly behind the concha cartilage with a 5-0 plain catgut. Setting back of the lobule with the cauda helicis may produce an elevation of the upper helix (one structure in continuity: lowering one end will elevate the other), in which case a small wedge excision of the helical rim above the cauda helicis may be necessary. In contrast to a Mustarde technique, the anterior scoring technique requires no permanent sutures to re-create the antihelical fold nor concho-mastoid sutures.

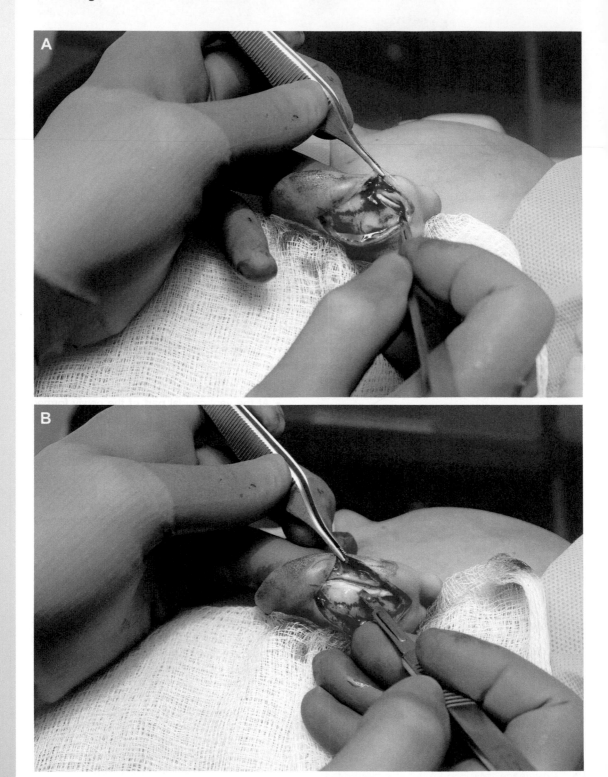

Fig. 10. (*A*) Cauda helicis and antitragohelicine fissure. (*B*) Transcartilaginous incision in the scapha.

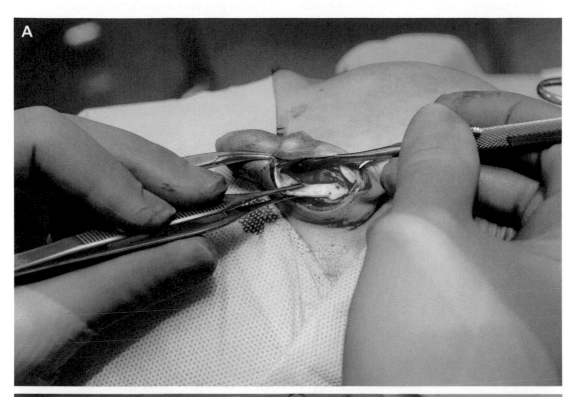

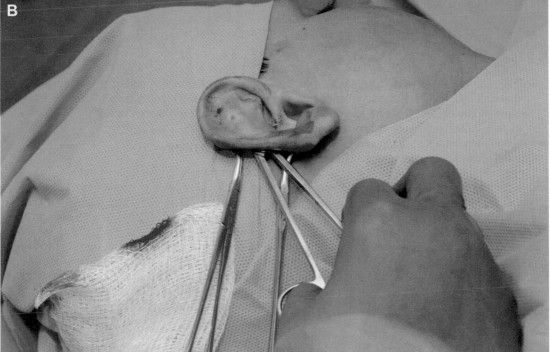

Fig. 11. (*A*) Elevation of the anterior skin and perichondrium to access the anterior surface of the concha and antihelix. (*B*) Anterior dissection completed with scissors.

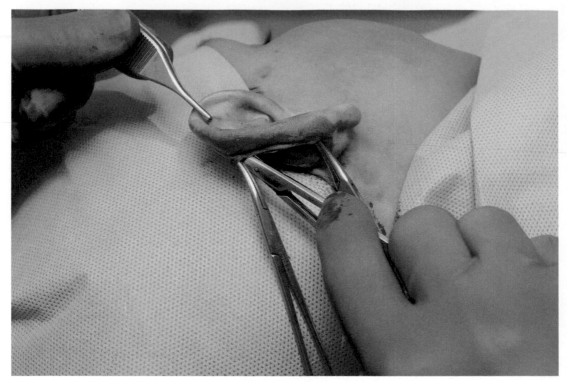

Fig. 12. Cartilage section in the scapha completed with scissors.

- The skin is closed with running horizontal mattress 5-0 plain catgut; the anterior flap is carefully molded on the cartilage framework and a 5-0 plain gut suture is inserted percutaneously from the fossa triangularis to the scapha to prevent any anterior displacement of the helical rim.
- A dressing is applied, starting with one thin gauze covered with xeroform dressing in the posterior auricular sulcus and one moistened elongated gauze to conform the concha, fossa triangularis, and scapha (**Fig. 17**A). Fluffed gauze (see **Fig. 17**B) and kling gauze complete the dressing (see **Fig. 17**C).
- Oral analgesics are used for the first 24 hours (acetaminophen and codeine).
- The dressing is removed after 7 to 10 days.
- The parents are then instructed to wash the child's hair, clean the incision daily, and apply a topical ointment to help dissolve the remaining sutures.
- The ears are left exposed during the day but a night cap (such as a lycra swimming cap) is recommended for sleeping during the first week.

- Follow-up is obtained 3 months later with either a clinic visit or a telephone interview, as preferred by the family.

COMPLICATIONS

This procedure under local anesthesia has been used by the author in more than 2000 children over the last 30 years and no major complications were encountered. A vagal response with hypotension was seen in less than 1% of the cases; no systemic treatment was necessary but the children were observed for an additional 30 minutes after the procedure. The surgical complications were reviewed in 500 cases operated over a 3-year period, as follows[1]:

Early complications were bleeding (2.6%) and hematoma (0.4%). There were no infections or ear necrosis. A 2- to 3-mm skin erosion on the anterior skin in 3 patients (0.6%) and one wound dehiscence (0.2%) were noted: spontaneous healing occurred in all cases. These complication rates compare favorably with the literature.

Late complications were keloids in 2 cases and inclusion cysts in 3 cases. Residual deformity was noted in 22 cases (4 %) and asymmetry in 28

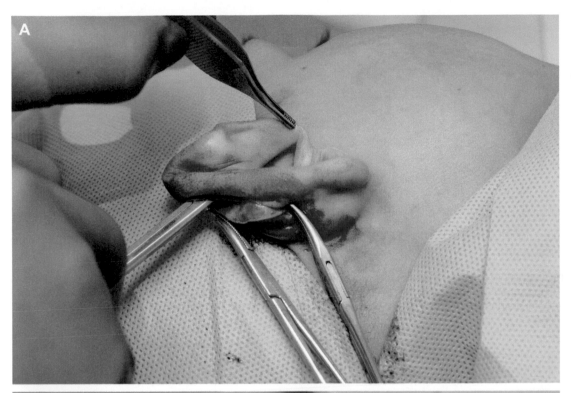

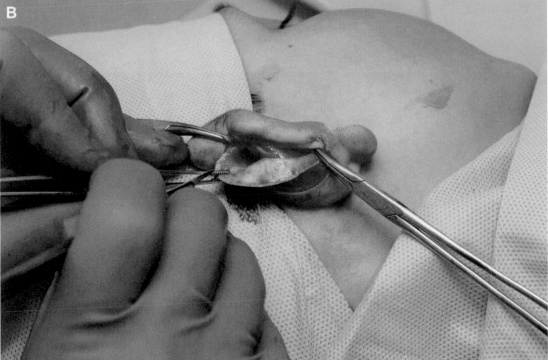

Fig. 13. (*A*) Origin of helix sectioned. (*B*) Scarifications/scoring (partial thickness cartilage incisions) with a number 15 blade.

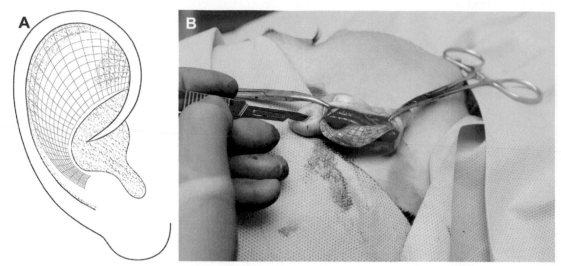

Fig. 14. (*A*) Scarifications on the anterior surface of cartilage. (*B*) Normal-appearing "fan-shaped" antihelix curving superiorly and posteriorly. ([*A*] *Modified from* Caouette-Laberge L, Guay N, Bortoluzzi P, et al. Otoplasty: anterior scoring technique and results in 500 cases. Plast Reconstr Surg 2000;105:506; with permission.)

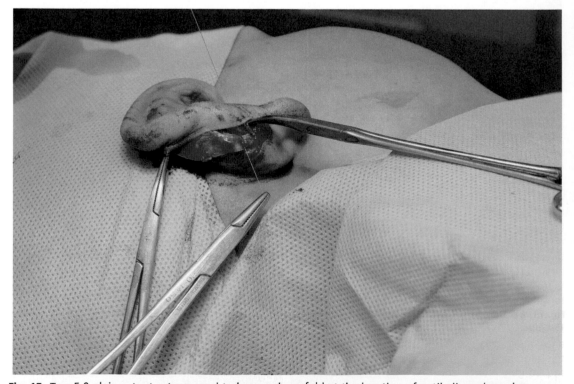

Fig. 15. Two 5-0 plain catgut sutures used to keep a sharp fold at the junction of antihelix and concha.

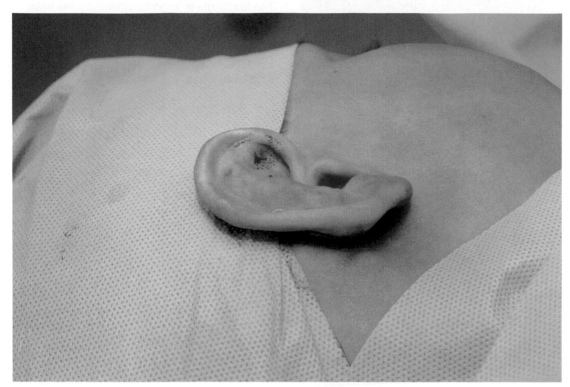

Fig. 16. Helical rim and anterior skin flap returned to their original position.

cases (5.6 %). Secondary surgery was performed in 6 cases (1.2%). A long-term follow-up was obtained through a questionnaire answered by 77.4% of the patients 2 to 5 years after the surgery: the satisfaction rate was 94.8%.

DISCUSSION

The use of local anesthesia for otoplasty in adults is well documented[2] but is seldom mentioned in a pediatric setting.[3] The author found that acceptance of local anesthesia by the patient and his family is very high: referrals are often directed precisely because the procedure is performed under local anesthesia. Because there is no cost for the families whether the surgery is performed under local or general anesthesia in Canada, the economic factor does not play a role in the acceptance of local anesthesia. The family, however, has more control on the date of the surgery and there is a shorter waiting time for procedures performed under local anesthesia. The children seem to appreciate their being in control and they tend to see the whole procedure as "their" decision and "their" achievement. Crying or yelling is not tolerated in the operating room: if a child refuses the surgery, he is simply sent home. Over the years, less than 1% of the children scheduled

under local anesthesia have had their surgeries canceled.

A calm and friendly environment, keeping the parents with the child as long as possible before the procedure and close to the operating room during the procedure, and covering the instruments and syringe are helpful to reduce the child's anxiety. Pirotte and Veyckemans[4] rightly point out that the children's reaction is much more related to stress than pain intensity. The absence of premedication or any systemic medication and the small amount of local anesthetic used make it unnecessary to install an intravenous catheter, cardiac monitor, or pulse oxymeter, keeping the setup as simple as possible. Should a child present an episode of vagal reaction, oxygen and all the necessary monitoring are readily available.

Many agents are available for local anesthesia, either amide or ester, with variable duration of anesthesia and with or without epinephrine; many dilutions are available. The author uses lidocaine 1% with epinephrine 1/100,000, a total of 10 ml or less. The recommended dosage of lidocaine with epinephrine (**Table 1**)[4-6] should not exceed 7 mg/kg; a 1% solution contains 10 mg per milliliter. Therefore, the volume used in a 5-year-old, 16-kg child, is safe (maximum, 11 ml). The anesthetic solution can be diluted (lidocaine 0.5% with

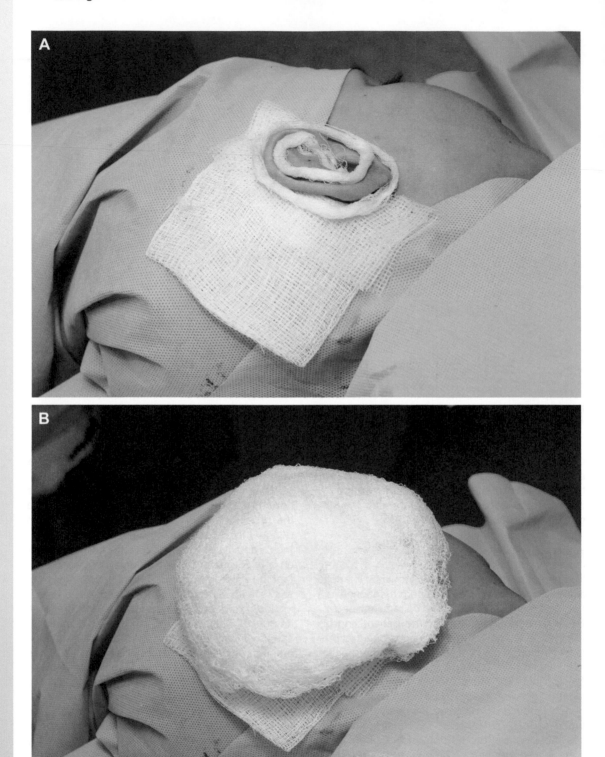

Fig. 17. (*A*) Thin gauze covered with xeroform in the posterior auricular sulcus; moistened elongated gauze to conform the concha, fossa triangularis, and scapha. (*B*) Fluffed gauze.

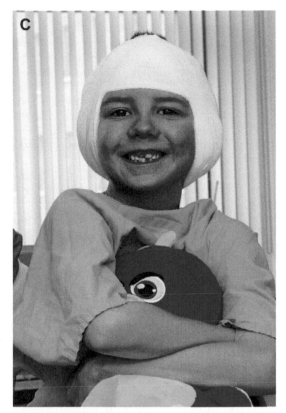

Fig. 17. *(continued),* (C) Dressing completed.

epinephrine 1/200,000) should the surgeon prefer to inject a larger volume.[7] No systemic complications have been encountered with this regimen and the bloodless field obtained with the local vasoconstriction makes the surgery easier. Many authors[4] have repeated the classic objection to the use of epinephrine in areas such as fingers, toes, ears, and nose. However, the concern for tissue necrosis because of the vasoconstriction has

Table 1 Maximal doses of local anesthetics in children (in mg/kg)[4–6] (different concentrations of solutions may be used: 1% is 10 mg per ml)		
	Without Epinephrine	With Epinephrine
Procaine	7	10
Chloroprocaine	10	20
Tetracaine	1.5	1 (?)
Lidocaine	5	7
Prilocaine	5	7
Mepivacaine	7	7
Bupivacaine	2.5	3
Ropivacaine	3	?

not been substantiated in fingers[8] and the author has not been able to find any report of ear necrosis following injection of local anesthetic with epinephrine in recommended dosages.

Even though lidocaine is a short-acting local anesthetic, the combination of epinephrine in the solution increases the duration of anesthesia significantly.[9,10] The anesthesia usually lasts for 4 to 5 hours, allowing the child to return home and start oral analgesia before the local anesthesia wears off. A combination of short-acting/rapid-onset and long-acting/slow-onset local anesthetics with epinephrine is also effective[11] and provides a longer duration of anesthesia. When a combination of anesthetics is used, the amount of each solution is proportionally reduced.

Attention to dosages is important in young children (see **Table 1**). Systemic absorption of the local anesthetic[12] may be significant particularly in a well-vascularized area such as the ear; however, the addition of epinephrine reduces the systemic absorption because of the vasoconstriction. The risk of intravascular injection is minimal because no major blood vessels are located within the auricle in the infiltrated areas. The surgeon should be aware of the early signs of systemic toxicity, such as headache, tingling of the lips, metallic taste, irritability, restlessness, and blurred vision. It is important to maintain good verbal contact with the child to detect these changes. High systemic levels cause agitation, tremor, convulsions, and arrhythmias; cardiac complications of bupivacaine are particularly difficult to manage. The signs and symptoms of toxicity are caused by the action of the local anesthetics on the sodium channels of excitable cell membranes such as seen in the brain and heart.

The use of topical anesthetic cream before skin puncture is recommended by some authors for skin anesthesia. The author has not found the addition of such cream to be a major benefit because the pain is mainly related to tissue distension, particularly the perichondrium on the anterior surface of the ear. The author routinely pinches the ear between 2 fingers next to the initial skin puncture to divert the child's attention and the skin puncture often goes unnoticed (see **Fig. 3**). The absorption of the topical anesthetic has to be taken into account in the calculation of the maximum dose of the injected anesthetic; therefore, the application should be limited to a small area (3 cm^2) on the posterior surface of the auricle with an occlusive dressing 60 minutes before the procedure.

The addition of bicarbonate to the lidocaine to correct the pH of the solution[4] may reduce the pain during infiltration; however, the author has not noticed a significant decrease in the pain of injection in the auricle, where the rate of injection/tissue distension is the most important component of the pain. Neutralization of the acidity may prove more important when a large amount of local anesthesia is used.

SUMMARY

Otoplasty in children as young as age 5 years can be safely performed under local anesthesia in a calm, reassuring, and friendly environment. The procedure is explained in simple terms and constant verbal contact is maintained with the child during a slow infiltration of the anesthetic. Children are amazingly cooperative and proud of their achievement. The surgery can be performed under ideal conditions in a cost-effective fashion.

REFERENCES

1. Caouette-Laberge L, Guay N, Bortoluzzi P, et al. Otoplasty: anterior scoring technique and results in 500 cases. Plast Reconstr Surg 2000;105:504–15.

2. Koeppe T, Constantinescu MA, Scheinder J, et al. Current trends in local anesthesia in cosmetic plastic surgery of the head and neck. Plast Reconstr Surg 2005;115:1723–30.

3. Lancaster JL, Jones TM, Kay AR, et al. Paediatric day-case otoplasty: local versus general anaesthetic. Surgeon 2003;1:96–8.

4. Pirotte T, Veyckemans F. Local anesthesia for children. In: Harahap M, Abadir AR, editors. Anesthesia and analgesia in dermatologic surgery, basic and clinical dermatology, vol. 42. New York: Informa Health Care; 2008. p. 133–62.

5. Tobias JD, Litman RS. Pediatric regional anesthesia. In: Litman RS, editor. Pediatric anesthesia: the requisites in anaesthesiology. Philadelphia: Elsevier; 2004. p. 171.

6. Polaner DM, Suresh S, Coté CJ. Pediatric regional anesthesia. In: Coté CJ, Todres ID, Goudsouzian NG, et al, editors. A practice of anesthesia for infants and children. 3rd edition. Philadelphia: Elsevier; 2001. p. 640, 133–62.

7. Gessler EM, Hart AK, Dunlevy TM, et al. Optimal concentration of epinephrine for vasoconstriction in ear surgery. Laryngoscope 2001;111:1687–90.

8. Lalonde D, Bell M, Benoit P, et al. A multicenter prospective study of 3,110 consecutive cases of elective epinephrine use in the fingers and hand: the Dalhousie Project clinical phase. J Hand Surg Am 2005;30:1061–7.

9. Liu S, Carpenter RL, Chiu AA, et al. Epinephrine prolongs duration of subcutaneous infiltration of local anesthesia in a dose-related manner. Correlation with magnitude of vasoconstriction. Reg Anesth 1995;20:378–84.

10. Cregg N, Conway F, Casey W. Analgesia after otoplasty: regional nerve blockade vs local anaesthetic infiltration of the ear. Can J Anaesth 1996;34:141–7.

11. Kakagia D, Fotiadis S, Tripsiannis G. Comparative efficacy of ropivacaine and bupivacaine infiltrative analgesia in otoplasty. Ann Plast Surg 2005;54:409–11.

12. Berde C. Local anesthetics in infants and children: an update. Paediatr Anaesth 2004;14:387–93.

Index

Note: Page numbers of article titles are in **boldface** type.

A

Abdominoplasty, full, tumescent anesthesia for, 605–606, 607
Abductorplasty, carpal tunnel release with, 576
Aftercare and management costs, favorable implications on, 532–533
Allergy, due to local anesthetics, 523
Amides, 515–516
Amino-amide and amino-ester local anesthetics, 516–517
Anaphylaxis, due to general anesthesia, 509–510
Anesthesia, for liposuction, 594
   general, cardiovascular complications with, 503–505
      complications of, **503–513**
      delayed discharge and unplanned admission in, 510–511
      neurologic complications with, 506–507
      renal complications with, 507–508
      respiratory complications with, 505–506
   infiltrative, 541
   intravenous regional, 523
   local, and intravenous, rhinoplasty with, **627–629**
      breast surgery under, **583–591**
      cosmetic face, neck, and brow lifts with, **653–670**
      costing procedures of, and plastic surgery, 532
      cubital tunnel release using, **557–565**
      for facial rejuvenation, 654–655
      for otoplasty in children, **671–686**
         maximal doses of, 685
         technique of, 673–677
      hand surgery using, **567–581**
      mechanism of action of, 517
      of foot, ankle block for, 553
   regional and general, costs of, **529–535**
   tumescent, 541
      anesthetics for, 522–523, 603, 606
      indications for, 603–606
Anesthesia-related metrics, 532
Anesthesia technique, manipulating intangibles through, 534
Anesthesiologist, plastic surgeon as, 533
Anesthetics, local, adjuvants to, 521–522
      administration of, 522–523
      after administration of, 541
      allergic reactions to, 523
      basic and clinical science of, 515–521
      complications and reactions to, 523–524

      duration of action of, 520–521
      effectiveness of, onset of, 519
      elimination of, 521
      for plastic surgery, primer on, **515–528**
      for skin grafting and local flaps, **537–549**
      for tumescent anesthesia, 522–523
      hair transplantation and, **615–629**
      history of use of, 515
      injecting of, major steps for, 539–540
      limitations of, 524
      lipid solubility of, 519–520
      liposomal encapsulated, 523
      metabolism of, 521
      mixing of, 516
      newer, 516
      physical properties of, 519
      potency of, 518
      potential future of, 518–519
      resistance to, 598
      safe dosage of, 520
      systemic toxicity due to, 524–526
      transcutaneous delivery of, 522
      warming of, 522
   local structure of, 516–517
Ankle block, for local anesthesia of foot, 553
Anti-inflammatory agents, nonsteroidal, 522
Arrhythmia, general anesthesia and, 504
Aspiration, general anesthesia and, 506
   risk factors and interventions for, 506
Atelectasis, general anesthesia and, 505–506
Awareness, under general anesthesia, 507
      risk factors for development of, 507

B

Basal cell carcinoma, of distal tibia, split-thickness skin grafts for, 542
   of nasolabial area, reconstruction of defect of, V-Y advancement flap for, 546
   of nose, full-thickness skin grafts for, 543
   of temporal region, full-thickness skin grafts for, 544
Bicarbonate, 521
Bier block, 523
Blepharoplasty, with CO_2 laser, for lower eyelid repair, 646–648
   with CO_2 laser in, 644–646
Breast augmentation, operative method for, 587–588, 589

Clin Plastic Surg 40 (2013) 687–690
http://dx.doi.org/10.1016/S0094-1298(13)00089-8
0094-1298/13/$ – see front matter © 2013 Elsevier Inc. All rights reserved.

United States Postal Service

Statement of Ownership, Management, and Circulation
(All Periodicals Publications Except Requestor Publications)

1. Publication Title	2. Publication Number	3. Filing Date
Clinics in Plastic Surgery	0 0 6 - 5 3 0	9/14/13

4. Issue Frequency	5. Number of Issues Published Annually	6. Annual Subscription Price
Jan, Apr, Jul, Oct	4	$466.00

7. Complete Mailing Address of Known Office of Publication (Not printer) (Street, city, county, state, and ZIP+4®)

Elsevier Inc.
360 Park Avenue South
New York, NY 10010-1710

Contact Person: Stephen R. Bushing
Telephone (Include area code): 215-239-3688

8. Complete Mailing Address of Headquarters or General Business Office of Publisher (Not printer)

Elsevier Inc., 360 Park Avenue South, New York, NY 10010-1710

9. Full Names and Complete Mailing Addresses of Publisher, Editor, and Managing Editor (Do not leave blank)

Publisher (Name and complete mailing address)

Linda Belfus, Elsevier, Inc., 1600 John F. Kennedy Blvd. Suite 1800, Philadelphia, PA 19103-2899

Editor (Name and complete mailing address)

Joanne Husovski, Elsevier, Inc., 1600 John F. Kennedy Blvd. Suite 1800, Philadelphia, PA 19103-2899

Managing Editor (Name and complete mailing address)

Adrianne Brigido, Elsevier, Inc., 1600 John F. Kennedy Blvd. Suite 1800, Philadelphia, PA 19103-2899

10. Owner (Do not leave blank. If the publication is owned by a corporation, give the name and address of the corporation immediately followed by the names and addresses of all stockholders owning or holding 1 percent or more of the total amount of stock. If not owned by a corporation, give the names and addresses of the individual owners. If owned by a partnership or other unincorporated firm, give its name and address as well as those of each individual owner. If the publication is published by a nonprofit organization, give its name and address.)

Full Name	Complete Mailing Address
Wholly owned subsidiary of	1600 John F. Kennedy Blvd., Ste. 1800
Reed/Elsevier, US holdings	Philadelphia, PA 19103-2899

11. Known Bondholders, Mortgagees, and Other Security Holders Owning or Holding 1 Percent or More of Total Amount of Bonds, Mortgages, or Other Securities. If none, check box ☐ None

Full Name	Complete Mailing Address
N/A	

12. Tax Status (For completion by nonprofit organizations authorized to mail at nonprofit rates) (Check one)
The purpose, function, and nonprofit status of this organization and the exempt status for federal income tax purposes:
☐ Has Not Changed During Preceding 12 Months
☐ Has Changed During Preceding 12 Months (Publisher must submit explanation of change with this statement)

PS Form 3526, September 2007 (Page 1 of 3 (Instructions Page 3)) PSN 7530-01-000-9931 PRIVACY NOTICE: See our Privacy policy in www.usps.com

---

13. Publication Title	14. Issue Date for Circulation Data Below
Clinics in Plastic Surgery	April 2013

15. Extent and Nature of Circulation		Average No. Copies Each Issue During Preceding 12 Months	No. Copies of Single Issue Published Nearest to Filing Date
a. Total Number of Copies (Net press run)		1124	874
b. Paid Circulation (By Mail and Outside the Mail)	(1) Mailed Outside-County Paid Subscriptions Stated on PS Form 3541. (Include paid distribution above nominal rate, advertiser's proof copies, and exchange copies)	595	518
	(2) Mailed In-County Paid Subscriptions Stated on PS Form 3541 (Include paid distribution above nominal rate, advertiser's proof copies, and exchange copies)		
	(3) Paid Distribution Outside the Mails Including Sales Through Dealers and Carriers, Street Vendors, Counter Sales, and Other Paid Distribution Outside USPS®	279	211
	(4) Paid Distribution by Other Classes Mailed Through the USPS (e.g. First-Class Mail®)		
c. Total Paid Distribution (Sum of 15b (1), (2), (3), and (4))	►	874	729
d. Free or Nominal Rate Distribution (By Mail and Outside the Mail)	(1) Free or Nominal Rate Outside-County Copies Included on PS Form 3541	73	130
	(2) Free or Nominal Rate In-County Copies Included on PS Form 3541		
	(3) Free or Nominal Rate Copies Mailed at Other Classes Through the USPS (e.g. First-Class Mail)		
	(4) Free or Nominal Rate Distribution Outside the Mail (Carriers or other means)		
e. Total Free or Nominal Rate Distribution (Sum of 15d (1), (2), (3) and (4))	►	73	130
f. Total Distribution (Sum of 15c and 15e)	►	947	859
g. Copies not Distributed (See instructions to publishers #4 (page #3))		177	15
h. Total (Sum of 15f and g)	►	1124	874
i. Percent Paid (15c divided by 15f times 100)		92.29%	84.87%

16. Publication of Statement of Ownership
☐ If the publication is a general publication, publication of this statement is required. Will be printed in the October 2013 issue of this publication. ☐ Publication not required

17. Signature and Title of Editor, Publisher, Business Manager, or Owner

Stephen R. Bushing – Inventory Distribution Coordinator

Date: September 14, 2013

I certify that all information furnished on this form is true and complete. I understand that anyone who furnishes false or misleading information on this form or who omits material or information requested on the form may be subject to criminal sanctions (including fines and imprisonment) and/or civil sanctions (including civil penalties).

PS Form 3526, September 2007 (Page 2 of 3)

Moving?

Make sure your subscription moves with you!

To notify us of your new address, find your **Clinics Account Number** (located on your mailing label above your name), and contact customer service at:

Email: journalscustomerservice-usa@elsevier.com

800-654-2452 (subscribers in the U.S. & Canada)
314-447-8871 (subscribers outside of the U.S. & Canada)

Fax number: 314-447-8029

Elsevier Health Sciences Division
Subscription Customer Service
3251 Riverport Lane
Maryland Heights, MO 63043

*To ensure uninterrupted delivery of your subscription, please notify us at least 4 weeks in advance of move.

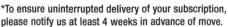

Printed and bound by CPI Group (UK) Ltd, Croydon, CR0 4YY

03/10/2024

01040370-0008